Praise for ANTHONY WILLIAM

"Anthony's understanding of foods, their vibrations, and how they interact with the body never ceases to amaze. Effortlessly he explains the potential harmony or disharmony in our choices in a way anyone can understand. He has a gift. Do your body a favor and treat yourself."

— Pharrell Williams, 11-time Grammy-winning artist and producer

"While there is most definitely an element of otherworldly mystery to the work he does, much of what Anthony William shines a spotlight on—particularly around autoimmune disease—feels inherently right and true. What's better is that the protocols he recommends are natural, accessible, and easy to do."

— Gwyneth Paltrow, Oscar-winning actress, #1 *New York Times* best-selling author, founder and CEO of GOOP.com

"Anthony is a trusted source for our family. His work in the world is a light that has guided many to safety. He means so much to us."

— Robert De Niro and Grace Hightower De Niro

"Anthony is a great man. His knowledge is fascinating and has been very helpful for me. The celery juice alone is a game changer!"

— Calvin Harris, producer, DJ, and Grammy-winning artist

"Anthony's knowledge on the food we consume, the impact it has on our body, and our overall well-being has been a game changer for me!"

— Jenna Dewan, star of *World of Dance* and *Step Up*

"Anthony is a magician for all my label's recording artists, and if he were a record album, he would far surpass Thriller. His ability is nothing short of profound, remarkable, extraordinary, and mind-blowing. He is a luminary whose books are filled with prophecies. This is the future of medicine."

— Craig Kallman, Chairman and CEO, Atlantic Records

"Anthony's books are revolutionary yet practical. For anybody frustrated by the current limits of Western medicine, this is definitely worth your time and consideration."

— James Van Der Beek, creator, executive producer, and star of *What Would Diplo Do?* and star of *Pose* and *Dawson's Creek*, and Kimberly Van Der Beek, public speaker and activist

"My family and friends have been the recipients of Anthony's inspired gift of healing, and we've benefited more than I can express with rejuvenated physical and mental health."

— Scott Bakula, producer and star of *NCIS: New Orleans*; star of *Star Trek: Enterprise* and *Quantum Leap*

"Anthony is a wonderful person. He identified some long-term health issues for me, he knew what supplements I needed, and I felt better immediately."

— Rashida Jones, producer and star of *Angie Tribeca*; executive producer of *Claws*; star of *Tag*, *Parks and Recreation*, and *The Office*

"What if someone could simply touch you and tell you what it is that ails you? Welcome to the healing hands of Anthony William—a modern-day alchemist who very well may hold the key to longevity. His lifesaving advice blew into my world like a healing hurricane, and he has left a path of love and light in his wake. He is hands down the ninth wonder of the world."

— Lisa Gregorisch-Dempsey, *Extra* Senior Executive Producer

"Anthony William is changing and saving the lives of people all over the world with his one-of-a-kind gift. His constant dedication and vast amount of highly advanced information have broken the barriers that block so many in the world from receiving desperately needed truths that science and research have not yet discovered. On a personal level, he has helped both my daughters and me, giving us tools to support our health that actually work. Celery juice is now a part of our regular routine!"

— Lisa Rinna, star of *The Real Housewives of Beverly Hills* and *Days of Our Lives*, *New York Times* best-selling author, designer of the Lisa Rinna Collection

"Anthony is not only a warm, compassionate healer, he is also authentic and accurate, with God-given skills. He has been a total blessing in my life."

— Naomi Campbell, model, actress, activist

"I had the pleasure of working with Anthony William when he came to Los Angeles and shared his story on Extra. What a fascinating interview as he left the audience wanting to hear more . . . people went crazy for him! His warm personality and big heart are obvious. Anthony has dedicated his life to helping people through the knowledge he receives from Spirit, and he shares all of that information through his Medical Medium books, which are life changing. Anthony William is one of a kind!"

— Sharon Levin, *Extra* Senior Producer

"I've been following Anthony for a while now and am always floored (but not surprised) at the success stories from people following his protocols . . . I have been on my own path of healing for many years, jumping from doctor to doctor and specialist to specialist. He's the real deal and I trust him and his vast knowledge of how the thyroid works and the true effects food has on our body. I have directed countless friends, family, and followers to Anthony because I truly believe he possesses knowledge that no doctor out there has. I am a believer and on a true path to healing now and am honored to know him and blessed to know his work. Every endocrinologist needs to read his book on the thyroid!"

— Marcela Valladolid, chef, author, television host

"I am a doctor's daughter who has always relied on Western medicine to ameliorate even the smallest of woes. Anthony's insights opened my eyes to the healing benefits of food and how a more holistic approach to health can change your life."

— Jenny Mollen, actress and *New York Times* best-selling author of *I Like You Just the Way I Am*

"Anthony William's God-given gift for healing is nothing short of miraculous."

— David James Elliott, *Impulse, Trumbo, Mad Men, CSI: NY*; star for ten years of *JAG*

"Anthony William is a gift to humanity. His incredible work has helped millions of people heal when conventional medicine had no answers for them. His genuine passion and commitment for helping people is unsurpassed, and I am grateful to have been able to share a small part of his powerful message in Heal."

— Kelly Noonan Gores, writer, director, and producer of the *Heal* documentary

"Anthony William is one of those rare individuals who uses his gifts to help people rise up to meet their full potential by becoming their own best health advocates . . . I witnessed Anthony's greatness in action firsthand when I attended one of his thrilling live events. I equate how spot-on his readings were with a singer hitting all the high notes. But beyond the high notes, Anthony's truly compassionate soul is what left the audience captivated. Anthony William is someone I am now proud to call a friend, and I can tell you that the person you hear on the podcasts and whose words fill the pages of best-selling books is the same person who reaches out to loved ones simply to lend support. This is not an act! Anthony William is the real deal, and the gravity of the information he shares through Spirit is priceless and empowering and much needed in this day and age!"

— Debbie Gibson, Broadway star, iconic singer-songwriter

"Anthony William has a remarkable gift! I will always be grateful to him for discovering an underlying cause of several health issues that had bothered me for years. With his kind support, I see improvements every day. I think he is a fabulous resource!"

— Morgan Fairchild, actress, author, speaker

"Within the first three minutes of speaking with me, Anthony precisely identified my medical issue! This healer really knows what he's talking about. Anthony's abilities as the Medical Medium are unique and fascinating."

— Alejandro Junger, M.D., *New York Times* best-selling author of *Clean, Clean Eats*, and *Clean Gut* and founder of the acclaimed Clean Program

"Anthony's gift has made him a conduit for information that is light-years ahead of where science is today."

— Christiane Northrup, M.D., *New York Times* best-selling author of *Goddesses Never Age, The Wisdom of Menopause*, and *Women's Bodies, Women's Wisdom*

MEDICAL MEDIUM

LIVER
RESCUE

ALSO BY ANTHONY WILLIAM

Medical Medium: Secrets behind Chronic and Mystery Illness and How to Finally Heal

Medical Medium Life-Changing Foods: Save Yourself and the Ones You Love with the Hidden Healing Powers of Fruits & Vegetables

Medical Medium Thyroid Healing: The Truth behind Hashimoto's, Graves', Insomnia, Hypothyroidism, Thyroid Nodules & Epstein-Barr

All of the above are available at your local bookstore, or may be ordered by visiting:

Hay House USA: www.hayhouse.com®

Hay House Australia: www.hayhouse.com.au

Hay House UK: www.hayhouse.co.uk

Hay House India: www.hayhouse.co.in

MEDICAL MEDIUM

LIVER RESCUE

ANSWERS TO ECZEMA, PSORIASIS, DIABETES, STREP, ACNE,
GOUT, BLOATING, GALLSTONES, ADRENAL STRESS, FATIGUE,
FATTY LIVER, WEIGHT ISSUES, SIBO & AUTOIMMUNE DISEASE

ANTHONY WILLIAM

HAY HOUSE, INC.
Carlsbad, California • New York City
London • Sydney • New Delhi

Published in the United States by: Hay House, Inc.: www.hayhouse.com®
Published in Australia by: Hay House Australia Pty. Ltd.: www.hayhouse.com.au
Published in the United Kingdom by: Hay House UK, Ltd.: www.hayhouse.co.uk
Published in India by: Hay House Publishers India: www.hayhouse.co.in

Cover design: Vibodha Clark
Interior design: Bryn Starr Best
Interior illustration design: Vibodha Clark
Recipe photos: Ashleigh & Britton Foster
Indexer: Joan Shapiro

Library of Congress Cataloging-in-Publication Data

Names: William, Anthony, author.
Title: Medical medium liver rescue : answers to eczema, psoriasis, diabetes,
   strep, acne, gout, bloating, gallstones, adrenal stress, fatigue, fatty
   liver, weight issues, SIBO & autoimmune disease / Anthony William.
Description: Carlsbad, California : Hay House Inc., 2018.
Identifiers: LCCN 2018034048 | ISBN 9781401954406 (hardback)
Subjects: LCSH: Detoxification (Health) | Liver--Care and hygiene. |
   Medicine, Preventive. | Self-care, Health--Popular works. | BISAC: HEALTH
   & FITNESS / Diseases / Abdominal. | HEALTH & FITNESS / Alternative
   Therapies. | HEALTH & FITNESS / Healing.
Classification: LCC RA784.5 .W53 2018 | DDC 613--dc23 LC record available at https://lccn.loc.gov/2018034048

Hardcover ISBN: 978-1-4019-5440-6
E-book ISBN: 978-1-4019-5441-3

10 9 8 7 6 5 4 3 2 1
1st edition, October 2018

Printed in the United States of America

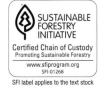

SUSTAINABLE FORESTRY INITIATIVE
Certified Chain of Custody
Promoting Sustainable Forestry
www.sfiprogram.org
SFI-01268
SFI label applies to the text stock

For the Medical Medium communities who wake up every morning
to spread Spirit's message with compassion in their hearts
and life-giving light in their hands.

For all the doctors and practitioners—past, present, and future—who
dedicate their lives to seeking out healing truth for their beloved patients.

And for Mom and Dad, who brought me into this world.

CONTENTS

Foreword xv
A Note for You xix

PART I: Your Liver's True Calling: Miracle Peacekeeper

Chapter 1: What Your Liver Does for You 3
Chapter 2: Your Adaptogenic Liver: Processing Fat and Protecting the Pancreas 11
Chapter 3: Your Life-Giving Liver: Glucose and Glycogen Storage. 19
Chapter 4: Your Medicinal Liver: Vitamin and Mineral Storage 25
Chapter 5: Your Protective Liver: Disarming and Detaining Harmful Materials 29
Chapter 6: Your Purifying Liver: Screening and Filtering Blood. 33
Chapter 7: Your Heroic Liver: The Liver's Immune System. 39

PART II: The Unseen Storm: What's Happening inside Our Livers

Chapter 8: Sluggish Liver 47
Chapter 9: Liver Enzyme Guess Tests. 55
Chapter 10: Dirty Blood Syndrome 63
Chapter 11: Fatty Liver 75
Chapter 12: Weight Gain 81
Chapter 13: Mystery Hunger. 87
Chapter 14: Aging. 93

PART III: The Call to Battle: More Symptoms & Conditions Enlightened

Chapter 15: Diabetes and Blood Sugar Imbalance 101
Chapter 16: Mystery High Blood Pressure 113
Chapter 17: Mystery High Cholesterol 117
Chapter 18: Mystery Heart Palpitations 121
Chapter 19: Adrenal Problems 127

Chapter 20:	Chemical and Food Sensitivities	135
Chapter 21:	Methylation Problems	141
Chapter 22:	Eczema and Psoriasis	147
Chapter 23:	Acne	155
Chapter 24:	SIBO	161
Chapter 25:	Bloating, Constipation, and IBS	171
Chapter 26:	Brain Fog	175
Chapter 27:	Emotional Liver: Mood Struggles and SAD	179
Chapter 28:	PANDAS, Jaundice, and Baby Liver	187
Chapter 29:	Autoimmune Liver and Hepatitis	193
Chapter 30:	Cirrhosis and Liver Scar Tissue	199
Chapter 31:	Liver Cancer	203
Chapter 32:	Gallbladder Sickness	209

PART IV: Liver Salvation: How to Care for Your Liver and Transform Your Life

Chapter 33:	Peace within Your Body	221
Chapter 34:	Liver Myths Debunked	225
Chapter 35:	The High-Fat Trend	247
Chapter 36:	Liver Troublemakers	259
Chapter 37:	Powerful Foods, Herbs, and Supplements for Your Liver	283
Chapter 38:	Liver Rescue 3:6:9	331
Chapter 39:	Liver Rescue Recipes	355
Chapter 40:	Liver Rescue Meditations	425
Chapter 41:	The Storm Will Pass: Peace Be with You	435

Index	443
Acknowledgments	455
About the Author	459

FOREWORD

Every time I read one of Anthony William's books or listen to one of his radio shows, I learn something new. Something that rings true that they don't yet teach in medical school. Not only that, I actually apply a great deal of what I've learned to my own life. An example is a smoothie from his first book, *Medical Medium*. In that book, Anthony gives recipes for breakfast smoothies that you can begin each day with as part of his 28-Day Healing Cleanse—something I followed several years ago. My variation of one particular recipe has become a "go to" staple for me, my granddaughter, and many of my friends. It never fails to elicit rave reviews. And now—after reading *Liver Rescue*—I am happier than ever that I enjoy this elixir regularly. Not only does it hydrate my tissues optimally, it also helps detox my liver each time I drink it.

I won't keep you in suspense. Here it is: 2 to 3 organic bananas, 1½ to 2 cups frozen wild Maine blueberries (I buy these in bulk and keep them handy), a scoop of organic frozen cherries. Then I add water to get the desired consistency (usually 2 to 3 cups) and liquefy it in a blender. This ends up making 2 large servings or 4 small ones. If I don't have guests, I pour the unused portion into a glass Mason jar and keep it for later.

Anthony's book *Medical Medium Life-Changing Foods* was, as the title says, life changing for me, just like his first book. From this beautiful resource, I learned all about the incredible energy, healing information, and spiritual lessons contained in all fruits and vegetables. This knowledge has made eating even the lowly potato (which represents grounding and humility) a far more enjoyable experience. I no longer mindlessly consume food. I now enter into a grateful relationship with it. (Not always, of course, but far more than I used to.)

And now, through reading *Medical Medium Liver Rescue*, I have more respect for my liver—and everyone else's—than I ever did before. As a medical doctor, my introduction to liver function was pretty much limited to newborn jaundice and cirrhosis of the liver in the many alcoholics I cared for as a young intern. I also witnessed the deadly effects on the liver of the first experimental bypass surgeries back in the 1970s. Many of those patients died of complications that included liver failure. Obviously bypass surgery has come a long way since that time.

But here's the thing. Medical science still doesn't appreciate what the liver actually does on a day-to-day basis—long before anything like elevated liver enzymes, fatty liver, or cirrhosis appears. When I wrote the first edition of *The Wisdom of Menopause* back in 2001, I knew full well that menopause, in and of itself, was not to blame for all the many symptoms that women began to experience at midlife, such as insomnia, hot flashes, and irritability. Indeed, *Medical Medium Liver Rescue* points out that, in large part, these symptoms arise from a beleaguered liver—not because a woman has reached a certain age and is now destined to deteriorate, but instead, because our lifestyles have compromised our liver function.

As Anthony points out, the liver offers us two levels of protection against environmental toxins of all kinds: disarmament and detainment. But these functions don't last forever if we continue to ignore our liver function. Anthony elaborates on a phenomenon that I have observed repeatedly over the years. When a woman is, on average, age 38 and a man, on average, 48, these abilities of the liver start to wane and symptoms such as weight gain and hot flashes start—including what we label "aging." For most people, by this time, liver detox capacity has fallen to 60 percent of what it could be. Basically the liver is saying, "I've taken care of you for decades and I can't keep this up unless you change something."

Sobering, isn't it? (And what a great word to use, given alcohol's effect on liver health.)

Here's what you need to know. The liver's job is screening and filtering. It separates the beneficial from the toxic. It cleans the blood that goes from the liver directly to the heart. It is the ultimate blood purifier. It also protects you by sequestering solvents, pesticides, and viruses deep in its core, where they stay out of your blood stream.

When the liver lets go of toxins, they can go to three places. One—they go to the colon via bile and the gallbladder and are eliminated in feces. Two—they go to the kidneys, where toxins are eliminated through urine. And finally, three—they are eliminated in the bloodstream as free radicals (but this is a last resort).

Now listen up. Everyone needs to know this part. We are living in a time when more people than ever are being diagnosed with atrial fibrillation, heart palpitations, and other heart problems. In fact, heart disease of all kinds is the number one killer of both women and men. Here's a large part of the reason, in Anthony's words, which you'll read later on in this book:

When your liver gets to the point of being unable to process all the unproductive material running through it, more free radical debris and toxic matter (and less toxic matter the liver didn't bury in its core) will be in the bloodstream, forcing the heart to pump harder to pull the blood up from the liver—like sucking pudding through a straw—resulting in high blood pressure. If your liver is clogged to the point where biofilm starts to break off into the blood, then you're likely to develop heart flutters as this jelly-like substance gums up heart valves, preventing the smooth flow of blood.

But regardless of where you are now in terms of your health, there's no need to throw up your hands and just accept diminished liver function as inevitable with each passing year. Instead, know that the minute you begin to take care of your liver, it will be far better able to take care of you. Our bodies have an almost miraculous ability to regenerate and restore health when we start giving them the materials and attention they need.

In *Medical Medium Liver Rescue*, you will learn about many of the functions and mysteries of the liver that medical science doesn't yet know about or understand. But most importantly, you will learn exactly what your liver needs to heal itself and perform the lifesaving functions it was designed for. You will learn about a special group of cells known as "perime" that the liver produces when its storage bins get too full, and also a system known as "hepa tracking" that the liver is capable of, producing supernatural ability and strength to prevent troublemakers from being expelled into your blood stream.

I swear, by the end of this book, you will be so grateful for your liver that you will feel compelled to do those things that will help it help you! Not only that, Anthony has included very specific instructions, complete with supplement lists, for supporting your liver in a wide range of situations, from daily maintenance to specific health conditions including acne, irritable bowel syndrome, adrenal problems, bloating, autoimmune disorders, constipation, diabetes, dark under-eye circles, eczema and psoriasis, fatigue, gallbladder infections, gallstones, gout, heart palpitations, high blood pressure, high cholesterol, hot flashes, jaundice, liver aging, Raynaud's syndrome, seasonal affective disorder, weight gain, and even varicose and spider veins. Finally, there is an entire chapter on Liver Rescue that anyone can use to rescue and restore optimal liver function.

In summary, *Medical Medium Liver Rescue* belongs in everyone's health library. Read it. Apply it—even if just a few of the suggestions—and enjoy the lifelong benefits of a healthy, happy liver. You won't regret it.

— Christiane Northrup, M.D., *New York Times* best-selling author of *Goddesses Never Age*, *The Wisdom of Menopause*, and *Women's Bodies, Women's Wisdom*

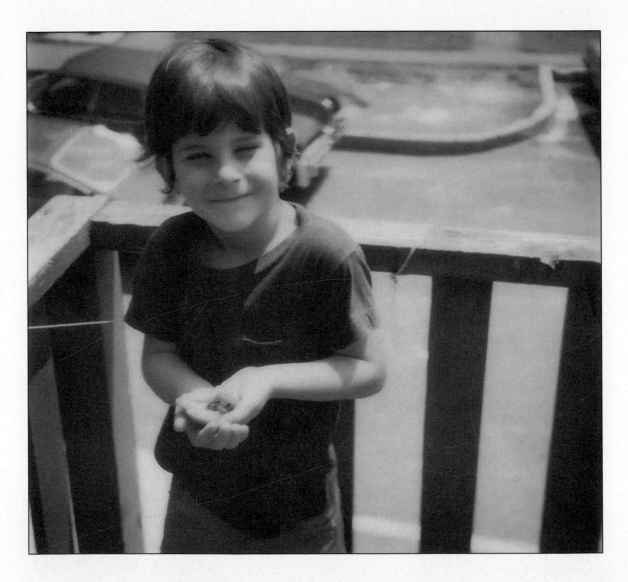

Anthony William, age 4, healing an injured baby bird

A NOTE FOR YOU

Treasure hunting has long been a part of human history. When people search for treasure, whether it's an old shipwreck filled with bounty or a chest of gold marked on a treasure map, it's common to get very close after years spent far away. The searchers have done their research, sometimes decades of it, spent all the money they could possibly spend, invested their time and energy, and then, as they're digging down, an earthquake sends the treasure toppling through a crevice so that they'll never reach it. The same can happen with a shipwreck. Ocean conditions must be just right for diving—a collapsed coral reef could block it, or shark-infested waters could make it too unsafe.

The truth about chronic illness has been so far away for so many decades, with good people researching and getting closer to answers. Famous neurologists get nearer and then can't keep going due to lack of funding. Just as we get close in this modern day of medicine, in which so many people have suffered and even lost lives with no answers, all progress is put on the shelf. Answers are only almost found. A theory such as the gene blame game puts the truth

further away, because it causes medical science to pour all its resources into researching genes instead of digging for the answers that would actually put a stop to the chronic illness madness that has been with us for far too long.

How many times have you seen something unfold that you knew could have gone differently if only others understood what you'd learned in life? For my whole life, I've watched the decades roll by while medical communities move along with steps and missteps, trying to figure out why people suffer. I've witnessed them almost stumble upon the answers to what causes chronic illness and then never quite pull through and succeed. My job is to deliver the answers to you. Are you ready to receive them?

In these pages, you'll find the truths that medical science and research have come so close to having in hand and then been thwarted from attaining. I've been given the answers about chronic symptoms and conditions so that you don't need to be held back anymore by the blunders and roadblocks in the way of medical advancements in chronic illness. Here, there's no fire-breathing dragon guarding the castle of answers or sea monster blocking the treasure chest. There are no funding deficits or agendas or grandfathered mistakes to stop you from discovering how to move forward, because I'm not shackled by a system. Freedom lives here in these words; it is attainable.

THE EPIDEMIC OF CHRONIC AND MYSTERY ILLNESS

Chronic illness is at an all-time high. In America alone, more than 250 million people are sick or dealing with mystery symptoms. These are people leading diminished lives with no explanation—or explanations that don't sit right or that make them feel even worse. You may be one of them. If so, you can attest that medical science is still puzzling through what's behind the epidemic of mystery symptoms and suffering.

Let me be clear that I revere good medical science. There are incredibly gifted and talented doctors, surgeons, nurses, technicians, researchers, chemists, and more doing profound work in both conventional and alternative medicine. I've had the privilege of working with some of them. Thank God for these compassionate healers. Learning how to understand our world through rigorous, systematic inquiry is one of the highest pursuits imaginable.

Most doctors have an innate wisdom and intuition that tells them that the medical establishment doesn't give them what they need in order to offer the best diagnosis and treatment plan when it comes to chronic illness. How many times have you heard, "There is no known cure for [fill-in-the-blank disease]"? Even at the best, most elite medical schools, there are doctors who graduated at the top of the class who are honest about the fact that they finished school unprepared to work with chronic illness patients. They had to become experts on their own. Then there are doctors who believe that they are given all the answers in school and for some reason think that their training supersedes the mysteries of chronic illness; they think everything else is nonsense and hocus-pocus, which is unfortunate, since they live in denial of the millions of people who are suffering with no real answers. Either way, it's not doctors' or researchers' fault that the medical industry hasn't been able to solve the mysteries of chronic illness. Every day, amazing, brilliant minds in science stumble upon discoveries that require a green light from investors and decision makers at the top in order to move forward. Thousands of discoveries that could really change people's lives for the better are kept from going anywhere, and individuals in the field of science are held back.

We sometimes treat medical science like pure mathematics, governed solely by logic and reason. Though at times intertwined, math and medical science aren't the same. Math is definitive; science isn't. True science applies to an outcome, a result of applying theory. You can use math in medical science; you can use it to make a drug, for example, though the drug shouldn't be deemed scientific until there's a proven result and the numbers make sense in the end. Science labs are play shops of people methodically slapping together different materials to test out different hypotheses and theories while investors apply pressure to rush a favorable outcome. Too often, theories are treated as fact before they ever get a chance to be proven—or disproven. That's especially the case with chronic illness. It's extremely rare in the medicine of chronic illness that you ever get a straight answer that's correct.

Wouldn't it be nice if science were the ideal we sometimes make it out to be? If it were a pursuit where money never mattered and only the truth won out? Like any human pursuit, medical science is still a work in progress. Think about the recent recognition of the mesentery as an organ. Here this active, mesh-like connective tissue has been in plain sight all along and even acknowledged along the way, and only now is it beginning to get its full due. There's more to come; new breakthroughs occur every day. Science is constantly evolving, and so theories that one day seem like the be-all and end-all can be revealed the next day to be obsolete. What this translates to is: science doesn't have every answer yet.

We've already waited 100-plus years for real insights from medical communities into liver problems—and the health problems no one knows are liver problems—and they haven't come. You shouldn't have to wait another 10, 20, 30, or more years for scientific research to find the real answers. If you're stuck in bed, dragging through your days, or feeling lost about your health, you shouldn't have to go through one more day of it, let alone another decade. You shouldn't have to watch your children go through it, either—and yet millions do.

A HIGHER SOURCE

That's why Spirit of the Most High, God's expression of compassion, came into my life when I was four years old: to teach me how to see the true causes of people's suffering and to get that information out into the world. If you'd like to know more about my origins, you'll find my story in *Medical Medium: Secrets Behind Chronic and Mystery Illness and How to Finally Heal*. The short version is that Spirit constantly speaks into my ear with clarity and precision, as if a friend were standing beside me, filling me

in on the symptoms of everyone around me. Plus, Spirit taught me from an early age to see physical scans of people, like supercharged MRI scans that reveal all blockages, illnesses, infections, trouble areas, and past problems.

We see you. We know what you're up against. And we don't want you to go through it a moment longer. My life's work is to deliver this information to you, so that you can be elevated above the sea of confusion—the noise and rhetoric of today's health fads and trends—in order to regain your health and navigate life on your own terms.

The material in this book is authentic, the real deal, all for your benefit. This book is not like other health books. There's so much packed in here that you may want to come back and read it again to make sure you get all the information. Sometimes this information will seem to be the opposite of what you've heard before, and sometimes it will be close to other sources, with subtle and critical differences. The common thread is that it's the truth. It's not repackaged or recycled theory made to sound like a new understanding of chronic symptoms and illness. The information here doesn't come from broken science, interest groups, medical funding with strings attached, botched research, lobbyists, internal kickbacks, persuaded belief systems, private panels of influencers, health-field payoffs, or trendy traps.

The above hurdles get in the way of medical research and science making the leaps and bounds it's meant to in understanding chronic illness. When outside sources have a vested interest in obscuring certain truths, then precious research time and money get spent in unproductive areas. Certain discoveries that would truly advance the treatment of chronic illness get ignored and lose funding. The scientific data we think of as absolute can, instead, be skewed—contaminated and manipulated—and then treated by other health experts as law, even though it's inherently flawed.

To go with the facts and figures about liver health in the pages to come, you won't find citations or mentions of scientific studies that have spawned from unproductive sources. You don't need to worry that this information will be proven wrong or superseded, as you do with other health books, because all of the health information I share here comes from a pure, untampered-with, advanced, clean source—a higher source: the Spirit of Compassion. There's nothing more healing than compassion.

If you're someone who only believes in what science has to say, know that I like science, too. Also know that unless we're talking about liver transplants (an area where science is phenomenally advanced), science still has a lot to learn about the liver's day-in, day-out functions, challenges, and needs. While we're in a great time, we're also sicker and more tired than ever before in history. If medical professionals had any idea how much of people's suffering traces back to an overburdened or neglected liver, there would be a revolution in the way we think about nearly every aspect of our health.

Unlike many other areas of science, which are strongly founded in weights and measures and math, scientific thinking about chronic illness is all still theoretical—and today's theories hold very little truth, which is why so many people are still dealing with chronic symptoms and conditions. If it keeps going like this, we'll reach a point where there aren't any studies at all in which agendas and interests aren't driving the outcomes against your favor. This trend is why the scientific establishment has let chronic illness communities down since the beginning, letting doctors down, too, and leaving hundreds of millions to suffer.

WE THE QUESTIONERS

Once upon a time, we lived by the rule of authority. We were told that the earth was flat, and then that the sun revolved around the earth, so we believed it. Those theories weren't fact, and yet people treated them like they were. People living back then didn't feel like life was backward; it was just the way life was. Anyone who spoke out against the status quo seemed like a fool. Then came the paradigm shift of science. The questioners—the committed researchers and thinkers—the ones who all along hadn't been content to take a "fact" at face value, finally proved that analysis could open the door to a much deeper, truer understanding of our world.

Now, science has become the new authority. In some cases, this saves lives. Surgeons now use sterile tools, for example, because they understand the risk of contamination that surgeons of old didn't realize. Just because of certain advancements, though, we can't stop actively questioning. It's time for that next paradigm shift. "Because science" isn't enough of an answer when it comes to chronic illness. Is it *good* science? What was the funding behind it? Was the sample size diverse enough? Big enough? Were the controls handled ethically? Were enough factors considered? Were the measurement tools advanced enough? Does the analysis stamped on the results tell a different story from the numbers themselves? Was there bias? Did an influencer of establishment power put a thumb on the scale? Some science will hold up brilliantly. Some will reveal holes: payoffs, kickbacks, small sample sizes, poor controls. We're handed the word *science* as though we're meant to bow down to it without question. It sounds a lot like an authoritative ideology, doesn't it? We haven't shifted out of that belief system as much as we think. Progress doesn't happen without the very framework being questioned—and in our society today, we're not allowed to question the scientific framework.

Trends don't always look like trends. They often disguise themselves as sound medical advice. So much of the health information out there is repetition or, worse, garbled whisper-down-the-lane. We must be wary of someone sending out a message with an agenda so that when it reaches us, it's twisted. Good primary sources used to be the gold standard. Now, in an enormous push for content, some research for health literature gets rushed, published based on one okay-enough-sounding source. We must look at the special interests of who's interpreting and posting. Even the research results themselves—can they be trusted?

Science is so often used as an attack mechanism. That label can be used to put a spin on everything possible. Take the food wars, for example. Vegans are battling paleos with science. Paleos are battling vegans with science. They're both using studies to justify their sides—because you can find a study to justify practically anything. (Eating liver to help your liver? There's a study for that. Cheese as a longevity food? There's a study for that. Are they right, or are they skewed? That's for you to decide as you read this book.) When even science isn't enough, food war participants go for the emotional aspect of the other's belief system. Vegans tell paleos they're killing animals. Paleos tell vegans they're starving themselves and their children. Getting better is not about choosing sides or what you have adopted as a belief system in that moment—even if it's a belief system based on reports you've read of scientific studies. It's about understanding our livers' responsibilities and supporting them in those.

We won't get there by treating science as God and treating those who question theories and findings as fools. Medical science looks out for medical science. While individual health-care providers can have the best of intentions, the greater industry is not about looking out for a person; it's about looking out for itself, since it has its authority to uphold. It's self-involvement in the most chronic way.

Let's be honest. Even today's science in those areas we think to be concrete sometimes shows cracks. If you've heard about recalls of hip replacement parts or hernia mesh, you know what I'm talking about. These are tangible items that were designed with exacting scientific standards, then went through rigorous scientific testing before being put to use, and even that highly scientific process wasn't guaranteed. Certain products developed unforeseen problems, and an area of science that seemed indisputable turned out to be fallible. Think, then, what kind of uncertainty remains in scientific understanding of chronic illness, the liver, and the liver's multitude of functions. This isn't a device that can be held in your hand, measured, and analyzed independently from the rest of you. It's an active part of the human body, and we all know the human body to be one of the greatest miracles and mysteries of life. Again, science is a human pursuit and a work in progress, especially when that work involves decoding the human body. It takes constant vigilance, receptiveness, and adaptability to keep that work truly progressing.

If you've never struggled with your health, suffering for years with no answers for your condition, or if you feel cemented within a certain medical, scientific, or nutritional belief system, I hope that you'll approach the chapters to come with curiosity and an open heart. The meaning behind today's widespread chronic symptoms and suffering is so much bigger than anyone has yet discovered. What you're about to read is unlike any information about the liver, chronic health issues, or healing you've seen before. This information has helped tens of thousands of people over the past decades.

ALL IN THIS TOGETHER

Since I first started to share Spirit's information, I've been so blessed to see it make a difference for these people. With the publication of the Medical Medium book series, I've been beyond moved to see this information reach the wider world and help thousands more.

I've also noticed that some of these messages have been manipulated as certain career-driven individuals try to climb the ladder of acclaim and notoriety. This approach gets at people's core, raw nerve of suffering and takes advantage of it.

This is not how the gift I was given was ever meant to be used. Spirit is a voice for the ones in need of answers, a source independent from a system filled with traps that have wasted so many lives along the way. We love it when people become experts on the health information I share and when they spread the compassionate message far and wide in the name of truly helping others. I am so thankful for this. What gets dangerous is when that information is tampered with—intermixed and twisted with trendy misinformation, changed just enough so that it sounds original, or blatantly poached and attributed to seemingly credible sources that are anemic of the truth. I say this because I want you to know to protect yourself and your loved ones from the misguidance out there.

This book is not repetition of everything you've already read. It's not about a belief system that blames your genes or says your body is faulty, nor is it about putting a spin on a trendy high-protein diet to keep symptoms at bay. This information is fresh—an entirely new perspective on the symptoms holding back so many people in life, and an entirely new perspective on how to heal.

I get it if you're wary. We react, we judge; that's what we do. It can be an instinct that protects us in certain circumstances; sometimes, it gets us through life. In this case, I hope you'll reconsider. You may judge yourself out of learning the truth. You could lose the opportunity to help yourself or somebody else.

So fasten your seat belts with me here. We are all in this together with getting people better, and I want you to become the new expert in liver health. Thank you for coming with me on this healing journey and taking the time to read this book. Learning the truth will change everything for you and the ones around you—now you'll finally hold the treasure.

"We see you. We know what you're up against.
And we don't want you to go through it
a moment longer."

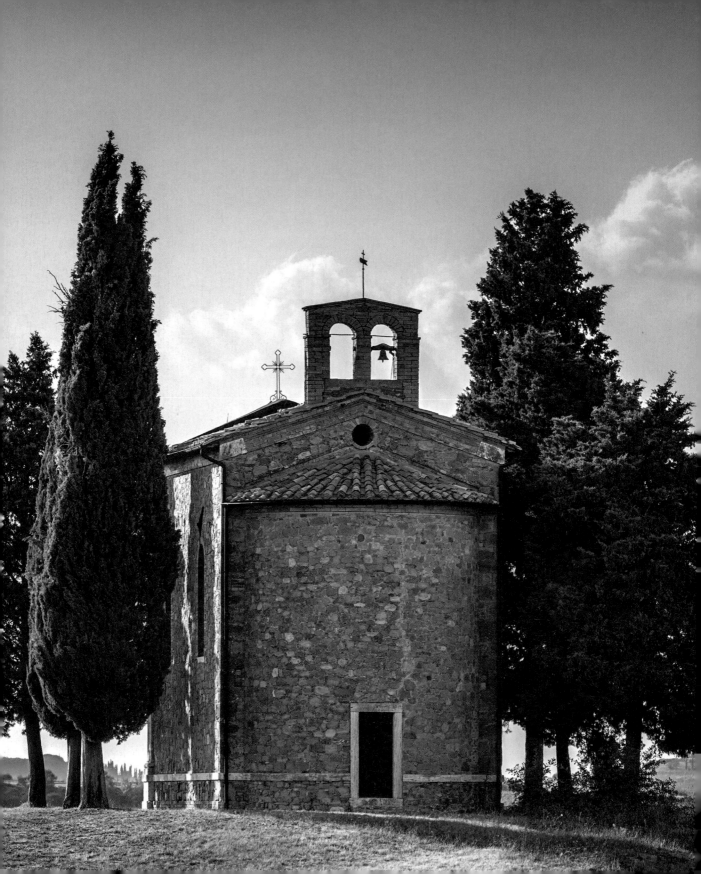

PART I

YOUR LIVER'S TRUE CALLING

MIRACLE PEACEKEEPER

CHAPTER 1

What Your Liver Does for You

A small crowd stands on the dock, waiting to board the boat that will take them to deeper water. Off to the side, the tour photographer perches with her camera, snapping photos of the soon-to-be-passengers. Their faces are expectant, though none are overjoyed. It's drizzling and chilly. A few people missed breakfast to get here on time, and it wasn't their idea, anyway, to spend the morning at sea—they're humoring friends and family members who insisted it was worth taking a few hours out of their busy lives to appreciate the natural world.

Out on the water, the mood starts to lift. The breeze wakes everyone up, and the farther the ship gets from civilization, the easier it is to forget earthly troubles. Several passengers lean against the sides, mesmerized by the endless ripples, wondering if they'll see what they came for or if this hope, like so many others before it, will elude them.

And then, it happens. The tour guide instructs the group to look out over the starboard side—a flipper has been spotted. Passengers gather along the railings, a few pointing to the spot where they saw it before it vanished underwater. The crowd stands waiting. A moment passes, then another. *Was it worth getting up from my seat?* a few of them wonder. They stare.

Finally, a wide expanse of slick skin begins to surface, and with it, an eruption of sacred ocean spray as the magnificent creature empties its lungs. The crowd inhales the tonic and collectively breathes out an *Oooooh*. Next comes an *Aaaaahh* as the whale comes up again and rolls over in the water, showing off another flipper before dipping back down. The blessed animal stays with the ship for a few moments longer, and the *oohs* and *aahs* continue. At last, the whale displays its tail high in the air before parting ways.

Every last passenger applauds. Every last passenger has just had a profound religious experience. Snap some photos of them as they step off the boat, compare them side by side with the "before" photos, and you'll see radically changed people, like they're floating on air and their souls have been infused with the light of God.

We all know that whales exist. Maybe we've watched some nature specials, seen an article or an inspirational poster here or there. We don't hear much about them in daily life, though. If whales are doing well or if their numbers are dwindling, if pollution is threatening them or if it's a great year for migration, it's not the main news of the day. Whales live out of sight, and we're a you've-got-to-see-it-to-believe-it—or you've-got-to-see-it-to-appreciate-it—kind of culture. To be changed by these gentle giants, we need to go out looking for them. To understand their value, it takes seeing them up close.

It's the way it is with so much of life. Think of the soon-to-be-parent standing in the ultrasound lab next to their partner, seeing an image of the fetus growing inside that pregnant belly for the first time. The level of realization is profound in a way that no amount of maternity clothes piling up in the closet or prenatal vitamins on the kitchen counter can conjure. Until that moment of seeing the baby on the screen, what was going on beneath the surface could only be imagined for the partner who didn't feel the growth happening inside; it wasn't as real.

Believe it or not, the workings of your liver are up there with these most profound, hidden miracles of the universe. That's right—sea creatures as big as dinosaurs, the phenomenon of birth . . . and your liver.

A REAL MISSING LINK

You wouldn't know it, because the liver doesn't get much attention. Of the organs, it's not Mr. Popular. We don't learn much about the liver in school, and it doesn't make headline news as, say, the brain does. With the brain, we can hook up some diodes and watch its waves. We know the difference between asleep and awake. We can feel directly when we're experiencing thought blockages, emotional issues, anxiety, or depression. We're familiar, too, with the effects of mental deterioration, on the lookout for symptoms of dementia. In so many ways,

we're reminded of our brains on a daily basis, down to common expressions like "brain food," "Use your head," "She has a good head on her shoulders," and pointing to our head and saying, "It's all in here."

The heart, too, makes a lot of headlines, because it's there in daily evidence. We feel it beat; we feel it race; we can tell if it's out of sync. We can see its patterns on a heart monitor and track whether our heart rate improves on an exercise program. We see "heart-healthy" labels at the grocery store, and from the time we were kids, we've known about broken hearts and heartaches and heart attacks, seen heart shapes plastered everywhere on Valentine's Day, made heart shapes with our hands, and loved from the bottom of our hearts. We say, "That warms my heart," and sing about "a little bit of my heart," and may tell a friend with a new boyfriend, "Don't give him your heart yet." The parent watching a child enter a first relationship prays that the child's heart is protected.

Other body parts, too, make themselves known. Our muscles get firmer and more pronounced when we exercise or smaller and softer when we spend our days stuck in bed. Our skin is a plain-to-see reflection of what's going on in our life, whether pale or peeling or rashy or broken out—or glowing. With the lungs, we can see the rib cage expand when we take a deep breath and shrink when we let it go. Though smoking was once an unknown threat, now public service announcements about the danger of smoking and lung cancer are everywhere. Our bladders are evident when they fill up; we analyze the color and amount and content of our urine; and pain and burning let us know of urinary tract infections. The gut is constantly reminding us that it's there, too. We can feel the stomach when it's full, we can feel it rumble when it's empty, and we can even examine the contents of what it expels. We know to place a high value on these and other critical body parts, because it's easy to pay witness to their hard work.

Then there's the liver—out of sight, out of mind. For all we know, it's not there; it's just a word we heard mentioned in a grandmother's kitchen as she made stuffing with turkey giblets. If we can't feel the liver the way we can feel the heart beating, then it can't be working all that hard for us. If we can't see it struggling, then there must not be a problem. And so the organ remains in that mystery category. What's it really doing in there? Anything? It's easy to forget the liver even exists.

Medical experts know *something* is wrong beneath the surface. They know something beyond what can be seen and felt is amiss. They witness health complaints on the rise. They witness patient after patient describing mysterious, chronic illnesses, and so they look high and low for answers. Trouble is, health trends often get in the way of finding the truth.

One recent trend has directed an enormous amount of time, energy, and resources toward the thyroid. We looked at this popular theory in my previous book, *Medical Medium Thyroid Healing: The Truth behind Hashimoto's, Graves', Insomnia, Hypothyroidism, Thyroid Nodules & Epstein-Barr*. The trend puts forth that an ailing thyroid is the explanation for everything from hair loss to miscarriage—and we looked at why that trend is wrong. While the thyroid is an incredible part of the human body, the gland itself is not the missing link in the explanation of chronic illness. So much of the time, when the thyroid gets the blame—or the heart or the gut or the genes—it's really about a liver in trouble.

Truth is, your liver is the best friend you've ever had. It performs over 2,000 critical functions that are undiscovered by medical research and science. It works hard for you night and day.

It prepares ahead when it knows you need extra support, and it's there to clean up the mess after your earthly mistakes. It's a storehouse, a filter, a processing center, a garbage service, and more. It shields you, it protects you, and it defends you from every angle. It's been looking out for you all along—dying out fires, defusing bombs, taking bullets for you, rounding up the bad guys inside of you, and preventing internal disasters. Your liver is the reason, after everything you've been through in life, that you're still alive.

Ask a surgeon what it was like to see a living liver for the first time. After all those classroom hours and all that textbook reading, after seeing picture upon picture, after months in the lab practicing on cadavers, what was it like to stand in the operating room with a patient's functioning liver exposed? The surgeon will probably describe disbelief. Maybe she or he couldn't even sleep that night from the buzz of seeing the majestic, mysterious organ in its element—just like witnessing a majestic, mysterious whale. That's with knowing only a fraction of what the liver does.

Now you get to see your liver in a whole new light, to have that surgeon's appreciation for the liver—and then some. That's why I wrote this book: so you could see inside your body and get acquainted with your greatest ally, the one that's been there for you all this time, the one working harder than anyone knows. To be wowed by the wonders of the natural world, we don't need to go to the farthest reaches of the globe; we need only to look inside ourselves.

THE ENDANGERED LIVER

What if you're too overloaded to examine miracles for miracles' sake? In the face of daily challenges, when we have a million pressing tasks to accomplish, what does it matter that the liver is a dazzling display of the intelligence of the human body? Why care about the liver?

We already have so much to worry about. Keeping our families safe and healthy; performing well at work; staying fit; avoiding the obesity epidemic, the depression epidemic, heart disease, early aging; living with chronic illness; inheriting a polluted earth; wildlife going extinct; an uncertain future . . . the list goes on and on. Up against all this, it takes enough energy to get through the day. So why add one more item to the list? Why burden ourselves with an extra concern—the liver, of all things—when we constantly hear that we're supposed to be de-stressing, simplifying, and learning the art of saying no to what we don't need?

Because our livers are in trouble, and we do *need* to take better care of them. Because discovering the power of your liver—and the power of caring for your liver—changes everything. Because what if there were one aspect of your well-being that you could focus on that would help with all the others—plus take care of the developing health problems you don't even know you have? If only we realized how many symptoms, conditions, and diseases are rooted in the liver—that it's not just about liver cancer, cirrhosis, and hepatitis—the liver would be front and center in the medical world.

Liver rescue is about your heart, brain, immune system, skin, and gut. It's about sleeping well, balancing blood sugar, lowering blood pressure, losing weight, and looking and feeling younger. It's about being clearer-headed, more peaceful, happier. It's about being able to adapt to our fast-changing times. Saying yes to liver support is the most efficient action on your to-do list. A healthy liver is the ultimate de-stressor, the ultimate anti-aging ally, the ultimate safeguard against a threatening world. It's

key to mental, emotional, physical, and spiritual well-being. Turning your attention to your liver is not the proverbial straw that broke the camel's back; it's the helping hand that lightened the camel's load and saved its life.

When people seek enlightenment, they focus on the brain and third eye, trying to reach higher consciousness by quieting the mind or to manifest the future through their thoughts. The liver gets completely ignored in the process. Meanwhile, we can glean more enlightenment from our livers than you would believe.

With all our focus on the health of the planet, we can't lose sight of our own climates. We each have an individual planet that we need to worry about: our body. For your whole life, you've carried around a whole world. And just as we know that the earth's delicate balance means that one weakened link can threaten the integrity of the whole, it matters how we take care of ourselves. Are creatures like those majestic whales important? Do we care if they go extinct? Of course— endangered species matter, and they deserve protection. So do our overworked, overburdened, maxed-out, stressed-out, threatened livers. Nobody wants a world with toxic oceans and species struggling to survive amid pollution. And nobody wants a body with toxic blood and a liver that's struggling to do its many jobs that keep you healthy.

Yet here we are, at a moment in history when our livers are endangered. Our own environments are mucky with the toxins we're exposed to in everyday life—in fact, our bodies are worse off than our planet—and our livers bear the brunt of the cleanup job. Envision your liver as a baleen whale and your blood as the ocean. If the ocean gets thick with sludge—think antibiotics, other medications, pesticides, fungicides, cleaning products, solvents, plastics, chronic dehydration, viral and bacterial waste matter, excess fat from unproductive foods, and more—it's harder for that whale to pull in nourishment. Without ever getting a break, the whale can get sickly over time. It can become difficult for it to even come up for air.

The world has liver issues. At this point, it's more common than not to have a compromised liver. If I walk into a crowd of 1,000 people, 900 will have hurting livers—and almost none of them will know it. That's because, as I mentioned, the liver is more important than anyone realizes. Medical science has dedicated relatively little research to the liver other than in the realm of transplants, so it isn't taught how connected the liver is to the state of ill health in the world. Medical communities haven't yet been informed about all that the liver does; how many of the health complaints, diseases, symptoms, and conditions of our time are actually symptomatic of liver trouble; or what the liver most needs to thrive, so they aren't able to pass along this critical knowledge. It remains a distant unknown, like the Great Pacific Garbage Patch before it was discovered. (Even that discovery remains a mystery as far as what truly festers deep within its murky, uninhabitable core.) Without realizing it, we're forced to push our livers to their absolute limits.

If we want to make a difference on this earth, we need to be able to function. Symptoms limit us. Brain fog, fatigue, weight gain, seasonal affective disorder (SAD), irritability, high blood pressure, high cholesterol, anxiousness, acne, bloating, and constipation are experiences so commonplace that you may not even think of them as symptoms of anything underlying—yet they're very often signs of a liver calling out for help. They're holding people back, coloring their view of life, and growing into more serious conditions if we don't know how to stop them. Liver trouble can be like a rotten tooth that keeps on getting ignored until it eventually creates a deep infection in the jaw.

Then there are the conditions that we know are serious and seem almost impossible to stop: ones like diabetes, depression, heart palpitations, gout, eczema, psoriasis, and methylation problems—it's also unknown that these are liver-caused. As for fatty liver, jaundice, hepatitis, cirrhosis, and liver cancer, the medical knowledge that they're related to the liver doesn't take away the mystery surrounding them. Not to mention that as our body's main filter and nutritional storehouse, the liver is essential for dealing with any health problem, period. So the fact that liver problems are rampant globally puts us at a precarious moment.

It's not an overstatement to say that if every person walking around on this planet right now had a healthy liver, the world would be a different place. Illness wouldn't have the hold it does on the population. Anger, rage, greed, and violence wouldn't fill the news. Fear wouldn't define the modern age. That's how tied into our beings liver health is.

Which is why our livers matter. Like a vortex of plastics in the ocean—or like a threatened species—the liver can't be ignored anymore just because it doesn't seem real. It can't be cast aside in the name of loftier goals like saving the world. Those lofty goals start with saving our lives first—and that starts with saving our livers.

LIVER 101

If medical research and science grasped the full scope of the liver's value, kids would be learning their liver basics right alongside their ABCs and 123s. In college, Liver 101 would be a required course for everyone, not just students aiming for medical school.

Instead, we inadvertently strain our livers from an early age. And what happens when we grow up and go off to university? To offset the stress, so many students experiment with drinking, maybe even drugs, while eating poorly, hyping themselves up on caffeine, and pulling all-nighters. This does a number on their livers without their knowledge—which is ironic, since knowledge is the goal of education. It's like college is one long anti-liver protest. We focus so much on the promise of a young person's mind and on developing the brain—anything to get the "right" grades and the "right" credits to have the "right" career someday—that it can come at the expense of the liver. What's that brilliant career if the liver gets overburdened and keeps you from performing at your best, or if your liver gets so bad that you lose the job that you fought so hard to land? All those credentials and stamps of approval can't help you out of bed when fatigue and other symptoms have flattened you.

We know in the backs of our minds that drinking too much can cause the liver harm; we've heard the terms *cirrhosis*, *hepatitis*, *liver failure*, *jaundice*, *liver cancer*, and *elevated liver enzymes*; maybe we've come across a mention of *liver heat* or been offered liver supplements by an alternative practitioner. And of course we've all heard of eating animal liver—which happens to be one of the worst things you can do for your own liver (more on that later). For many of us, that's the extent of what we associate with the liver. The liver got more attention in ancient mythology than it does is modern medicine.

There's still so much of the nitty-gritty left to be discovered. In medical school, not very much time is spent teaching doctors-in-training about the anatomy of the liver and its working parts, unless you're planning to be a surgeon or hepatologist or opting for an elective on liver transplants. Even then, you don't learn about its essence. You don't learn about how to truly take care of one. The resources available are like a few grains of sand on an entire beach.

What would we learn if we did get the liver education we're meant to receive? To begin with, we'd discover that the liver is a workhorse, performing thousands of functions, the most critical of which we'll explore in the remaining chapters of Part I, "Your Liver's True Calling: Miracle Peacekeeper":

- Processing fat and protecting the pancreas
- Glucose and glycogen storage
- Vitamin and mineral storage
- Disarming and detaining harmful materials
- Screening and filtering blood
- Guarding you with its own personalized immune system

In all of this, your liver's job is to keep you balanced, which is a pretty tall order in a world that's so imbalanced. Do you work hard in life, to the point of feeling overworked? Do you ever feel under heat? Do you feel like everything you do is behind the scenes, so you never get credit? Multiply it all by 20 and we've just described your liver. You could be working off-the-charts hard, with five jobs and 100 responsibilities, and your liver's working harder. Appreciating the liver for this feat is a huge part of moving forward with it in harmony—like finally being acknowledged by your partner for the endless household tasks you usually do without thanks.

In the ideal liver education, we'd also discover that the liver is a warhorse. As we'll explore in Part II, "The Unseen Storm: What's Happening inside Our Livers," and Part III, "The

Call to Battle: More Symptoms and Conditions Enlightened," it's ready to fight for you at any moment and works constantly to shield your other organs. In fact, it's probably in battle for you right now, up against poisons and pathogens such as the Unforgiving Four (radiation, toxic heavy metals, DDT, and the viral explosion), which we're often exposed to in daily life, along with the unproductive foods and ingredients that sneak their way into our diets. These liver battles often show themselves in the form of symptoms and conditions, so it's all about decoding what that elevated blood sugar, high blood pressure or cholesterol, or brain fog really mean. Understanding, for example, that unexplained weight gain is a sign of a clogged liver, not laziness or a permanently slow metabolism, can radically change your outlook on life. If you're struggling with ailments such as eczema, gout, or diabetes, know that it's not your fault. Take away the mystery, and it takes away the struggle's power over you.

Finally, as part of our ultimate liver training, we'd find that the care and feeding of the liver is paramount. Has there ever been a time in your life when you felt run ragged? When you needed a rest? When you needed to be soothed and pampered while you recovered from life's battles? That's exactly what the liver is crying out for, so in Part IV, "Liver Salvation: How to Care for Your Liver and Transform Your Life," we'll look at how to restore peace to your liver when it's overwhelmed—and simple yet potent ways to care for it in everyday life, so you can prevent health problems before they start. The liver has incredible powers of healing and regeneration, and they're yours to harness.

YOUR BEST FRIEND FOR LIFE

When you become your own liver expert, life becomes bright and shiny and new. It's not only the relief of feeling like you're in control again and rediscovering your ability to heal; it's also because your liver is intimately tied to your emotional well-being, which we'll also explore more in this book. Getting in touch with your liver is how you get in touch with who you are on a soul level. It's not the lesson we're taught as we grow up, and yet it's the gem: for more wonder and magic and happiness, liver harmony is key. Since your liver is your best friend, there's a back-and-forth. How we feel affects that friend, and how that friend feels affects us. Without knowing it, we've been putting a strain on that friend. We've been getting in its way, and that's been bringing us down. Work with your friend, not against it, and that all changes.

If you're tired and frustrated and sometimes feel alone, if you drag through the day, if your back is always against the wall, remember that your liver is on your side, fiercely loyal and waiting patiently for the moment when you see its true value. You're about to learn more about the liver—and what it can do for you—than you ever thought possible.

So hang on for this ride. It's time to push off from shore and witness what's deep down inside of us, waiting to reveal itself so we can better understand the nature of life. It's time to repay the debt to this most giving of organs. It's time to rescue your liver, so it can rescue you.

CHAPTER 2

Your Adaptogenic Liver

Processing Fat and Protecting Your Pancreas

Your liver is the only organ in your body that's truly adaptogenic. While the brain has amazing adaptive abilities in certain situations when mind, body, spirit, soul, and environment all come together for the right person, it doesn't matter who you are or where you are with the liver—when it's well cared for, your liver has the ability to adapt to your every situation.

Have you ever been in an interaction where no matter how hard you tried, you couldn't get a concept through to someone? That's because some people's brains can't adapt to certain situations. It's why a little while after a new employee has started, a manager who's observed what clicks and what doesn't will often assign her or him to stick to certain tasks. As much as we think of the brain as adaptive, you really have to work to get it to adapt, and some people's adapt more easily than others'. It's why you'll hear the expression "Get this through your thick head."

The liver is more adaptive. On the spot, on a dime, on time—*bam*, it adapts without your even realizing it. Nonstop, it's switching job responsibilities hyper-fast and performing its different chemical functions, no questions asked. That employee at a new job will take weeks to adapt, asking a million questions, coming up against challenge after challenge in getting her or his brain to adapt. Simply taking a new route to work could take months of adjustment. Not so with the liver. You won't need someone yelling at you, "Get this through your thick liver!"

When it's supported, your liver has the ability to release and withhold at will. If you get cold, your liver will create heat to warm you; if you get hot, it will take on heat to cool you. If you run a marathon, your liver will release every bit of stored glucose to help you cross the finish line. If you drink too much water and dilute your blood composition, your liver will absorb the excess water like a sponge. If you breathe in cigarette smoke, your liver will absorb the smoke's chemicals from your bloodstream. If you eat a 12-ounce steak with French fries and chocolate cake, your liver will process and break down those denatured omega-6s and trans fatty acids to protect you. If you're swimming in the ocean and a rogue wave starts taking you out to sea or a riptide pulls you under and won't let go, your liver will release its storage banks of adrenaline to give you superhuman strength and a chance at saving yourself.

Not only that—your liver is also a memory bank. Your liver is like your third brain, alongside your body's second brain, your thyroid. It's a memory organ in its own right, equal to the brain in power. If on the first Friday of every month you go out with your friends and treat yourself with drinks, chicken wings, and tiramisu, your liver remembers when your splurge day is and prepares ahead of time. If you eat pizza every weekend, your liver knows. If your eating habits seem unpredictable, your liver tracks the sporadic nature of this behavior. Your liver has a longer memory than you do. So what may seem to you like a random food choice in the moment—for example, without realizing it, downing a double bacon cheeseburger on the first cold day of the year or, without realizing it, taking your family out for all-you-can-eat barbecue on the day you receive your tax rebate—likely fits into a pattern that your liver has recorded over years and years in its memory membranes, which remain undiscovered by medical research and science. You can't trick your liver, you can't outsmart it, and you can't out-remember it. Your liver's memory is not like the brain's memory, which can often play tricks on you. (*You sure you parked your car here, Tom? Or was it over there, in that parking lot?*) The liver's memory never falls short or deceives you. What may feel like a new path may really be a repeat of a food plan you tried five years ago and forgot—and your liver holds the data. If a certain choice is truly random—maybe, for the first time in your life, you eat a bacon cheeseburger for breakfast—then we're back to the liver's adaptogenic nature that makes it ready to respond to your needs at a moment's notice. At the same time, it documents this new, random breakfast and waits as long as necessary

to draw on that information for the next surprise breakfast.

PROCESSING FAT

Good fat, bad fat, high fat, low fat, nonfat, saturated fat, unsaturated fat, trans fat, healthy fat, omega fatty acids—it's enough to make your head spin. We know fat is one of the most important health topics out there, and yet with so many fat-related buzzwords over the years, and so much contradictory advice, how are you supposed to know what's right for you and your family? Looking back at the long history of health fads and trends that have misguided people in so many ways, are we supposed to think that the popular idea of today suddenly has it all figured out? If we leave it to the fads and trends to inform us, we'll never get a reliable answer, because the tide of public opinion will change tomorrow and the next day and then again and again and again.

So if we really want to understand the truth of how to make the right decisions, we need to step onto solid ground and spend some time examining how the body actually processes fat—and that means looking at the liver. That's because your liver is a processing center for virtually anything that comes into your body, and processing fat is one of its main jobs. Whenever you eat fat, your liver releases bile to break it down and deliver the fat to your body as an energy source.

This is more complicated than it sounds. Different amounts and complex compositions of bile are needed for different foods and different levels of fats, so your liver has to draw on its powers of memory and adaptation to prepare and respond to your fat intake at every meal. Keep in mind that when bile raises, it helps you in the moment, though it's not what you want to have happen repeatedly in the long run. It's the beginning of weakening a liver that could already be challenged by other troublemakers (toxins, poisons, and pathogens). Your liver's levels of alert fall into the following categories:

- **Code Green:** This is the bile composition required for a diet composed of 15 percent or less of fat, all from healthy sources such as avocados, nuts, seeds, olives, certain oils (such as olive, coconut, and hempseed), coconut meat, coconut milk, some varieties of fish, wild game, and raw dairy. (Even though you may have read in my other books that dairy feeds viruses, this doesn't mean the liver isn't geared to break down some types of it properly.) Code green also means that the rest of someone's diet includes ample fruits, leafy greens, vegetables, potatoes, squash, and, if desired, millet and some legumes. In this mode, the liver is able to create the necessary bile composition in its normal course of action, not in a state of panic, struggle, and distress.

- **Code Yellow:** This is when someone's diet is composed of 15 percent or less of fat, with some of those fats from the unproductive sources we'll look at in Chapter 36, "Liver Troublemakers." In this mode, the liver goes into a low level of alert, raising its bile production by up to 5 percent, at the same time adjusting bile composition to create a more acidic blend, with even higher sodium levels, amino acids, and enzymatic chemical compounds. This chemical function, unknown to medical research and science, creates a degreasing agent.

- **Code Orange:** When someone's diet is composed of 15 to 30 percent fat, all of it from the healthy sources mentioned in Code Green, the liver's state of alert goes up a level, recognizing that this amount of fat consumption is not sustainable for optimal health. Bile levels rise by up to 10 percent to protect your pancreas from the stress that may eventually be placed on it and to safeguard your longevity.

- **Code Orange-Plus:** When the diet is 15 to 30 percent fat, with some fats from unproductive sources, the liver increases its efforts to keep up, increasing bile production by up to 15 to 20 percent.

- **Code Red:** A diet that's 30 to 40 percent fat, all of it from healthy sources, prompts the liver to work nearly as hard as it can to adapt with more bile fluid and bile salts to allow for fat breakdown and digestion in the name of trying to guard your longevity. At this point, bile production increases by up to 20 to 25 percent, and the liver sends out a chemical compound as a warning request for extra sodium from the bloodstream, so it can adjust its bile composition to include more of the degreasing agent. The liver also releases calcium into the bile to protect the linings of the duodenum and the rest of the small intestinal tract from this stronger degreaser.

- **Code Red-Plus:** What happens when a diet is 30 percent or more fat, and when some of it comes from fried foods, rancid everyday cooking oils (such as canola oil, palm oil, and corn oil), lard, bacon grease, saturated fat, and the like? This launches the liver into all-out adaptogenic mode, where it draws on all of its reserves to produce epic levels—an increase of up to 50 percent or more—of the most dynamic bile fluid possible so your blood doesn't get too thick from the fat intake. Your liver licenses itself to go to war and come up with an endless supply of bile if needed. It's like that old saying, "everything but the kitchen sink"—and in this case, it's everything *including* the kitchen sink that gets thrown into this bile. That's why it's Code Red-Plus, a step beyond Code Red. It's common when someone is on a ketogenic diet. Ketogenic could mean plant protein–based or animal protein–based; it's not about choosing sides in today's food wars. Regardless of what type of diet you subscribe to, your bile situation is about the liver's needs and the liver's response to a diet that's designed to starve the body of glucose by using mostly fats as the calorie source. In this scenario, your liver is taking bullets for you, doing everything it can to thin your blood by breaking down and disposing of all those fats to prevent damage to your heart and pancreas. Your bile reserves eventually become exhausted, as do your liver's bile production capabilities and its ability to perform certain chemical functions, such as forming extremely acidic degreasers and then expelling large amounts of calcium to protect linings from damage. Over time, your liver loses its calcium reserves along with many other precious mineral reserves.

As you can see from this list, it's not all about "good" fat versus "bad" fat. While choosing fats from healthy sources is a great first step, it's not the only safeguard—levels of fat matter, too. And it's not all about your body size, either. Even if you're slim and you exercise regularly, it's possible to be in the Code Red-Plus category if fats dominate your diet. Your liver is still forced to exhaust itself producing the bile necessary to protect you from hurting yourself, and you can end up paying the price with weight gain in your older years and other liver health complications that arise along the way.

How would you feel if, after waking up in the morning, taking time to get washed up and dressed nicely for the day, you walked down to the kitchen and a bucket of oil spilled all over you? Your hair, your face, your clothes—drenched. You'd have to stop everything, go back upstairs, take another shower, and change your outfit, and only then would you be ready to face the day again. Then say you went to work and come noon, someone threw another bucket of oil at you. You'd have to go home and get cleaned up—starting from the beginning for the third time that day. *Then* how would you feel if, in the evening, just as you were settling down to a nice dinner, another bucket of oil doused you? Dripping with sludge, you'd have to stop what you were doing and slip-slide yourself back to the shower to peel off your soiled clothes and scrub the mess away. That would not be a fun day. It would be awful. You'd spend more than half of it cleaning up messes, and by the time night came, you'd be overworked, overstressed, and irritable.

That's your liver when every meal is filled with excess fats. A fried, greasy breakfast, followed by a lunch salad laden with high-oil dressing capped by a dinner of roast chicken, pizza, grilled cheese, or a BLT gives your liver a lot to do. It doesn't matter if that breakfast is two slices of conventional bacon with two antibiotic-treated chickens' eggs cooked in hormone-treated cows' butter with white buttered toast on the side or if it's two slices of organic, farm-raised bacon with two organic free-range eggs cooked in organic coconut oil, ghee, or grass-fed butter. When it comes to fat-processing, the liver doesn't care. It cares for other reasons about pesticides, hormones, and heavy metals; in terms of fat ratios, it doesn't matter. Whether the fat content of a meal is through the roof from conventional, organic, or wild sources, the liver's going to be overburdened.

By the way, one of the great food industry blunders is the measurement of how much fat is in food. The fat content of your favorite foods is not what you think it is; if you had your own way to test how many grams of fat are in a serving in your own kitchen, you'd be quite surprised. For example, no two chickens are the same. Every package of a company's chicken is going to list the same nutrition information, though, not that exact chicken's spot-on fat measurement. No piece of pork, no can of tuna, no jar of nut butter, no container of hummus is identical to another; what you see on the label is a generalized ratio of how much fat is in what. You may think you're getting 6 grams of fat when really you're getting 12 grams or more. When it comes to fat measurement, it's like a soccer game with no rules, which means we end up consuming more fat than we realize. It's another old-rooted, systemic mistake.

Processing some healthy fats is all in the name of duty for the liver. Anything more, and it gets strained—it's not a whistle-while-you-work situation anymore. Your liver doesn't wake up in the morning and say, "It seems like a great day to process high levels of fat"—just like you don't wake up and say, "It seems like a great day to take four showers and ruin three sets of clothes." The bombardment of a high-fat diet takes time and energy away from the liver performing its other duties, because it's constantly in cleanup-in-Aisle-Three mode. This is over and over and over and over, year after year after year. That's why your liver needs to use a brain-like mentality to think ahead of you. When it knows you're about to break some of your food laws, it can gather high reserves of potent bile to deal with the mess. Cleaning up messes all the time is still not ideal, and yet preparation is one of the only ways your liver keeps itself going—and prevents the rest of your body from breaking down. As you'll learn in the chapters to come, the liver can be pushed only so far.

PROTECTING YOUR PANCREAS

Which brings us to the "why" of all this fat-processing: Why does your liver put itself through all this? Why doesn't it just take a rest once in a while? Why doesn't it pass on some of the work to another organ? Your liver performs this function even when it takes nearly all of its reserves, all of its energy, and all of its vitality, because it has a higher goal: saving your life.

It starts with oxygenation. Your liver senses whether you're in Code Green, Code Red-Plus, or in between by staying highly attuned to the oxygen levels in your bloodstream. The more radical fats we consume—that is, when the majority of a food's calories are derived from fat, whether healthy or unhealthy—the more radical fats in our bloodstream, the less oxygen in our blood. When the liver senses those lower levels of oxygen, it goes into bile production mode to break down and disperse those fats and thin the blood—in large part because oxygen feeds your brain and heart. Without oxygen, these organs can't perform with ease; they labor. So when we adhere to a food belief system and try one of those high-protein diets—which are also high-fat (almost every high-protein diet is high in fat, whether you're told it is or not, regardless of whether the diet is vegetarian, vegan, based on animal protein, or anything in between)—without realizing it, we're also starving the brain and heart of oxygen, regardless of how much exercise we get, and straining the liver beyond belief.

There's more. Another major reason why your liver is committed to doing this work is to protect your pancreas. While your liver is a workhorse and a warhorse, your pancreas is a delicate flower. One of this flower's functions is to produce its vital nectar, the hormone insulin, to regulate blood sugar. Your liver tries to protect the body from excess fat because otherwise, the pancreas takes the heat, forced to produce more and more insulin over time, eventually becoming erratic in its hormone production and maybe even losing the ability to produce insulin at all. Without insulin, we end up with diabetes.

Your liver works hard to break down and distribute fats as fast as it can to keep lingering fat out of the bloodstream so it won't get in the way of organ function or the nervous system, or indirectly hurt or hinder the pancreas, leading to diabetes. With the overabundance of radical fat in almost everyone's diets, the liver can't protect us from excess fat entirely. Overwhelmed, the liver distributes some extra fat to the lymphatic system. This protection mechanism for the brain and heart puts the fats in suspension in the lymph fluid, though it's not all roses. When fats are pumping through the lymphatic system, the immune system weakens and white killer cells can't battle viruses, bacteria, and toxins as well as needed inside the lymphatic system. It's not the liver's or the immune system's fault; it's the radical fats we've been trained to eat throughout our lives.

The more fat hanging around in the bloodstream, organs, digestive tract, and lymph fluid, the more insulin is needed to try to force sugar through and around the fat saturation so it can enter into the cells and the body can function. With the bloodstream filled with fats, for example, the nervous system starts to starve, since it runs on sugar (plus mineral salts), and glucose can't easily find its way past fat to nerves. Trying to get life-sustaining glucose into organs, muscles, and the nervous system while meeting resistance from excess fat is the true, unknown meaning of the term *insulin resistance*.

The pancreas doesn't only overproduce insulin in those moments when sugar and carbohydrates are consumed. If you have very high blood fat from a high-fat diet and you're running on fats, vegetables, and green juices, your pancreas will still produce just as much insulin, and insulin resistance will still be there, even without the carbs. It's just that the symptom won't show itself until you get a craving and reach for pasta or bread or something sweet and that carbohydrate enters the bloodstream, in which case a blood sugar test will indicate a problem. Everyone will say that carbs are the instigator, when the reality is that healthy carbohydrates are not the problem; they're like a forensic team's UV light that *reveals* the real problem. You know the kind I'm talking about? The blue lamp that makes visible the blood on the walls and bodily fluids on the floor? Turn it on, and suddenly, you could go from standing in what seems to be a pristine hotel room to standing in the middle of a crime scene. No one blames the lamp. We know it's the light of truth working for us to solve a mystery, not working against us, when it reveals a secret. That's how we need to think of healthy carbohydrates: the heroes, not the bad guys. They reveal when high fat has created a crime scene.

If the fat ratio in a diet were lowered, and more foods like pumpkin, sweet potatoes, potatoes, squash, zucchini, berries, and other fruits were consumed, insulin resistance would reduce and blood sugar would become more balanced. The pancreas would also be saved from pumping out extra insulin. Remember: natural, healthy sugars and carbohydrates are not the enemy; they're friends. It's excess fat that becomes the bully on the school playground.

FREEING YOUR LIVER

Have you ever fought for a person or a cause in your life that was important to you? Now you have the perspective to see that your liver is of just as much import. When you know that every day, your liver fights for you, you can start to fight along with it. It's not an invisible battle anymore. Maybe you can even fight *for* your liver, in which case it's not an invincible battle, either.

You can take away some of the circumstances that put it on the defense in the first place, and you can give it a rest here and there with some of the suggestions we'll explore in Part IV, "Liver Salvation." You don't need to change your whole lifestyle. You don't need to become obsessive about fat. Awareness is everything. Knowing that a certain food choice has a certain effect, you can move forward on your own terms—fully informed. Choice by choice, you can make your own decisions, rather than relying on the competing opinions out there that are based on trends, not the truth.

The truth is that it's not a chore to take care of our livers; it's an honor and a privilege. When your liver doesn't have to spend quite so much time and energy shielding your pancreas from fat intake, it frees up vitality to perform all of its other critical and amazing functions. You start to look better, feel better—because your most loyal companion is able to look out for you better than ever before. That begins with holding on to critical reserves of glucose for your times of need, reserves that can mean the difference between having a nervous breakdown when faced with a challenging stressor and calling it a bad day while keeping your cool. It's the difference between night and day.

CHAPTER 3

Your Life-Giving Liver

Glucose and Glycogen Storage

Do you have a drawer or a closet in your home where you stow items for later? Maybe it's your pantry, filled to the brim with extra snacks and ingredients that you know will come in handy if something prevents you from getting out for a fresh supply of food. The liver is like that storehouse for your body. It likes to hoard—in a good way, and for a few different reasons, one of which is so that it can bring out certain nutrients later for your body to absorb anew. (Another is so that it can store troublemakers to shield your organs from them and protect your life; we'll get to that in Chapter 5, "Your Protective Liver.") Storing glucose is a critical function of your liver; it's how you stay alive. Yes, sugar actually keeps you alive.

BLOOD SUGAR BALANCE

Liver glucose storage is a huge piece of protecting us from conditions such as diabetes. Think about when you're out all day running around, dropping off and picking up kids, attending meetings, getting groceries, and you don't get a chance to eat for five or six hours.

All that time, the blood sugar you got from your last meal is slowly dropping until it's all used up. Your liver—if it's in good condition—will then release stores of glucose to save your behind. It's taking that precious sugar that you got from a smoothie one day last week, or a baked sweet potato, and it's giving it back to you so you don't get too hypoglycemic and have a pancreas and adrenal crash.

Your liver stores most glucose as glycogen, in small, sometimes microscopic, pockets of special storage facility tissue around the outside of the liver that medical research and science have not yet discovered in its full scope. (Medical research and science don't yet know what all liver tissue does.) The liver can systematically craft and hone concentrations of chemical compounds far more technically advanced than what human scientific methods offer at the moment. Even the respected science of a lab technician playing around with solutions and dilutions in 1 part per million or 4 parts per billion would be the equivalent of preschool compared to the doctorate degree the liver has in keeping you alive.

This storage system is also how the liver stows away concentrations of other nutrients (which we'll look at in the next chapter) as well as hormones, biochemical agents, and other chemical compounds. Any helpful component like this that the body may need at a moment's notice, the liver keeps in storage banks close to its exterior, where there are plenty of blood vessels for ready reabsorption when it gets discharge signals from sources such as your brain or thyroid. As needed, the liver brilliantly breaks down glycogen back into glucose, using stored water molecules combined with a chemical compound it produces to reconstitute and release glucose into the bloodstream at just the right balanced and measured levels. The liver also keeps some readily available glucose that's not stored as glycogen so it can be released even faster.

Blood sugar is how we function; the human body depends on it. We all know that jittery, lightheaded, irritable feeling we get when it dips—how it feels impossible to concentrate, be active, or get anything done. Blood sugar drops would happen all the time if not for this key role of the liver—or, if your liver is not in top condition (and almost everyone's liver is not at its best), then if not for the adrenals, which pump out adrenaline and cortisol to fill in for glucose when it's not available. You don't want to be relying on your adrenals for this function, though, because these glands are already over-worked in our stress-filled age; plus, an excess of stress hormones has a caustic effect on your system. True blood sugar support is all about a well-functioning liver that's well stocked with glucose and glycogen. When we're deprived of blood sugar long term, we lose the ability to walk, run, exercise, think—to function.

The liver plays a role in athletics like nobody's business. If marathon runners and other athletes knew how hard the liver works, and how responsible it is for getting you to your goal—that you can have the most agile muscles in the world and yet hit a wall if your liver runs out of stored nutrients such as sugar—physical training would rise to a whole new level. The liver releases all the stored glucose it has to get you to the finish line. Know that, and you have a whole new perspective on caring for your body for optimal performance.

YOUR LIVER'S FAVORITE FUEL

Glucose isn't solely useful for keeping your blood sugar under control; your liver itself needs it, too. In the ideal liver training, we'd learn from birth that our livers live on oxygen, water, glucose, and mineral salts. Glucose—that is, sugar—is the real fuel. Now, isn't *sugar* a bad word? While protein and fats are celebrated much of the time, we're very often taught to fear sugar instead. Here's the truth: our first food, breast milk, has a high ratio of sugars—because a mother's body knows that her child will thrive on glucose. It's glucose that builds muscles in a child and allows for the development of organs such as the brain, liver, and especially the heart. As we grow up, that need for glucose doesn't go away. It's critical for cooling the brain when we're in confrontation, being challenged, or even in a simple debate at work or school. Without glucose, we can't cope with any pressure or stress. We need it to maintain healthy muscles, a healthy brain, and a healthy heart. And it's imperative for the liver's function and its ability to support your entire body.

Not that all sugars are beneficial. Sweeteners such as table sugar and high-fructose corn syrup, which aren't attached to nutrients, aren't doing anyone any favors—they're a drain on health. Certain sugars, though—natural sugars from whole foods, like those found in fruits, coconut water, raw honey, sweet potatoes, and the sugars you get from digestion of good carbohydrates like squash and potatoes—are wildly beneficial.

That may sound scary or flat-out wrong, given the common anti-sugar advice out there. Maybe you have fruit fear. That's probably because you've been told at some point that the sugars in fruit feed everything from *Candida* to cancer. You might have heard, too, that the condition fatty liver can be caused by sugar, so you should therefore avoid fruit. Well, you don't need to live with that burden anymore. The truth is that you need those natural sugars—and all the other nutrients you get from fruit—to function at your best. (You'll find plenty more about why it's okay to trust fruit in my books *Medical Medium* and *Life-Changing Foods*, and we'll examine the real cause of fatty liver in Chapter 11 of this book.) When you hear that you should stay away from every sugar possible, know that doing so will hurt your liver. When you hear that sugar turns to fat in the body, understand that it's really fat turning to fat. What no one realizes is that nobody eats a diet with just sugar in it; they also eat a lot of fat to go along with it, and that's what's problematic. I don't care how strong the trend is—this is about you, and what you need to thrive. It's critical that you know the truth, which is that getting high-quality, bioavailable glucose from healthy sources such as fruit is one of the best actions you can take for your liver.

So why all the confusion? Why the saying that "sugar is sugar," as though your body can't distinguish between the sugar in a grape and that in a gumball? Because medical research and science have not yet developed tools advanced enough to fully analyze the true value of natural sugars from whole-food sources. Remember: as institutions, research and science look out for research and science. If they don't have the tools to analyze and distinguish different types of sugar, they protect themselves by saying that all sugar is the same, and all sugar is bad. As I said at the beginning of this book in "A Note for You," I'm not talking about the noble individuals who devote their brilliant, tireless minds to science and stumble upon amazing discoveries in the lab; I'm talking about the establishment, the investors, the decision makers at the top who decide which potential advancements to greenlight and which to stifle or sweep under the carpet.

This means that the ill effects we all witness of table sugar and high-fructose corn syrup on health continue to get grouped with the effects of the sugars in something like bananas—and that's a major loss for everyone, because that natural sugar is (1) bonded to critical nutrients that you can't get any other way and (2) a missing piece in liver health. Much of the time when sugar gets the blame, what scientific observation is truly picking up on—without realizing it—are the ill effects of the *combination* of processed sugar plus fat. We covered this a bit in the previous chapter, and we'll look at it in much more detail later.

It's not only that the nutrients happen to be bonded to sugar; the liver *needs* nutrients that are surrounded by sugar, because sugars help it do its job. Sugar is how other nutrients propel through the bloodstream and enter into organs; without sugar, a nutrient can't drive itself where it's needed. Fat doesn't work this way. The fats we eat don't carry an antioxidant, vitamin, or other nutrient for delivery in the body; they don't drive nutrients into organs and tissue. That doesn't mean that healthy fats don't hold nutrients—it's that they don't deliver them the way sugars do. A healthy fat will indeed contain vitamins, minerals, and other nutrients, and that's the basis of the scientific belief system that fats are so beneficial. What medical research and science don't realize is that as healthy as a given fat source may be, as much as it may have to offer, it's a microscopic fraction of what sugar has to offer in the way of actually getting nutrients to their destinations. Radical fats' nutrients are hard to access, because they're suspended and encapsulated in globules of fat that aren't easily broken down.

On top of which, excess fats in the bloodstream are like a school bus driving in front of a mail carrier for an entire delivery route. It doesn't mean the school bus is all bad; it's filled with wonderful children, and the bus driver's duty is to travel at a measured pace. Still, the bus does slow down the mail carrier (the sugar delivering nutrients). It holds up deliveries, some of which are critical, like the refund check that will allow you to take your daughter out and get her the soccer equipment she needs. While fat is just trying to do its job, too much of it keeps sugar from doing its own vital duty.

It takes work for the liver to process vitamins and minerals and antioxidants and the like—and all that work generates heat. The liver is the organ that runs hottest to begin with; as the heater of the body, it's there to help you stay warm when the temperature drops. It generates additional heat doing its many jobs; the more fat and toxins it has to process especially, the harder it has to work, and the hotter it gets. The only way the liver keeps from overheating is with sugar; along with the right blend of water and mineral salts, glucose is what helps the liver keep its cool. Like a cooling agent for a car's engine, glucose keeps it running.

Glucose also feeds the liver. As I said, it's fuel. While the liver is made up of two main lobes and also includes the smaller caudate and quadrate lobes, it has tiny lobes internally, too, called lobules, which you can think of as elves in a toy factory. Those elves are busy. All day long, they sort through material deliveries (everything you're exposed to, from food and drink to what you breathe to what goes on your skin), deciding what's a useful building block and what needs to go to the trash heap. The elves bundle up the good and bad and send them on their separate paths—and this work makes them hungry. They need to be fed at regular intervals, and glucose is what they crave. It's yet one more reason why your liver's backup supply of glycogen is so precious. Otherwise, the liver can't function. It can't process critical nutrients, it can't protect you from fats, and it can't do anything else that we're looking at here in Part I.

When you take fuel away from the liver for too long, it not only runs out of steam; it begins to fight for its life—and yours. It may even send out soldier elves—that is, chemical compounds that act as agents to gather minuscule sources of glucose from throughout the body and then bring them back to the liver. It's something like robbing Peter to pay Paul. This is one of those times when the liver shows itself to be like another brain, because it keeps a record of the glucose it takes from other parts of the body—a record that cannot be weighed or measured, a record of intelligence. With cellular information, it documents the glucose stolen from Peter so Paul can make sure he pays him back along the way: When the liver gets restocked with an adequate amount of glucose, it will then release not just the normal, regulated amount of glucose that Peter needs; it will release a little extra. The liver tags the extra glucose with a hormone that allows for quick, easy usage—paying back Peter in a very efficient manner that not only satisfies him; it makes him forget he was ever robbed.

You'll notice that today's high-fat diet trend throws in little bits of sugar now. If it didn't, and a diet were only fat and protein long term, it would create a tragic situation of the liver scraping by to survive. It would also cause the robbing Peter to pay Paul situation to go on way too long. And so, because experts have observed that an all-fat-and-protein diet leads to negative health effects, they're allowing pints of berries in a diet or bringing in apples, pumpkin, or avocado or adding hidden sugars in their protein bars.

Avocados, by the way, were thought to be poisonous until very recently, with experts of yesterday calling them dangerously fattening and terrible for health. Now they're in vogue, though no one even realizes just how wonderful they are for health. Along with fat, avocados contain very valuable, viable sugar. Before you worry that their fat-sugar combination is a problem, know that an avocado is a rare, random exception to the fat-sugar issue; the avocado's fat content is so infused with its sugar that it's designed not to let the sugar get in the way and to keep the liver balanced, unless you eat avocados in high quantity day in and day out. So while you don't want lots and lots of avocado, the liver won't cry out so much when avocado's fat is coming through; its viscosity is easier on the organ, making it a healthier source than many others. Avocados are good for you.

Now back to the diet experts: note that they haven't been bringing avocados and other low-sugar sources into diets because they understand that the body is desperate for glucose. It's because they've seen that the old model wasn't getting people anywhere in the end; they weren't improving. If diet experts knew that the liver was literally starving on a high-fat diet, considerations would be made and today's diets would be different. They'd

realize that a high-fat diet is accidental cruelty to the liver. With any other living thing, we know it needs to be fed, and that feeding it the wrong food would be inhumane. We know, for example, to feed a horse or a hamster or a pet bunny rabbit this and this and not that. With the liver, medical research and science aren't there yet—so we need to be the ones who know how to look out for our livers.

REAL RESTORATION

So many trends over the years have convinced so many of us that carbs and sugar are to be feared. If you're on a diet with no sugar, though—no carbohydrates like fruit and squash and potatoes and sweet potatoes and millet and raw honey—then your liver will starve slowly, and you'll age rapidly over time. If you do eat carbohydrates and they're always accompanied by fat—think a twice-baked potato with sour cream and bacon bits, a banana split, or even meals we're taught to think of as healthy, such as whole-milk yogurt with fruit and granola; a salad with grilled chicken, hard-boiled eggs, and a whole wheat roll; or a turkey sandwich with lettuce, tomato, and mayonnaise—your liver can also starve for glucose. Shielding the pancreas from the fat in a meal prevents the liver from getting all the precious glucose it can out of the food, and the result can be a constant, nagging hunger that won't go away no matter how much you eat. (More on this in Chapter 13, "Mystery Hunger.") Whether on a high-fat, no- or low-carb diet, or a diet where all carbohydrates are accompanied by fat, the liver never gets restored. Any little bits of downtime the liver gets don't feel like real rest—it's like when you take a three-day weekend thinking it will be the perfect opportunity for restoration, and at the end of it, you don't feel fully rested. Has that ever happened to you? That's how the liver feels with fat always blocking glucose.

Give your liver what it needs, on the other hand, and it will support you like nothing else can. With bioavailable glucose in the diet from healthy sources plus a stockpile of glycogen for times of need, your liver can give you energy, slow down the aging process, and help shield you from disease. It can easily adapt to your needs on a moment-by-moment basis without a fight, and, as we'll see in the next chapter, it can act as the ultimate conversion tool and medicine chest.

CHAPTER 4

Your Medicinal Liver

Vitamin and Mineral Storage

When a doctor tells you that you have deficiencies in certain vitamins and minerals, what she or he should really be saying is, "Your liver has some problems." Just as your liver is meant to store glucose, it's also meant to stow away every single vitamin and mineral, as well as other nutrients, so that even if you're not getting enough of a certain nutrient in your current diet, your body can draw on the reserves that your liver held on to from an earlier time. If you're running low on vitamin D or B$_{12}$ or deficient in any other vitamin or mineral, it means your liver carried you for quite a while, and now its life-giving well of vitality and prosperity is finally running dry.

The liver's ability to store nutrients is vast, and it's organized in a complicated structure—it can catalogue by level of importance, with the most critical items most readily available. A liver in top condition is able to support you with a medicine chest full of nutrient therapies.

Mainly, the liver stores nutrients that the stomach and intestines have converted during digestion into forms your body can use. That's the beginning phase, the couple of rocks you step over on your way to the mountain you're

trying to climb. It's a biochemical conversion that happens in the gut that goes beyond weights and measurements documented by medical science and research. It's far more involved than a chemical process that turns A into B; it's a process that takes a given nutrient, alters it for a specific use in the body, and adds to it—brings life to it—so that, when the time is right for your liver to receive the nutrients through the bloodstream, it can take on those nutrients. Then, they must be altered once again, this time by the liver, through a chemical process that's like a baptizing of the nutrients. This creates in the nutrients a life-sustaining mission and prepares them for their crusade with a protective shield and armor that the liver produces from specific antioxidants gleaned from certain healing fruits. The liver bubbles the chemical compound around the nutrients as part of this miraculous baptismal process, so that as they travel on their journey, they're not destroyed by toxins or held up too long by an overabundance of fat in the bloodstream.

Finally, nutrients are ready for the liver to release them into the bloodstream so they can be delivered as precious, vital resources to organs and tissue throughout your body in forms they can easily accept. The delivery here is key. It's sort of like holiday gift giving. If you stick a present in the mail with no wrapping, bow, or even box, it's not going to survive the trip or get where it's supposed to go. If you wrap it up, on the other hand, and put some ribbon on it, nestle it in a shipping box with bubble wrap, seal it with packing tape, and carefully write the address on it, the present is ready for the trip. Write "FRAGILE" on it, and carriers will be even more mindful to take care of the package and get it safely to its destination.

THE BACKUP PLAN

Normally, the liver holds on to upgraded nutrients as the gut provides them, and then the liver re-dispenses them as needed. Sometimes, your gut is in distress, with intestinal linings scarred and damaged by long-term, chronic strep; low hydrochloric acid causing bad acids to rise up and create acid reflux; or intestinal inflammation from viruses, other pathogens, and the foods that feed them. When that happens, the gut's not capable of absorbing, altering, and delivering nutrients that are critical to life—so your liver is there as a backup conversion tool. To keep you alive, your liver overuses its conversion method, *methylation*.

For example, your ileum, a section of your small intestine, is meant to hold elevated biotics (microorganisms from fresh foods that are undiscovered by medical research and science) that both create vitamin B_{12} and convert B_{12} from other sources to more methylated, bioavailable forms. When the ileum is weary, your liver is the backup conversion tool. It takes over the job that the intestinal tract can't do anymore and keeps you feeling vital and healthy.

Even with an intestinal tract that's really struggling, your liver will overcompensate so much that you don't discover your irritable bowel syndrome (IBS), small intestinal bacterial overgrowth (SIBO), *Candida* overgrowth, gas, or bloating, and they're not even on your doctor's radar, because your liver is masking the situation with its assistance. When the liver is pushed too far along the way and becomes stagnant, sluggish, or fatty—too weakened to be a backup tool—then the digestive problem or nutrient deficiency starts to reveal itself.

Because we're not taught how to take care of our livers, we often overburden them faster than we do our stomachs and intestines. This means that if your gut gets to the point where it's having trouble converting nutrients, there's a good chance your liver is already sluggish and weakened, so even though it can still do a great job as the conversion understudy, it has trouble doing so. It can't absorb, alter, and deliver to its full capacity, and when that diminishes even more, it will translate to your doctor telling you you're lacking certain nutrients. On top of which, a stagnant liver can get so clogged up with toxins that it starts to leak them back into the body, which weakens the digestive tract, meaning it's further reliant on the liver's conversion ability—a vicious cycle. How many vicious cycles have you come across in your life? Maybe in a friendship or relationship, an emotional conflict became a vicious cycle. A child building a dam in the mud during a rainstorm will find that the very need for the dam—the rain—also keeps undermining the project as more and more water builds up behind the barrier, breaks through, and turns everything back into a pile of mud. It's the same principle behind nutrient conversion—when someone has a digestive disorder, which can come about because of a compromised liver, it takes longer to heal because an out-of-commission liver undermines the gut and vice versa.

EVERYTHING WE NEED

A strong liver is critical to gut health for reasons beyond nutrient conversion. It's also about storage—because the more the liver's storage banks are saturated and overcrowded with toxins that the liver has collected to save you, the less room the liver has for vitamin and mineral storage. The organ is faced with a decision: to keep the "nuclear waste" containment system in place to protect the body, or to let out the poisons so it can store more vitamins, minerals, and other valuable materials that can help repair the gut and the rest of the body. As vital as nutrient storage is, saving you from toxic matter wins out. It's a critical, lifesaving function of your liver, and one you'll discover more about in the next chapter.

This dilemma is another reason why taking care of our livers is one of our highest callings: because saving our livers saves them from this nearly impossible choice. If we're helping our livers cleanse troublemakers (those rascally toxins, poisons, and pathogens) as well as protecting them from avoidable troublemakers in the first place, the liver has the room it needs to fully support us with both its medicine chest of nutrient storage and its masterful waste containment. The liver gets everything it needs—and that means that we get everything we need.

CHAPTER 5

Your Protective Liver

Disarming and Detaining Harmful Materials

Your liver has been rescuing you with its neutralization abilities since Day One. If we had real awareness of just how important that is, we'd celebrate it like nothing else: "Hey, I just got exposed to something toxic, and I'm going to survive because my liver's looking out for me!"

Instead, we ingest the aluminum particles from mac and cheese baked in a foil container, or the mold hidden in a piece of chopped meat that got old in the fridge, or the pesticides from a highly sprayed crop of corn, or the plastics from a microwaved dinner, or the preservatives in a fast food meal, or the bacteria or mercury in a bad batch of shellfish, and we keep going about our lives, never realizing that the liver stepped in and kept us safe from what could have been a health disaster. We get exposed to something like radiation from a CT scan, and we don't stop and say "thank you" to our livers for shielding us.

The occasions we know to celebrate—the birthdays, the graduations, the promotions, the so-called clean-bill-of-health visits to the doctor—tend to be marked with indulgences that give our livers even more work: hormone-filled conventional ice cream from antibiotic-fed cows, for example, or cocktails made with mixes full of MSG, dyes, and synthetic fruity flavors. Instead of getting to party alongside us, our livers need to work even harder than usual to keep us free from harm.

Our livers get no respect. In fact, the liver is one of the most disrespected organs in the body. When the great Aretha Franklin recorded "Respect," she could well have been singing from the perspective of the liver. A real celebration would be drinking green juice or maybe just eating a few steamed potatoes to give the liver a break and help it restore its disarming abilities.

TROUBLEMAKER NEUTRALIZATION

Those abilities are powerful. Harmful substances such as synthetic pesticides and herbicides, pathogens, molds, plastics, toxic heavy metals, and other troublemakers have an ionic charge that's destructive to the cells in our bodies. It's a charge that makes them magnetically "sticky." As these toxins float along in our bloodstream, lymph fluid, and even spinal fluid, they create a reckless path of destruction, endangering nutrients, sucking the life out of oxygen itself, and even injuring immune system cells. The toxic ionic charge can also injure red blood cells, sort of like when a meteorite enters our atmosphere and starts falling to earth, mowing down tips of trees until it lands at its final destination in the side of a mountain.

As toxins float toward the liver, they tend to keep that toxic ionic charge. A healthy liver, though, one that hasn't been compromised or clogged up and isn't sluggish or stagnant or diseased, can discharge that charge. As toxins travel into the liver like pieces of candy on a factory conveyor belt, the liver can neutralize these harmful materials so they don't carry the same destructive force. Picture a line of workers standing over the conveyor belt, at the ready to collect defective candy—candy canes with cracks and gobstoppers that have broken in half—so they don't end up packaged as treats.

The liver also releases an amazing chemical compound into the bloodstream to disarm troublemakers' damaging ionic charge and keep them from getting ignited when they're still out in the wild yonder of your body. Your body is not only filled with electricity; it *is* electricity. It's why when someone has a heart attack, emergency responders use electricity to try to waken the heart. It's also why we need this chemical compound from the liver to float around the body and do its job of coating toxins, suffocating them, shorting out their charges, and keeping these troublemakers dormant, so that the body's electricity won't ignite them. It's an extraordinary job that a liver can do, and do well if it's healthy.

Since medical research and science haven't scratched the surface of all the liver does, though, we don't know much about it, so we can't be the cheerleaders the liver needs. If your liver is struggling, it will only be able to release small amounts of this undiscovered disarming chemical compound, which means toxins can escape its reach and slowly wreak havoc.

TROUBLEMAKER STORAGE

If your liver is too run down or overloaded to neutralize and repackage a certain toxin in a safe manner, or to produce its disarming chemical compound and release it into the bloodstream, then the liver will stow away toxins that enter it in order to protect you. There are two types of storage facilities in the liver. The first type is what we looked at in the previous two chapters: pockets of glucose, glycogen, vitamins, minerals, and other nutrients (as well as other phytochemicals and helpful hormones) in porous, sponge-like areas along the outside of the liver, easily accessed through the pores themselves and not just sent out through main avenues like the central veins.

Then there are the storage pockets for harmful materials. Because this is the secondary method for dealing with toxins—the liver's first line of defense is to get those toxins out of your body—these aren't storage bins set aside ahead of time for this purpose. They're more like heaps at a trash dump that arise out of necessity: scrap metal goes in one heap, rotted wood in another, old tires in another, dishwashers and washing machines in another, while hazardous waste like old batteries, refrigerators, and microwave ovens get grouped in a contained area. The liver drives toxins deeper and deeper into itself depending on how damaging they have the potential to be—it's closest to the center of the liver where it likes to push materials that include petroleum products, dioxins, DDT and other pesticides, aspartame, MSG, viruses and viral waste matter, conventional cleaners, certain pharmaceuticals such as opioids, and toxic heavy metals.

This is all in the name of protecting you. With the most destructive substances as deep as they can be, you're able to go about your life for as long as possible. Why hoard harmful materials in its deep, inner core when they can eventually cause liver sickness there? Because the liver has a responsibility to make sure that those poisons aren't free-floating and able to head to the brain and heart, where they could do extensive damage and shorten your life span. The liver takes the hit instead, patiently waiting hour by hour, day by day, year by year, for its chance to cleanse or detox the items in the way it needs to. (More in Part IV, "Liver Salvation.")

The liver is not just one static mass. It ebbs and flows and practically shapeshifts, which it owes to certain undiscovered cells that I call *perime cells*, for those times when the liver's storage bins get too full. These perime cells are produced and released by liver lobules. While research and science have correctly documented lobules as six-sided, they're not aware of these perime cells, nor the fact that perime cells cluster in groups of sixes and nines (for example, a larger group of 33 perime cells would be considered a six) to form tissue that can adhere and release as needed, block certain areas, pad other areas, and be disassembled and reconstructed to allow for storage bin expansion in the liver. By shapeshifting like this, perime cells help prevent the release of toxins that would be harmful to the liver and other organs into the bloodstream.

Free-floating perime cells, part of the liver family's cell structure, can't live outside the liver, and medical research and science aren't aware of them because researchers can't live inside a liver for a day to witness what's really happening. A cadaver's liver won't exhibit all that a

living liver has to show, and any living liver, such as one being prepared for transplant, must be treated with the utmost care, not poked, prodded, and damaged. And so the liver remains in large part a mystery to medical communities; medicine is still far from understanding all of its inner workings.

TAKING ON THE WORLD'S MISTAKES

These two levels of protection—disarmament and detainment—don't always last forever. When a woman is, on average, age 38, and a man is, on average, age 48, these abilities often start to wane, and symptoms such as hot flashes and weight gain start to crop up—symptoms that often get mistaken for menopause or aging. This is not because the liver naturally loses power midway through a person's life. It's because of all we're up against in the way of pathogens, pollutants, poisons, and diet that overburden the liver over time if they aren't cleansed, so that at a certain point, the liver sends out default warning signs in the way of symptoms. It says, "I've taken care of you for decades. I can't keep going at this rate."

Unfortunately, since it started—coinciding with the hormone replacement movement of the 1950s and '60s—this cry has been misinterpreted. When the liver cried out for help during this first wave of women experiencing liver trouble, the liver got slapped in the face by agenda-driven opportunists in the medical arena. (More on why these symptoms started to arise at that time in history in *Medical Medium*.) The liver still gets misunderstood. This punishment the liver has faced is something like your daughter trying out for swim team as a way to ease the emotional challenges of adjusting to a new school and not making the cut because she wouldn't buy the expensive swimsuit that the coach, unbeknownst to you, was obligated to sell at quota due to an athletic department contract. Your daughter's real needs in this scenario, like your liver's, go ignored.

At this point in human history, because of the toxins we inherit at conception and in utero, we don't come into the world with livers working at 100 percent. So we start out at a disadvantage—and then there's everything we're exposed to after we're born. You can be mindful of your health, watch what you eat, exercise, keep your immune system strong, and follow your doctor's orders with prescriptions, and if you don't tap into the basics of liver rescue that we'll look at in Part IV, it's common to have a liver working only at 60 percent of its intended protective capacity by the time you've reached age 40. Even normal antibiotic use as a child can be enough to result in a weakened liver by a person's late 20s if steps aren't taken to detox and restore the liver in the interim.

BACK FROM THE BRINK

There's so much that we deal with in this world. Viruses, bacteria, mold, pesticides, herbicides, fungicides, engine oil, gasoline, exhaust fumes, plastics, synthetically scented products, toxic heavy metals, radiation, hidden ingredients, high-fat meals, high-stress jobs, and more—it's a constant onslaught, and our livers do everything they can to defend us from the world's mistakes for long as they can. The liver is the most grounded organ in the body. That's why it's able to withstand so much for so many years, pushed to the degree that it is without support. Silently, gracefully, like an undercover spy, the liver detects threats and neutralizes or detains them—that is, until it becomes overpowered and cries out for your help.

When it can no longer keep up with the processing of fat, with the glucose, glycogen, vitamin, and mineral storage, with the toxin defense, and with the screening and filtering of blood that we'll look at in the next chapter, then it starts to take on fat, becoming a fatty liver. Or it begins to grow a cyst, hemangioma, or tumor inside. Or scar tissue begins to develop rapidly, sending you into cirrhosis. Or gout, diabetes, eczema, psoriasis, or other symptoms and conditions you weren't aware were liver-related begin to cause problems. Or undetected viruses proliferate, leading to viral issues in the body labeled as autoimmune, with pathogens eating up tissue and breaking down cells, causing pain and chronic mystery illness.

When we support the liver, though, when we bring it back from the brink, or when we're proactive about protecting it before it needs to send those emergency signals, then a world of possibility opens up to us. We get to make the calls, and in doing so, we change our destiny.

CHAPTER 6

Your Purifying Liver

Screening and Filtering Blood

Your liver is one of your busiest organs, with a highway of blood running through it. As you've seen in the previous chapters, this blood is rich with nutrients from the food you eat and also filled with medicines you take, the occasional alcohol you may drink, toxic heavy metals and chemicals you come into contact with, excess adrenaline that you may constantly be up against, as well as various hormones, some of which come from toxic, detrimental sources and some that are essential for the liver to be able to mass-produce cells so it can mend and heal any of its burned-out tissue.

As your body's central processing center, your liver must be masterful at separating the bad from the good—the poisons, pathogens, and excess fat from the nutrients, essential hormones, and other beneficial elements that can help you thrive—all while trying to maintain the proper oxygen balance with so many different materials in the blood. Monitoring the blood begins with the liver's immune system: white blood cells that are very wise and quick to react at any given moment, standing guard at the hepatic portal vein—the main entrance to the liver—on the lookout for viruses and bacteria. (More on that in the next chapter.) Then, the blood branches out into smaller vessels and enters the liver itself, where it's the task of the liver lobules and Kupffer cells to sort and distribute the helpful elements while screening for toxins or pathogens that slipped by the guards.

GOSPEL OF PURIFICATION

It's helpful to think of these lobules once again as elves in a toy factory, stationed in front of a conveyor belt of raw materials coming in from the outside. Is that a piece of hearty pine that will make a sturdy rocking horse, or some lightweight balsa that will be perfect for a toy plane? Does that log have an infestation of bugs that will wreak havoc if they get loose in the workshop? Is that plank contaminated by pesticides? It's all for the elves to decide, and to sort and distribute accordingly. Kupffer cells, configured like sweeping apparatuses, are the brooms the elves use to clean up their workshop. As elves (lobules) get hungry and find food (glucose), life enters the brooms (Kupffer cells) so they can perform their job.

You and I know that these "elves" and "brooms" aren't really magic. Funny thing is, they may as well be for all that medical research and science have discovered in the way of how liver lobules and Kupffer cells truly interact and the roles they play in deciding what to do with all of the different materials coming through your bloodstream. While science is aware of certain cells being part of a cleansing process (such as discarding old red blood cells), how the liver's cells communicate and how the liver performs for its own needs while simultaneously keeping the rest of you in mind are a whole other story. Medical research and science haven't gotten to the point of decoding the complex, precise chemical functions that allow for intercommunication of liver cells or how lobules decipher what's good and bad. As far as the medical establishment is concerned, it may really be magical creatures deciding which unhelpful materials get disarmed, thrown out, or stored where they can't cause harm, which helpful materials get organized and put away by category, and which go straight to the elves who build toys, pack them up, and send them out.

It's especially important that your liver do a good job of separating the beneficial from the toxic, because after it leaves the liver, blood moves to the heart. The blood that reaches the heart is meant to be clean, and it is if your liver is in good condition. Your liver uses all of its reserves and power to fend off and dispose of toxic threats, knowing that if they escape the liver, they'll do you harm. As you've already read, it buries the most toxic threats such as solvents and pesticides in its core and has a particular awareness that viruses must be harnessed deep inside, because that's safer than viruses making a run for the brain or heart.

Before it ever gets to that point of stowing away troublemakers, though, the liver will try to dispose of them as part of its screening and filtering process. If it can get troublemakers out of your body safely, it will. For the most part, that means allowing for less-toxic debris to leave in a "taking out the trash" process so it has more strength to contain the more dangerous toxins. When the liver lets go, toxins get released to three possible places: the colon (sometimes via the bile and gallbladder), where they're eliminated through the feces; the kidneys, where they're eliminated through urine; and, as a last resort, loose in the bloodstream, where they become free radicals. A truly healthy liver, one that's clean and isn't struggling, will only send troublemakers to the colon and urine for elimination. Even a liver that's in poor condition will do everything it can to prevent serious threats from going free in the bloodstream.

As for those troublemakers that the liver has deemed safe to send out, the liver lobule elves package them with chemical compounds that identify the neutralized troublemakers' destinations, like tracking information on a parcel, and carry them toward either the colon or the kidneys. The sponge-like nature of the liver plays a role in how it releases debris, as it excretes most of these toxins through the pores in its underside when the liver is in trouble—highly toxic, sluggish, and stagnant—and unable to release the toxins through the bile duct. It becomes an emergency excretion tactic that doesn't always go perfectly. Once squeezed out the bottom of the liver (you can picture the bottom of the liver sort of like the underside of a mushroom cap), many of these poisons that have been screened, filtered, neutralized, and packaged with an identifying chemical compound can absorb into tiny micro blood vessels on the outside of the colon wall that catch debris and guide them to larger veins so they can enter into the colon for elimination.

When the liver is sluggish, weak, and struggling, the elves get tired and overworked and don't always wrap the troublemaker "presents" too well on their way out. Without the chemical compound packaged properly with it, a toxin released from the liver becomes a free radical package with no stamp, tracking number, or address saying where it's supposed to go. It heads out a hepatic vein and up to the heart in this unidentified, untethered form, cycles through the rest of the circulatory system, and in many cases gets returned to sender—coming back to the liver when the bloodstream's path brings it there.

The liver has a second way of sending troublemakers to the colon for elimination, and that's through the bile. This is its preferred process for disposing of more heavy-duty debris. While still microscopic (and even beyond microscopic; a microscope could only find half of these troublemaker particles), these are the poisons your body most wants to shield you from as it delivers them out of your body. It's another reason why dysfunctional livers with diminishing bile are such a big problem—because bile is a big part of our detox process. In good condition, with plenty of bile, the liver can send toxins out through the bile duct directly to the intestinal tract, or through the hepatic duct to the gallbladder, to be released next time it's called for to aid with digestion. On the other hand, if the liver is stagnant, burdened, clogged, and beaten down, not only does it lose the elves' packaging help and the volume of bile to flush out plenty of toxins; it also has less oxygen to aid with the delivery process. It must hold on to these serious troublemakers instead.

When your liver gets to this point of being unable to process all the unproductive materials running through it, more free radical debris and toxic matter (the less-toxic matter that the liver didn't bury in its core) will be in the bloodstream, forcing the heart to pump harder to pull that blood up from the liver—like sucking pudding through a straw—resulting in high blood pressure. If your liver is clogged to the point that clumps of biofilm start to break off into the blood, then you're likely to develop heart flutters as this jelly-like substance gums up heart valves, preventing smooth flow of blood. (More in Chapter 18, "Mystery Heart Palpitations.") Those are just two of the side effects of a clogged liver. You'll read about others—such as weight gain—in Part II, "The Unseen Storm," and Part III, "The Call to Battle."

If we knew about all of this from birth, we would grow up with reverence for our livers' filtration abilities, and we'd honor them accordingly. Instead, we hear more about the liver's role in detoxification—the breaking down of harmful chemicals and agents, including drugs and alcohol, so the body can process them out. We hear that over time, processing of these types of substances can cause scarring and hardening of the liver tissue. This is about as far as medical communities' understanding of detox goes.

In reality, it's just a fraction of one of the most powerful functions your liver performs: protecting you from dangerous substances. What's off the radar of medical research and science is the full extent of the liver's miraculous ability to screen and filter even when your liver is sluggish, stagnant, overburdened, or sick. When researchers truly discover what your liver is doing here and report it in the medical journals, doctors and medical universities will herald it as gospel.

ONE PRECIOUS LIVER

Another way you can think of this screening and filtering process is as a vetting and inspection process for poisons and toxins in your blood. As you've seen, the liver's filtration system catches as many of these toxins as it can so they can't make mischief in your body. As part of its storage system, the liver throws the specific troublemakers that are too dangerous to release in the moment into liver cells such as hepatocytes, waiting for the day when that person's lifestyle changes so they can be cleansed safely. Over time, these cells stretch to make room if they get crowded, then eventually harden to prevent the cell walls from bursting and letting loose the poisons. For the less aggressive toxins, the liver uses those shapeshifting perime cells to trap them temporarily until it can neutralize and then excrete them, allowing the perime cells to then move along, re-gather, and regroup according to what they're needed for next.

It's a chemical function that creates hepatocyte hardening for the more dangerous troublemakers—a chemical substance naturally created by the liver that saturates a cell and cell membrane, entering into the cell prison and gluing the poisons and toxins together, creating microadhesions that become scar tissue over time. This is where a doctor may point out scar tissue in your liver, citing it as a bad thing. In fact, that scar tissue, while not ideal for liver function, is better than the alternative of troublemakers flowing freely, plaguing whatever they like, beginning with the heart—for example, by causing plaque to gather there or creating a viral infection inside your heart. The scar tissue is a sign that your body is trying to protect you. This cell hardening process is for the more dangerous troublemakers that the liver can't afford to let loose in your body; scar tissue is a sacrifice it's willing to make to protect you from

the worse outcome, which would be those troublemakers heading to your brain or heart.

Another chemical function that the liver performs is to produce a chemical compound that gathers up the white blood cell guards to act together as a softening agent on hardened hepatocyte "prison" cell walls. The white blood cells can then enter the hepatocytes and destroy any viruses hiding within their scar tissue. It's also a technique that the liver employs when we give it a chance to detox—the softening agent can free poisons from hardened cells deep within the liver. Next, the liver lobule elves will repackage and prepare the troublemakers for excretion through bile, absorption into the colon, or elimination through the kidneys.

Alternatively, you can think of your liver as a filter on a cigarette catching some of the tar, chemicals, and nicotine from cigarette smoke before it enters your lungs. As we know well by now, that cigarette filter isn't enough to stop all of the smoke's harm; toxins still get through to the lungs. Similarly, the liver can't stop every harmful element from getting past it when there's a stream of them, which is why the deactivation and detainment process you read about in the previous chapter is so important. What the liver *does* do to screen and filter is miraculous. It stands between us and tremendous suffering from the world's pollution, pathogenic activity, and poisons that we don't even realize we're exposed to in everyday life. It keeps us alive. Without it, we'd all have toxic blood.

And yet the liver doesn't hold a place of honor in our lives. Instead, our standard reference point for filters is that they're replaceable—disposable, even. Vacuum cleaner bags, water filters, air conditioner filters, aquarium filters, oil filters, pool filters: when we see that they get full or worn through or black with waste and buildup, we can take them out and empty them or throw them away. What if you had to keep using the same coffee filter over and over for five years? What if you took your car to the auto shop for a tune-up and the mechanic said, "No can do. We can't replace that transmission filter"? You'd want to learn everything you could about how to preserve, maintain, and clean out the filters you use every day.

In the end, the liver is no cigarette filter, good for one use, that we'll soon toss on the ground and step on, knowing there's a new filter attached to the next smoke. We only get this one liver, this one precious filter. It is an organ in your body, and you can't replace it, except in the extreme scenario of a transplant. The liver you're born with is the one you're granted for life. It's one of your most intelligent organs, with many intricate and complex responsibilities and techniques, and it can only do its best work when it isn't constantly thwarted.

TROUBLE AHEAD

The last thing your liver wants is to release a reckless group of venomous snakes into the wild of your bloodstream and body. When toxins slip by the liver's primary filtration and neutralization processes, the perime cells you read about in the previous chapter (which look very much like normal hepatocytes) provide secondary, backup neutralization by releasing a disarming chemical compound that shocks rogue poisons, stopping them in their tracks and preparing them to be filtered out through the efforts of the lobules and Kupffer cells.

Sometimes, if the liver becomes too compromised, it's down to its last line of defense. When the liver senses that its normal screening, filtering, disarming, detaining, or disposal processes won't be enough to address a crowd of

troublemakers, and that as a result those troublemakers are on the verge of escaping unchecked, the liver sounds an alarm bell—an undiscovered chemical process that I call *hepa-tracking*. Essentially, the liver takes adrenaline that it has absorbed from daily stressors, recycles it, and adds it to a chemical compound tonic for the liver cells and lobule "elves" to consume for supernatural ability and strength in order to prevent the troublemakers from escaping. The tonic also helps direct all other cells within the liver to waste management of these troublemakers that haven't been processed, packaged, or disarmed properly. Because poisons start to escape only when the liver is already toxic and overloaded with troublemakers, when this alarm bell rings, it tends to ring a lot. Pandemonium can set in, like a fire alarm going off in the toy factory three times a day, halting the production line and keeping the elves from doing their normal jobs over and over and over again.

HEALING ACTIVATION

If you're taking care of your health—choosing natural products as often as possible instead of products like plug-in air fresheners and conventional household cleaners that expose you to harmful chemicals, steering clear of the fad diets that overload the liver with fat and clog up its filtration abilities, and employing safe liver cleanse techniques like those we'll look at in Part IV, "Liver Salvation"—this will reflect itself in your liver. You'll make your liver's quality control manageable: instead of bursting at the seams with toxins, liver cells will have the resources to screen, disarm, and neutralize troublemakers so that they can release and dispose of toxins without causing harm—before cells become overcrowded and scarring occurs.

And if scarring is already under way, you can harness the power of diet to activate a healing function of the liver that's undiscovered by medical research and science: When you consume antioxidants—those found in wild blueberries, red pitaya (dragon fruit), and red apple skins especially, as well as in other fruits, vegetables, herbs, and spices—the liver releases a chemical compound that adheres to the antioxidants. Together, the liver's chemical formulation and the healing foods' antioxidants form a hybrid biochemical compound that acts as a softener similar to the one that white blood cells create when needed. The difference is that the white blood cell compound is formulated to enter prison cells and destroy viruses.

This antioxidant-based softener performs a rescue operation for hardened, burdened scar tissue and other damaged tissue, membranes, and lobules—in particular, this softener brings life back to scarred, damaged lobule "elves." Softening hardened adhesions and scar tissue allows new cells to grow, making liver restoration and resurrection possible. This translates to you getting better.

As you can see by now, the liver is one of the smartest, most underestimated organs we possess. With brilliant techniques to draw upon, it has your back like nothing and no one else can. That's never truer than when it's enlisting its dedicated team of defenders—its own personal immune system—to protect you from invaders.

CHAPTER 7

Your Heroic Liver

The Liver's Immune System

When we hear the term *immune system*, we tend to think of our bodies' defense against sniffles, runny noses, fevers, sore throats, and coughs—and rightfully so. Protection against colds and flus *is* a critical function of the immune system. That's why we learn as kids to help out the process with plenty of fluids, rest, and vitamin C.

Evidence of invaders isn't always so obvious as these symptoms, though. Viruses and bacteria sometimes wage attacks far beneath the surface, on our organs and glands. In truth, conditions such as fibromyalgia, multiple sclerosis (MS), rheumatoid arthritis (RA), myalgic encephalomyelitis/chronic fatigue syndrome (ME/CFS), lupus, shingles, Lyme disease, Hashimoto's thyroiditis, hypothyroidism, and dozens more all get their start from viruses taking up residence in the liver. More than we know, we rely on immune defenses that happen deep beneath the surface to protect us from illnesses that have a much more lasting impact than the common cold. The liver doesn't like viruses (and bacteria) residing inside of it, so when it can't stop them from entering, it does everything it can to keep them contained as deep within itself as possible. Then it will send killer cells after the viruses to try to keep them at bay and guard the deep, internal fabric of the liver. When a virus starts to get out of control or tries to leave the depths of the liver, special white blood cells are there to destroy it. The liver also brings in white blood cells randomly and periodically to control any viruses living deep within it. Why doesn't the liver send its white count to out-and-out destroy all viruses and other pathogens in the liver? Because the liver is already putting a tremendous number of resources into trying to fight off new pathogens entering in through the hepatic portal vein and hepatic artery—trying to kill them off before entry so that they don't need to be buried in the first place.

These are the immune defenses of the liver—the liver's personalized immune system, a network of white blood cells that protect you from pathogens that threaten to harm the organ and take a toll on your health. Much of the sophistication of the liver's immune system is still unknown to medical communities, which is why we don't hear about it in our everyday world. It's like a secret recipe we all enjoy without realizing it. We eat the cake; it makes our lives better. Still, we don't know all the ingredients yet, or just how special those ingredients are.

BLOOD CELLS AT WORK FOR YOU

It's unknown to medical science and research that your liver's immune system is made up of six main units. *Hepatic vessel white blood cells*, *hepatic portal vein white blood cells*, and *hepatic artery white blood cells* are three of those units, and they're soldiers that stand watch over all blood that enters the liver.

While produced by the liver, hepatic vessel white blood cells don't actually live there. They're sent on a long journey down the hepatic portal vein—against the current—and then spend their lives away from home, guarding the blood vessels that lead to the portal vein.

Hepatic portal vein white blood cells monitor the portal vein itself. This is the main highway into the liver, past the point of any more on-ramps; exits from here on out will all be within the liver. Mainly, these white blood cells stay at the vein's entryways, like security guards or the TSA. Blood coming through the hepatic portal vein is filled with both nutrients and poisons. This is the hotspot for any kind of troublemaker trying to make its way to the liver, since it's the path for the majority of the blood to the liver and it comes unfiltered from the digestive tract; viruses, bacteria, pesticides from the foods you eat, everything else unproductive that goes into

your stomach, and, in turn, your intestinal tract can flow through this vein. Their specialized white blood cells stand watch over all of it.

Hepatic artery white blood cells are stationed at the other circulatory entrance to the liver, the hepatic artery. Because this blood is coming from the heart, it has higher levels of oxygen than the blood that enters from the hepatic portal vein; it also travels at a higher velocity. Hepatic artery white blood cells, therefore, are adapted to completely different oxygen levels and blood flow. Whereas hepatic portal vein white blood cells can survive being nearly suffocated from lack of oxygen, and speed doesn't need to be their game, hepatic artery white blood cells must swim aggressively while worrying less about oxygen.

Under a microscope—if these immune cells were on the radar of, or of interest to, today's medical research and science—these immune cells may look the same. In reality, their subtle differences mean everything. All three of these white blood cell types are incredible swimmers, with a rare ability to go against blood currents in their pursuit of pathogens. Athletes to the highest degree, they have a special shape that science and research have yet to discover that allows them to hover in an area of rushing blood, much like a grizzly bear wading against dangerous rapids to snatch migrating salmon.

Pathogens that escape these secret service agents at the liver's entryways find themselves up against the liver's next defense, *lobule white blood cells*. These are the personalized guards of those liver lobule elves; they have their own special size and shape geared toward protecting the lobules' safety. Lobule white blood cells border the capillaries and other blood vessels within the liver, on the lookout for invaders such as the Epstein-Barr virus (EBV), which is the unknown creator of hepatitis A, B, C, D, and E as well as of undiagnosed autoimmune conditions of the liver and a host of chronic illnesses that can result from chronic, low-grade viral infections in the liver that go undetected by medical communities. These white blood cells have license to kill, though their job is more difficult than that of the white blood cells guarding the liver's entryways. That's because your liver is your body's filter, so it can be filled with any number of built-up toxins that get in the way of the white blood cells' work. It's much like soldiers on a battleground unable to see clearly from the smoke of burning buildings. Heavy metal runoff, viral and bacterial waste, old pesticides like DDT, and other troublemakers muck up the liver, obscuring the lobule white blood cells' true targets: active pathogens. (It's one of the many reasons why keeping your liver clean and healthy is a critical part of protecting yourself from disease—not just liver disease, *all* disease.)

Because bile production is one of the top functions of your liver, there are unknown, special *bile duct white blood cells* assigned to watch over the bile duct system. These cells are the only part of the immune system that can withstand bile's harsh nature; that's made possible by their protective covers, undiscovered by medical science and research, which act as shields—like hazmat suits or firefighters' gear. The bile duct white blood cells look for passersby in the bile that may cause infection of the liver, gallbladder, duodenum, or intestinal tract—or even travel upward and invade the stomach— and nab them before they can cause trouble. Occasionally, a pathogen will slip by, at which point a signal will go out and a single bile duct white blood cell will launch a kamikaze attack, following the invader out of the liver and into the gallbladder, duodenum, and the rest of the small intestine, a path that will never let it return to the liver. By the end of the journey, this path ultimately destroys and kills the bile duct white blood cell by burning away its protective cover. For a little while, though, the cell's protective cover means it's able to withstand hydrochloric acid from the stomach and toxic substances that someone may ingest as part of food and drink, so as it goes on its suicide mission of pursuing the pathogen, it can stay intact at the outset.

Sometimes, if the threat is high, a few bile duct white blood cells will launch out of the liver together. These brave white blood cells know their time will soon end. In order to gain super-cell qualities and make their mission worthwhile, they take the same adrenaline that the adrenal glands produce to help digest food (one specific blend out of the undiscovered 56 different blends of adrenaline your adrenal glands produce) and absorb it so they can delay their own death to hunt down the pathogens they're pursuing. If someone has weak adrenals that aren't producing this specific adrenaline blend, the liver will release deposits of the blend that it has stored away in the hopes that the white blood cells will find it and put it to use. "A few" bile duct white blood cells may not seem like a lot; keep in mind that there are not many of these blood cells to begin with. The ones that do exist are powerful, and the soul of the liver considers them heroic.

Finally, there are *liver lymphocytes*, which patrol the outer region of the liver. These white blood cells tend to stay on the outside of the liver, from "watchtower" positions in and around the lymphatic vessels there, though they can enter the liver if it becomes necessary. They, too, have license to kill, especially when they come upon EBV cells trying to enter the liver through lymph fluid and establish itself as mononucleosis. Liver lymphocytes are also primed to protect against other herpetic viruses such as human herpesvirus 6 (HHV-6), HHV-7, and the undiscovered HHV-10, HHV-11, HHV-12, HHV-13, HHV-14, HHV-15, and HHV-16; the cofactor *Streptococcus*; various bacterial and viral mutations; and even dangerous superbugs such as *C. difficile* and methicillin-resistant *Staphylococcus aureus* (MRSA).

When a liver is too overburdened with toxins—such as from the environment, an already present viral load, or unproductive foods that someone eats regularly—its filtration system gets backed up and these poisons often leach into the lymphatic system. This makes the job of liver lymphocytes much harder. Their watchtowers become saturated with poisons, and they're forced to leave; they're also slowed down as they try to join forces with each other and reach pathogens, because the lymph fluid is filled with sludge and debris that make it harder for the liver lymphocytes to swim through. This can become treacherous, because when pathogens such as EBV are in the lymphatic system, they're especially aggressive, in a war stage, trying desperately to take up residency in organs such as the liver. Sometimes, the pathogens gang up on the lone lymphocytes and destroy them, winning the battle—though not the war, if you give your liver and lymphatic system the support they need.

THE LIGHT OF KNOWING

When you were born, your mother's liver sent a message to your own: that it could take care of itself. Going back thousands of years in the history of humankind, it has been ingrained in our livers that we don't always offer them a helping hand as we go through life. And so the knowledge is passed along, liver to liver, that it fends for itself.

Not that it couldn't use help. It does face limitations over time as it weakens and breaks down from lack of support. When we don't know what the liver is doing for us, it's completely on its own. The liver's immune system doesn't get the outside help it needs and deserves. And so, as the liver loses strength and grows toxic through the years, the liver's immune system becomes a tattered army out in the field and trenches, with holes in its boots and tears in its uniforms. Food and water, in desperate demand, are rationed, and the ammunition supply is down to its barest bones.

We can shift this course; we can do something about it. We can heal and avoid disease. We can protect the liver's reserves and its precious immune system. We can change direction from being sick to recovering. We can alter what many believe upon falling ill: that sickness is our destiny. We can use our free will to make choices that were never available before, back when we weren't aware of our livers' grace—now the choices are there for us to make. We can change our ways without needing to change who we are.

We need our livers, and our livers need us. Knowing this is the missing piece of the puzzle. While our livers came into the world with the directive to forge ahead without us if need be, they do call out for love and appreciation. When we simply think about the liver in a caring way, the spirit of the liver's immune system can feel it and even recharge from it. Providing our liver with the next level of assistance takes more than that. When we give our liver nutrients and nourishment like mineral-rich foods, we provide for the liver's physical needs, and the liver's immune system can strengthen. When we combine both spiritual and physical, our liver's immune system can do the work it's meant to do. Your liver can heal and function the way it's meant to, taking the mystery and misunderstanding of illness and replacing it with knowing, truth, and the answers that your liver's personalized immune system holds. Your liver's white blood cells carry intelligence; each cell knows what it's up against: which bacterium, virus, or even toxin it's battling. When we treat the liver with intelligence, we assist it with the true miracle of healing. While medical denial can keep us in the dark, we can play it smart by knowing that the liver's immune system is always kept in the light of knowing.

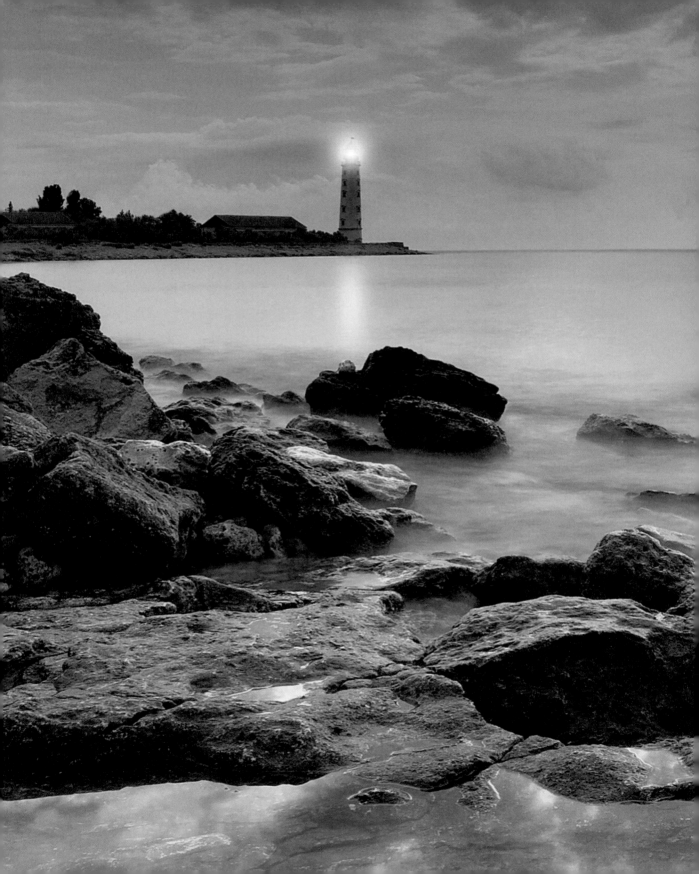

PART II

THE UNSEEN STORM

WHAT'S HAPPENING INSIDE OUR LIVERS

CHAPTER 8

Sluggish Liver

You've just taken a tour of some of the liver's essential functions. If we'd gone into detail on *everything* your liver does for you, we'd still be here decades from now, cataloging the multitude of minute tasks your liver performs. What matters is that you connected with some of the primary roles of your liver—roles that are life-changing to discover, because they give you a window into the soul of the liver, which should be just as legendary as witnessing the fin, tail, and eruption of sacred spray from a visiting whale on a trip out to sea. It was enough, I hope, to appreciate that the liver is our constant companion, tirelessly working for us.

You also started to get a picture of what the liver's up against. Viruses, bacteria, molds, pathogenic waste, toxic heavy metals, radiation, DDT and other pesticides, herbicides, fungicides, solvents, pollutants, drugs, medications, alcohol, excess adrenaline, high-fat diets, and more take a toll on the liver as it works to protect us on a daily basis. And it's not just what we're exposed to in our lifetime. We can also inherit pathogens and toxins from our parents, who got it from their parents, who got it from theirs, meaning that some of the mercury or DDT or EBV that our livers struggle to contain comes

from yesteryear. It's a big job, and the liver does it gloriously.

And then at a certain point, it can become too much. We don't learn how to give our livers a break every once in a while, the way we learn to scrub our dishes and wash our cars and empty our vacuum cleaner bags and launder our clothes. We don't learn to go easy on our livers in the first place, either. So instead of being able to function freely, the liver gets burdened as everything that we're exposed to builds up and up and up. It all amounts to a condition I call *sluggish liver*.

THE HIDDEN STRUGGLE

In order to truly understand sluggish liver, we need to relate to the organ as if it were a person. Knowing that the liver is living and breathing and highly active, that it engages in over 2,000 responsibilities related to storing, delivering, processing, expelling, cleaning, creating, and manufacturing that we caught a glimpse of in Part I, we can get some perspective on what it's like to *be* the liver. Every day, it's busy working for you, and every night, it's elevating you—selflessly striving to keep you healthy, all for your own benefit and the benefit of the people around you. If you're doing well, the ones closest to you will prosper, too.

The liver is meant to be your body's peacekeeper. It's meant to be the rock, the member of the family that makes everything okay, even when that's a challenge, like the go-to sibling who has the calm, composure, and reason to talk loved ones off the ledge before a situation escalates. It sacrifices itself to protect you from alcohol poisoning, dirty blood, high blood pressure, and much more. In most people, the liver serves this function for decades. Then, like any person, if it's pushed past its limit and taken for granted for too long, it reaches the point where it can no longer keep the peace. It becomes sick, congested, disgruntled, frustrated, and even angry, pushed over the edge and into battle.

The first of those battle modes is sluggish liver. If it's not caught at this stage, bigger and fiercer battles can arise that show themselves as bigger and fiercer symptoms and conditions like the many you'll read about in the chapters ahead.

What are your jobs and responsibilities? What are your chores? Your challenges? How do you feel every day as you're trying to win your battles? Are you tired? Do you struggle? Have there been times in your life when a challenge, great or small, wore you out? Broke you down or ate you up and spit you out? Have you ever run a race, or raced to meet a deadline, and then dragged for the next few days? That's how a sluggish liver feels.

Sluggish liver is so common that 9 out of 10 people deal with it. In 15 years, it will be 10 out of 10 for anyone who hasn't learned the truth about sluggish liver and how to protect themselves. It's the precursor to practically anything else that goes wrong with the liver—sluggish liver explains so much of what ails us today—and yet it's not on the radar of medical research and science. Cirrhosis, hepatitis, jaundice, fatty liver, liver cancer: these big-name conditions get all the attention when it comes to this organ. They are, of course, important conditions—and burdensome, sometimes heartbreaking, conditions for those forced to deal with them—and they're ones that we'll uncover in this book. They didn't start out as full-blown problems, though. A person doesn't just wake up one morning with cirrhosis or any of the others. First, sluggish liver develops: slowly, quietly, and over time, if we're not aware it's happening and how to counteract it, the liver gets overloaded. As a result, the liver becomes underactive, it can't protect you as well anymore, and illness is able to take advantage.

The symptoms and conditions that result from a compromised liver aren't only the ones you'd expect or the ones medical research and science have documented. Contrary to popular belief, for example, eczema and psoriasis actually arise from a particular type of overloaded liver. Acne, too, a problem we're told is only hormonal or skin-related, is a sign of a liver under a different type of duress. Mystery high blood pressure, mystery heart palpitations, type 2 diabetes, seasonal affective disorder (SAD), dark under-eye circles, chronic dehydration, varicose veins, weight gain, chemical sensitivities, bloating, constipation—it's unknown that these and more originate at the liver. And before any of them bloom into identifiable health issues, they begin as a liver given too much to handle with too little support. They begin as sluggish liver.

Which is why it's critical to arm yourself with knowledge about this unknown condition. You can't thrive without knowing how to protect yourself. And you can't protect yourself from what you were never warned exists.

A SLUGGISH LIVER BY ANY OTHER NAME

"Sluggish" is just one way to describe the liver when it's in this state of overload. "Stagnant" is another word that can help us see it for what it is. We learn in school that stagnant water is a breeding ground for pathogens and disease-carrying insects—we know that stagnant water in the Amazon can even harbor brain-eating amoebas! So we take care to keep our yards free of standing water; we know that otherwise, mosquitos will take advantage and multiply. Meanwhile, we don't learn that our livers can stagnate, too. And yet now, with this mental image, we can see that the last thing any of us wants is a liver that's grown stagnant, with toxins and bugs pooling inside of it, unable to keep up the normal flow that would flush out these unwelcome guests.

Alternatively, we can think of a sluggish liver as a misbegotten trash service. Nobody likes to be mistreated, dumped on, forgotten, or ignored, least of all the waste disposal folks who deal with trash day in and day out. Have you ever been taken advantage of? It's one of the worst experiences we can have, both emotionally and physically. If it's happened to you, it was probably disheartening and stressful, and possibly injurious. You've probably taken pains not to do it to someone else. So we're mindful to pay someone to haul our trash away, or we pay our taxes that fund the municipal service, or we haul it ourselves and pay the fee at the transfer station. We bag up our trash properly, get it ready on a regular schedule, and wash out our trash cans when they get grimy. Even before

all that, we recycle and compost as much as we can first to reduce the waste that anyone needs to process.

And yet again, with all that, we forget about the liver, our own internal trash service. Throughout my life, I've known people whose kitchens didn't contain a single crumb and whose carpets didn't hold a speck of dirt, yet their livers were a mess. Breaking a sweat and going to the bathroom aren't all it takes to process out the junk we're exposed to—not in today's world. We don't learn how to support the liver in its self-cleaning, nor do we learn the "reduce, reuse, recycle" equivalent rules of tempering the liver's load in the first place. The result is that we accidentally take advantage of our livers, assuming everything's going like clockwork when in reality, operations are screeching to a halt. It's like we're sending trash down the chute to a dumpster over and over again, never realizing that the garbage service has gone on strike and for the past several weeks, no one's been coming to pick it up. Sluggish liver is the liver's form of going on strike. Knowing as you do now how the liver always has your back, you can know that it's always a reasonable, sensible strike. It points us to a bigger picture: that we need to be just as engaged with our body's elimination processes as we are with taking out the trash. Otherwise, we prime pathogens—which have a monkey-see, monkey-do style of opportunism—to follow our lead and take advantage of our livers.

One last way to think of an overburdened liver is as the house of an accidental hoarder. Imagine the crowded home of someone who's inherited a collection of family heirlooms made of lead and asbestos; it's just like how we come into the world with livers already hindered by the pathogens and pollutants of our forebears. This hoarder tries to keep his home organized and neat despite the challenge, and for a while, it's possible. Now imagine that he has a series of impolite houseguests. These visitors trek mud and even gasoline through the house; bring piles of luggage filled with garbage; throw moldy clothes in the closets; carry with them mice, fleas, and bedbugs that infest the furniture; and to top it all off, they gobble up his special provisions that he keeps in the pantry for emergencies. One by one, the houseguests wear down the host. With each passing day, it's harder to keep up with the housework, and in the end he's forced to go into triage mode, letting some chores go so he can keep the house from falling apart and shield the neighborhood from the mayhem inside.

It's an experience that most of us could hardly bear. And yet it's a pretty close comparison to a liver that's become overrun with unwanted bugs and poisons from our everyday encounters, forcing out the liver's precious stores of backup nutrients in the process. We're not taught along the way that our livers battle viruses such as EBV, bacteria, heavy metals (everything from the aluminum foil used in the kitchen to mercury exposure), herbicides, and DDT plus its newer pesticide cousins—and more. Our livers, meant to purify and filter and hold on to the good we'll need later, become hoarders of the bad in order to protect us. Symptoms develop as warning bells, and because we don't know their true cause, we go on medications to put a damper on them, giving the liver yet one more task—to process the prescriptions—in its already dark hour.

All of this while we put great care into the world around us: getting rid of unwanted belongings, organizing the items we keep, running air filters, and perfectly arranging furniture in the name of having a clean and peaceful home. We have no idea that at the same time, we're trashing our livers and never giving them a break. People keep their homes spotless, scrubbing down surfaces and shampooing carpets with toxic cleaners, and plug in dangerous air fresheners to keep everything smelling fresh and clean, never realizing that in their very attempts to purify their surroundings, they're hurting their livers.

So that's sluggish liver: a selfless peacekeeper pushed too far; stagnant water; a trash service on strike; a home overrun with dirt, bugs, and chemicals. It's not a situation any of us would choose in our environments, much less inside our own bodies. Before now, because you didn't know it was happening, you didn't have any say in sluggish liver. Now, it's a whole new world. You're no longer forced to let it happen and suffer mysteriously as a result—because now, you're in on the secret.

LIFESAVING SYMPTOMS

Before we continue, let's make one more point clear: sluggish liver is not something that should make us feel less-than. A sluggish liver should never be confused with a lazy liver. Your liver will never be lazy; it can't be.

You know that feeling when you're under the weather, so you push through the day with that much more effort? It's true of a sluggish liver, too. When it has obstacles to overcome, it works harder—in fact, in sluggish condition, the liver works two or three times as hard to make up for its underactive state. No matter what, even when it's at its most stagnant, your liver finds a way to push through and labor with intensity. It learned to do this when you were still in the womb, through chemical communications from your mother's liver, and it will do this for the rest of your life.

Your liver holds the soul of courage within it. Its bravery and grit in defending your life are unparalleled. It will do anything to protect you: like a warhorse defending the soldier it's carrying, your liver will take any number of hits to try to keep you safe.

Taking those hits does put it in a compromised position. For one, it starts to lose its memory. Given that the liver is the third memory bank of the body (along with the brain and the thyroid), this is a big deal. It means that as the liver becomes saturated with heavy metals, pathogens, byproduct, debris, and poisonous chemicals, it can't help the body as much as it needs or wants to. It starts to lose the ability to identify, absorb, catalogue, alter, and deliver critical biochemical compounds and hormones.

It also starts to lose the ability to neutralize those substances that your body doesn't want. As we covered in Part I, many of the liver's over 2,000 functions exist around detoxification. When the liver is clogged or overloaded, it gets too beaten down to convert these substances as well as usual and instead ends up storing them, which slows down filtration even more. If you picture an aquarium filter that's slick with fish waste or a vacuum cleaner bag bursting with dust and dirt, you get the idea of how impeded a liver can become. Because the liver can't filter in this state as well as it's meant to, waste matter escapes and starts to back up into the bloodstream, causing some of the problems we'll look at here in Parts II and III. It's an ongoing cycle: the more pesticides and other toxic chemicals, viruses, bacteria, radiation, alcohol, antibiotics, drugs, toxic heavy metals, plastics, and high blood-fat levels the liver is exposed to, the more sluggish the liver gets, the less it can neutralize harmful materials and screen blood effectively. Toxic, dirty blood can translate into

dark under-eye circles, hot flashes, and more, which we'll cover in the next chapter.

It can also translate to liver heat. Just as an engine finds its parts warming up and is forced to work harder when it's running on old oil that's lost its viscosity, so too does the liver generate heat when it's got too much sludge to handle. This can translate into symptoms such as hot flashes and a sensation of "running hot," which we'll look at in the coming chapters. (Or, if the liver isn't entirely overloaded yet, you can feel perfectly fine. More on that in a moment.)

Does heat mean the liver is being lazy? Absolutely not. Trying to contain that heat is just one more job on top of cleaning up 50 other messes. Do you ever take the heat in your life? Take on blame and responsibility, whether they're rightfully yours or not? Not just heat—do you ever take a hit for someone, take punishment, take abuse, in the name of protecting someone else? That's your liver's daily life, and that someone it's protecting is you. It's constantly picking up the slack of our overpolluted, overstressed, overstimulated, undernourished lives.

The liver also has an anti-sluggish emergency alarm response. It's a chemically induced response that brings in new, vital energy to break up stagnancy. The response is a liver spasm. This spasm can result in a tingle, a twitch, a slight ache, warmth, heat, pulling, bloating, a prick, a stitch in the side, or—much of the time—no feeling at all. It usually occurs quietly, with little or no discernable sensation, though it does bring renewal to that portion of the liver that spasmed and allow the liver to temporarily regain some control.

One of the key reasons your liver goes into battle is, as you read about in Chapter 2, "Your Adaptogenic Liver," to protect a vital gland: your pancreas. If someone is eating a high ratio of fat calories that surpasses the limit of how much bile the liver can produce to break down the fat, the liver gets taxed. The liver needs to find alternative ways to absorb and process the fat to take the hit away from the pancreas. It's one of the reasons why the liver must be adaptogenic. The more the liver gets beaten down, the more its glucose reserves drop and drop and drop. When the liver doesn't have enough glucose in reserve, it can't release it to the pancreas to stop the insulin resistance process. As a result, your doctor may say your A1C levels are elevated or even off the charts, resulting in a diagnosis of prediabetes or type 2 diabetes. We'll get to that in Chapter 15, "Diabetes and Blood Sugar Imbalance." Your liver is so responsible for the pancreas that it also releases a chemical compound just for the gland, a Band-Aid chemical signature to the pancreas to help mend and heal wounds there.

Another precious part of you that your liver is trying to protect is your heart. Your liver processes and filters toxins out of your blood so that your heart doesn't become asphyxiated from poisons crowding out oxygen, so that plaque doesn't build up in the heart's valves or in the arteries, and to thin the blood so the heart doesn't have to work as hard.

There's so much more that can happen when the liver is under too much stress: scarring, cysts, tumors, a weakened immune system, enlargement, inflammation—all of which we'll cover in the coming chapters.

It's also common to have a sluggish liver and experience no symptoms at all for a long time. That's another miracle of the liver: it will hold out, shielding you from its burden, for as long as it possibly can. You probably know the feeling, what it's like to be faced with endless tasks while coming under siege from all angles, and yet not wanting to let down anyone in your life by showing how much you're struggling. You soldier on,

doing as much work as you can without complaint, and only when it's physically impossible to keep it up anymore do you make a peep.

The liver's soldiering-on is why it's very common for people not to exhibit their first symptoms of sluggish liver until their late 30s or into their 40s—at which point, in women, it's often mistaken for menopause. What seems like the sudden onset of hot flashes, irritability, and insomnia actually isn't sudden at all. It's the result of a lifetime of sluggish liver building up and up and up and just now making itself known after decades. This remains unknown to medical research and science due to the hormone replacement mass market and the hormone blame that to this day keeps women in the dark about what's really causing their symptoms.

Exactly how the liver becomes silently burdened depends on each individual's life circumstances; there are different combinations for everyone. Sluggish liver can be a result of a long-term, chronic, and low-grade infection of EBV, for example, or a low-grade infection from any one of a number of other viruses. The liver can be sluggish from toxic heavy metals that have gathered along the way; from prescription pharmaceuticals taken periodically; from celebratory alcohol imbibed over many gatherings; from a few decades of unhealthy, fatty foods; from tons of coffees, lattes, and cappuccinos; and from many emotional ups and downs that have triggered the adrenals to saturate the liver with adrenaline due to fight-or-flight responses throughout your lifetime.

No matter which particular challenges your liver faced, it miraculously built bridges and died out fires over the years, protecting you from all manner of threats and preventing you from suffering. Then, finally, the day came when it couldn't cope on its own anymore. It gave you symptoms—night sweats and brain fog, a bad night's sleep, a small bout of rosacea or eczema, for example—as a cry for help, hoping that someday you would be able to understand what was going on and offer relief. The world isn't there yet. Symptoms and illnesses aren't properly linked to the liver, never mind to the unknown condition sluggish liver.

We think of symptoms as pesky, as signs of our bodies turning against us, when in reality they're incredibly helpful clues about something going wrong deep within. We don't get annoyed at smoke, saying that it's a sign of the air having it in for us that day. Rather, we know that smoke is a sign of fire, so we give thanks for the signal and follow it to its source.

FIVE VARIETIES OF SLUGGISH LIVER

Just as different types of smoke can alert us to different types of fires, particular symptoms can clue us in to what's wrong with the liver. One way to help figure out what's going on is to learn about the five varieties of sluggish liver. That's right—sluggish liver is not all or nothing. The whole liver doesn't become sluggish at once; it may be only part of your liver that's sluggish while the rest functions fine. Many people have a combination of sluggish areas. Here's a look at the five areas of liver sluggishness. Keep in mind that you could have a sluggish liver in one or even all five of these areas and not experience a single one of these symptoms.

- **Middle of the liver:** A liver that's sluggish in its deepest part is most likely to reveal itself with symptoms such as hot flashes, night sweats, prediabetes, swelling, fluid retention, body temperature fluctuations, low energy, weight gain, brain fog,

dark circles under the eyes, hypoglycemia, hyperglycemia, fatigue, rashes, anger, frustration, irritability, a sense of loneliness, depression, anxiety, anxiousness, poor skin tone, skin pigment issues (including Raynaud's syndrome), and excessive thirst.

- **Bottom of the liver:** A sluggish lower liver can make you toss and turn in the night, result in other sleep disturbances and insomnia, and/or give you constipation, a feeling of unease, sensations of hot and cold when neither makes sense for your environment, jealousy, or a quick-to-get-hurt manner that gets you labeled as having a "thin skin."

- **Top of the liver:** Poor digestion, acid reflux, bloating, gastritis, pressure in the abdomen, irritability, frustration, stiff shoulder, shoulder ache, tongue sores, canker sores, corner-of-the-lip sores, other mouth sores, body temperature fluctuations, and a bulging, protruding, or hardened upper belly are all possible symptoms of a sluggish upper liver.

- **Left side of the liver:** When the left-hand side (the left lobe) of the liver is sluggish, feelings of weakness in the left leg or arm, nausea, anxiousness, lack of hunger, insatiable hunger, random stomach pain, moodiness, irritability, emotional sensitivities, and backaches can result.

- **Right side of the liver:** The right-hand, larger side (the right lobe) of the liver becoming sluggish can lead to brittle and/or discolored nails (from zinc deficiency), stitches in the right-hand ribs, mild weakness on the right side of the body, leg spasms or cramps, mild tongue discoloration, a raw tip of the tongue, sensations of inexplicable hot and cold, and difficulty warming up.

CRACKING THE CODE

Put another way, symptoms are like a foreign language, one none of us learned in school or even at home. It's our job to interpret for the body—in this case, the liver—so that it can finally get its point across. So many of the symptoms and illnesses that the world teaches us are signs of a faulty body are, in fact, a sluggish or damaged liver asking for assistance: If you experience fatigue, the doctor may say it's because you're too stressed out, when really it could be an infection of EBV inside the liver. If you experience hot flashes, you'll hear that it's hormonal and a sign of perimenopause, menopause, or postmenopause, when the truth is that they happen as a result of a liver that's been holding on to a virus, heavy metals, or toxins long term. With mysterious weight gain, a practitioner may say that you overeat or you don't eat right or

you need to exercise more; meanwhile, it's really a sign of a liver burdened with viruses, excess adrenaline, and other troublemakers. And if acne plagues you, the diagnosis will be puberty or another hormonal shift, when the reality is that it's from strep bacteria thriving in a congested liver, causing the lymphatic system to become overloaded, too. None of these issues mean your body is falling apart; they're your liver saying, "Please help me."

This part of the book, "The Unseen Storm," is all about interpreting what our livers are trying to tell us. It's about tracing the smoke to the fire. It's about decoding the puzzling messages that most of the time we don't even realize are coming from our livers—so that we can finally move forward. In the coming chapters, we'll take a more in-depth look at liver-related symptoms and conditions, some of which you'd expect, such as hepatitis, and others you may not connect with the liver, such as prediabetes, eczema, psoriasis, and SIBO.

No longer do you have to dislike or distrust your body. It's not out to get you. It's not letting you down. It's not weak. Your body is on your side. Let's stop thinking of the health problems we're about to look at as genetic life sentences, as our bodies disappointing us, or as autoimmune ticking time bombs that self-detonate beyond our control. Let's start seeing the hidden blessing that the liver cries out for help. After all, when the liver shows its struggle, it gives us the opportunity to respond, to bring it back to health, and to reclaim our lives.

CHAPTER 9

Liver Enzyme Guess Tests

Say a man named Noah goes to the doctor for a routine physical. The doctor draws some blood, and several days later, Noah receives a call saying the blood work came back from the lab. "Your liver enzymes are elevated," the doctor tells him.

"What does that mean?" Noah asks.

"Why don't you come in? I'll run some additional tests and we'll talk about it."

When Noah arrives for his appointment, he asks again, "What does it mean to have elevated liver enzymes?"

This time, the doctor says, "Well, we really don't know. We just know that it indicates *something* is going on with the liver. It could be liver damage."

"How could I have damaged my liver?"

"It could be a liver condition or a disease developing, although you seem very healthy on other counts, so I doubt that. Do you consume a lot of alcohol? Are you under a lot of stress? Look, Noah, it might not be anything at all. Or it could be inflamed liver cells. We'll have to take some more blood and run some more tests."

Thousands like Noah go through this experience of mystery elevated liver enzymes: it's obvious that something's going on with the liver, though no one, including the experts, knows precisely what. One common outcome would be if Noah received a CT or PET scan, MRI, and ultrasound of his liver, none of them displaying any problems worth investigating further. With no reason to biopsy the liver, Noah would receive the instructions "Eat a little better, keep your stress in check, and get more sleep. Come back in three months and we'll test it again."

Another possible outcome would be if Noah *did* have something apparent on one of his scans, such as extreme, visible inflammation, scar tissue, or cystic activity. Then, in the doctor's eyes, there would be a match for why the liver enzymes were elevated.

Many cases are like the first one, where liver enzymes are elevated with no real indication otherwise of a problem. This leads medical research and science to believe that an enzyme test is a guessing game, fallible and inaccurate. There are cases where someone has a cyst or scar tissue and an enzyme test comes back normal. You could have a fatty liver, too, with enzymes either elevated or not. Even when scans show something visible happening to someone's liver, an enzyme test doesn't say what it is or what to do about it.

That's why the title of this chapter is "Liver Enzyme *Guess* Tests." Here, we'll explore what's really happening when liver enzymes are released, and how these tests are still valuable, even though they're not the be-all and end-all. I don't want to devalue liver enzyme tests, because I do think they have their place. One of the many items graduates aren't given when they finish medical school is an oracle. Instead, they need to work with what is available within their means. So, really, it's a miracle that we have liver tests to help them along. These tests are important indicators that give doctors permission to go with the gut and use some intuition in giving guidance to their patients.

What I most like about liver enzyme tests is that they make doctors and patients aware that there could be a liver problem when otherwise, they'd have no idea. When people hear that they have elevated liver enzymes, it's a signal to some of them to change their lifestyles. It's that prompt for the doctor to tell Noah to take better care of himself. Chances are, Noah is going to think more about what he eats now, even lowering his chances of a heart attack. Even if his doctor or a trendy article gives him the wrong direction about what to eat, he'll likely end up getting some more productive food in himself one way or another, and he'll be a little more mindful about his health. That's worth a lot.

THE REAL MEANING OF ENZYMES

The two enzymes most commonly tested for are *alanine transaminase* (ALT) and *aspartate aminotransferase* (AST). Other common enzymes tested for are *alkaline phosphatase* (ALP) and *gamma-glutamyl transpeptidase* (GGT).

Doctors also commonly order blood tests to analyze levels of *albumin*, a blood protein that's believed to transport important nutritional components and possibly hormones throughout the bloodstream. If a test comes back showing you have low albumin, chances are the doctor will think you're eating poorly; medical research and science believe it's an indicator of bad nutrition. If it comes back high, then medical communities use it as license to move forward with further investigation into whether something, somewhere could be wrong in the body, such as a bacterial infection or an injury of some kind. Like the enzyme tests, this one doesn't pinpoint anything. (What elevated albumin really indicates is a viral flare.)

Doctors may also find elevated *bilirubin* in the bloodstream. Bilirubin is created when the liver breaks down and detoxifies red blood cells. There are two kinds of bilirubin, one created within the liver itself and one that's floating through the bloodstream that the liver must collect and convert so it can be used as viable liver bilirubin. If bilirubin is elevated in your blood work, it can indicate a pancreatic problem, a liver condition developing, a bile duct issue, or even a tumor in the bile duct.

All of these tests are accurate in that when the results are abnormal, there's a very good chance that something *is* wrong with the liver, though what that is often remains completely unknown to medical communities. While today's liver testing can catch problems before they're at their worst, it doesn't catch problems at their earliest. When any liver testing indicates a problem, it really means that the patient was dealing with a liver condition long, long before testing showed anything. If an adult's test results show elevated enzymes or bilirubin, it usually means that something could have taken root in the liver way back, 10 or 30 years ago or even longer—sluggishness, an old viral infection, so-called autoimmune inflammation, the early stages of hepatitis C, or another issue could have started to develop decades ago. (For an infant or a child, it's a different story. See Chapter 28 for information on juvenile liver problems.) The only reason that a liver problem would show up quickly on an adult's test would be if it's an acute infection. To diagnose that, doctors would also go by inflammation rising fast within the liver as well as other signs of the immune system reacting to an infection, such as elevated white count and symptoms such as fever, weakness, nausea, or skin discoloration.

The tests remain basic. When future tests are invented way down the road, then they will pick up on early signs of liver problems—because there is more to detect. For example, there are more than four enzymes that show up in the blood as indicators; there are dozens of undiscovered enzymes. There are also hundreds of chemical compounds yet to be discovered that will help medical professionals identify definitively what's really happening in the liver and where. Is it hepatitis A, B, C, D, E, or one of the numerous other forms of hepatitis that medicine will eventually identify? (More on hepatitis in Chapter 29.) Are pesticides and herbicides building up in the liver and hampering it? Future testing will be able to determine these answers, because the enzymes and chemical compounds that the liver releases are special, specific signals; each enzyme and chemical compound holds a cipher.

For true progress, it will take a bridge to connect the medical establishment with the land of honesty. This will mean the medical world acknowledging the prevalence of toxic heavy metals and where they come from as well as how dangerous the herbicides, fungicides, and pesticides we encounter in our everyday lives—such

as mosquito sprays dropped from the sky—are to the liver. Once this honesty develops, the door may finally open to discovering the enzymes and chemical compounds that the liver sends as flares. Only then will researchers discover that certain liver enzyme emergency flares actually contain information that illuminates why they're being released. They'll decode how certain flares signal certain insecticides while others match mercury and aluminum—that every toxin and every pathogen has a connection to a different liver enzyme coating, and that far from random, they actually create a comprehensive picture of the particular struggles of someone's individual liver.

Research and science aren't allowed to go there yet. Connecting those dots would mean exposing the influence of the pesticide world and the heavy metal world. It would mean being honest about the industries that put these into our everyday lives and how the medical machine is hand in hand with them. It's well known, for example, that drugs and pharmaceuticals can contain heavy metals, so how can we build the bridge yet to their effects on the liver? Pesticides, fungicides, and herbicides, too, have ties to the medical industry—another reason why we can't build the bridge yet. We won't be allowed to go there for a very long time. It will take a major shift for a doctor to be given the data and training to be able to say, "Whoa, this one enzyme is signaling that your liver is dealing with a virus, and hey, wait a minute, this other enzyme is triggered by a chemical in fungicides that's used on all kinds of products. And here's another enzyme coming from insecticides that your town drops to control the mosquito population." It's better for medical industry relationships that we stay in the dark: "You've got high liver enzymes? Let's never study which one's coming from what."

By the way, we just touched on one reason why the liver releases enzymes when it's inflamed or damaged: as emergency flares. If you were having trouble out at sea, the captain of your ship would shoot off a flare gun in the hope that someone would see and come to the rescue. Your liver's enzymes and their coatings are even more specialized than that. Its signals are like a boat sending up a red flare if it started to sink, an orange flare if it got stranded far from land, and a purple flare if pirates attacked. Whose attention is the liver trying to catch, though? Not the doctor's. Unlike when you take your poodle to the vet and the dog can see what's going on and tell that the vet is trying to help, the liver doesn't have eyes. It doesn't even know what doctors are. What the liver knows is how you work internally. The flares in the form of enzymes and chemical compounds are for other parts of the body to receive; they're warnings to other organs and glands that a liver condition is occurring. While symptoms and conditions are clues to *you* that the liver is hurting, the liver's enzymes and chemical compounds are clues to the rest of the body. The beauty is that when medical research and science eventually discover the various meanings of these emissions, they'll be able to read the liver's signals just as the body can.

In the meantime, today's blood tests pick up on only a tiny fraction of what's happening. For comparison, think of a sample of stagnant pond water. We know this stagnant water is probably infested with hundreds of problematic contaminants, among them parasites, bacteria, unproductive fungi and algae, amoebas, protozoa, and environmental toxins. Now, imagine if the water test came back showing that there were only four very similar microbes and that otherwise, it was fine to drink. You wouldn't trust the results, because the state of water

testing is further along than that. You'd know it was one shoddy test and that another sample would need to be taken and evaluated to get the real picture. And yet the incomplete picture is the stage we're still at with blood testing for all chronic health conditions. We can look at it as glass half empty—that we're that far behind—or glass half full (of contaminated water), that we're not yet far enough along.

Back to the enzymes and chemical compounds. Signals from the liver are not only cries for help; they're little blessings—messages to the other parts of the body to self-prepare. One of the organs they signal is the brain; they provide critical messages to the central nervous system. It would be awesome if they were messages that took control and got us to drink more celery juice! In reality, they're even better and, in fact, miraculous: these communications that we can't feel or see are directions to the nervous system to support the liver. For the adrenals, the signals forewarn them that there's a problem brewing, so the glands should slow down their engines a bit. The pancreas also gets a message to be mindful of its enzymatic output. (The digestive enzymes produced by the pancreas are not to be confused with the liver's warning enzymes.)

After signaling, the liver's enzymes and undiscovered chemical compounds have a second active role—a job they're assigned upon release—and that's to act as cleaning agents and devour toxic substances that are still active. That is, when a toxic substance does damage to the liver and then escapes, the enzymes and compounds are released with license to hunt down the escaped particles, chemicals, and toxins, feverishly seeking them out like scavengers and devouring them. Essentially, the enzymes neutralize what the liver and its perime cells couldn't because the liver had become too stagnant, sluggish, or overburdened.

This is an important point to revisit: usually, the liver will only release waste items if they've been disarmed and inactivated. The liver has a self-monitoring and self-collecting ability. It can choose what "garbage" it wants to package and release to the bloodstream for exit through the colon or kidneys or to send through the bile to the gallbladder. That is, unless, the liver is slowing down and can't perform its normal functions. If the liver is sluggish and some troublemakers escape without being disarmed, that's when it sends its liver enzymes to go chase after the un-neutralized particles. When a rogue virus such as EBV or HHV-6 is in residence in the liver, producing neurotoxins and other poisonous waste, that's another time when the liver will call on its enzymes. (While a stronger liver will disarm neurotoxins to a degree, even a disarmed neurotoxin remains toxic. A weaker liver has an even harder time neutralizing neurotoxins, and so enzymes become even more important, though they're not guaranteed to deactivate the neurotoxins.) In their mission to chase after waste matter, liver enzymes also have the ability to collect it again and bring it back to the liver, where it can be contained in a storage bin.

Keep in mind that you can have an early liver condition that's not accompanied by elevated liver enzymes—on a test. In truth, the liver enzyme flares are still present; even with the mildest of liver preconditions, the liver is sending out enzymes. Today's blood tests just don't pick them up unless they're really elevated. And remember: tests are only geared to detect a few enzymes, when there are really dozens. Another factor that can keep enzyme levels lower in the blood is when the liver calls for enzymatic activity to devour toxins inside of it. By taking care of the problems at the site, the liver has only

minor needs to send enzymes out looking for escaped materials—so they don't show up on blood tests.

Given that liver enzymes (and the undiscovered chemical compounds) are highly active, it means the liver doesn't consider them waste. When it lets them go, it lets them go for a reason. Medical research and science, meanwhile, believe that liver enzymes are only released when liver cells are broken, damaged, or exploded, or when they die—without even understanding why cells become disturbed, injured, or otherwise damaged. They usually cast it off as a natural liver process and enzymes as byproduct, when the truth is that there's much deeper meaning behind it. They don't realize the complex signaling and scavenging that's really going on.

By the way, liver enzymes are not released solely when the liver is hurt, which explains why you can have elevated liver enzymes with no apparent injury to the liver. You could have no symptoms, no liver damage, no condition or precondition developing at all, and yet you could get a reading of elevated enzymes out of nowhere because a toxic buildup of waste escaped the liver and it released enzymes to do their scavenging and cleanup.

If this were a 10,000-page book, we'd have the space we need to describe the ins and outs of the liver's enzymes and specialized chemical compounds in full detail.

WHAT ENZYME TESTS HAVE TO OFFER

I support testing for liver enzymes because it can indicate that someone's dealing with a hidden liver condition that otherwise no one would know about, even if it leads to a misdiagnosis or the best treatment plan isn't offered. When considering test results, though, we need to be aware that the testing remains extremely basic. For one, the test results don't come back saying *what* is wrong, ever. Doctors are left to look for visible signs of an issue, and if scans don't come back showing an obvious obstruction, growth, or pocket of scar tissue in plain view, they're stuck in a guessing game.

I've also seen hundreds of cases over the years of people who got back elevated enzyme results and did display something physical going on with their liver—whether a tumor, cyst, or scar tissue—and yet that issue wasn't really what was causing their symptoms. To understand why they had fatigue, aches and pains, vertigo, weakness, depression, or anxiety, they had to understand what we're exploring in this book.

For early signs and symptoms of liver disease, look no further than prediabetes or type 2 diabetes, hypoglycemia, blood sugar imbalances, eczema and psoriasis, weight gain, chemical sensitivities, brain fog, SAD, accelerated aging, methylation issues, hormone imbalances, bloating, gout, dark under-eye circles, varicose and spider veins, cellulite, fluid retention, lymphedema, swollen hands and feet, SIBO, and even low hydrochloric acid in the stomach. These are all liver-related, and there are so many more—like the numerous symptoms of a virus camping out in the liver. Some people I've talked with who had these symptoms and conditions got back elevated enzyme results, and some showed enzymes at normal levels. A lot of people with type 2 diabetes don't show elevated enzymes and a lot of people do; either way, diabetes stems from the liver. Gout is a serious liver condition, and it's a crapshoot as to whether elevated enzymes will appear on tests or not. Many people dealing with weight gain do show elevated enzyme levels, and many people don't, even when they have a pre-fatty or fatty liver.

Elevated enzymes can come and go even within a week or a month, all of it hinging on what the liver is dealing with in a given moment. If liver enzyme tests were taken for days in a row, one test could barely show them, a test three days later could show a drastic elevation, and then two days later they could be gone. The results you get on your liver enzyme test depend so much on which day you walk into the doctor's office—is it the day they're up, down, or in between? Since it's a one-and-done situation, with no readings on consecutive days for comparison, you can't know.

Despite all this, we can't discount the use of liver enzyme tests. As I said, when tests come back showing elevated enzymes, it's an indication to look more carefully and take better care of our livers, through whatever avenue we choose. What we need to keep in mind is that like all testing, it's never 100 percent flawless and accurate. We've learned this with testing for Lyme disease and human immunodeficiency virus (HIV). Many people are given a positive for HIV, get tested again, and receive a negative— it's commonplace. Lyme testing is the same. (For more on this, see *Thyroid Healing*.) It's similar with lupus and rheumatoid arthritis (RA) testing, too. They're tests geared to look for inflammation or an elevated immune system without identifying *why* the immune system is in overdrive or *why* inflammation is occurring. You could end up with the wrong conclusions, because interpreting the test results is guesswork.

THE EARLY BIRD GETS THE HEALTHY LIVER

Even when the tests do their job of showing something amiss, we can't rely on them as the only indicators of liver trouble. We can't live our lives like Noah, hoping everything's fine, relying on a liver enzyme test to be our wake-up call. And we don't want to be worse off than Noah, either, living with a liver condition that never shows up on a test and never gives us a wake-up call. You don't want to be that patient with diabetes, weight gain, gout, or even a chronic and low-grade viral infection such as EBV that can create ME/CFS or Hashimoto's thyroiditis, who doesn't start taking care of herself or himself until getting a reading of elevated liver enzymes at age 50, 60, or 70. Rather than waiting and wondering what pesky or life-threatening health problems could arise for us, we need to be proactive and self-reliant. We need to learn to read the signs and symptoms of liver-related distress. We need to beat the tests to the punch. When it comes to the liver, we want the early-bird special.

CHAPTER 10

Dirty Blood Syndrome

Almost everyone on the planet is mildly to chronically dehydrated throughout childhood and adult life. The body has an amazing ability to adapt to this. Or rather, one hardworking organ inside the body that we live most of our lives ignoring has an amazing ability to adapt. Not that it's easy for the liver to get us through decades of dehydration. A person who's chronically dehydrated walks around always on the verge of exhibiting serious and immediate symptoms because the liver is so overextended. Whether those symptoms come to pass depends on the individual's constitution.

What makes a good constitution, though? You'll hear it chalked up to genes—that someone with a weaker constitution didn't luck out in the gene lottery and someone with more robust health did. That's not how it works. That reasoning only distracts us from what a good constitution really depends on: fewer toxins in the body contributing to stronger organs, creating fewer health vulnerabilities and compromises. A weak constitution is the result of more toxins in the body contributing to struggling organs, creating more vulnerabilities and compromises.

If someone has a buildup of toxins in the body and one or more low-grade viral or bacterial infections, chronic dehydration will create more of a strain for that person's system. They'll set someone up to cross that fine line where chronic dehydration suddenly becomes life-disrupting.

For example, if you have a low-grade bacterial infection of strep (which you may not know you have), chronic dehydration could be the difference between feeling fine and developing another urinary tract infection (UTI), sinus infection, case of gastritis, sty, SIBO, or even a breakout of acne. Medical communities remain unaware that strep bacteria are chronic in so many, and that these conditions are strep-related. If you have a low-grade viral infection (again, which you may not be aware you have), chronic dehydration could also mean the difference between going about your life as usual versus suddenly developing a bout of serious fatigue, aches and pains, tinnitus, vertigo, tingles and numbness, dizziness, confusion, or heart palpitations.

Why should you care about chronic dehydration if you feel okay? If you don't have a known liver problem, a low-grade viral or bacterial condition, allergies, migraines, or any of the numerous other symptoms and conditions that dehydration can worsen, why should it matter to you? First, because you may not know you have a problem; medical testing doesn't yet detect every issue under the surface. And second, because when we're not careful, chronic dehydration gets everyone in the end. It's the straw that breaks the camel's back, causing a stroke at age 65 when the blood gets too thick and polluted after too little hydration over too many decades. It's that tip over the edge that causes a heart attack even though you've exercised your whole life. You felt good, went on cruises, played golf, had fun, worked hard, became successful—and after all that, the stroke or heart attack triumphed over you. Chronic dehydration won. Well, we can't let chronic dehydration win in the end.

The type of dehydration I'm talking about is not a once-in-a-while type, like forgetting to bring a water bottle with you on a long walk. This is an everyday type of dehydration. It happens all the time to students rushing between classes, workers busy at the office, and people running around on errands. At times, it will rear its head—take, for example, teenagers who spend a day shopping. Not eating for three to four hours or more, they'll start to get dizzy and confused with headaches, blurry eyes, slightly faint feelings, and even the shakes, since chronic dehydration can cause blood sugar to drop radically. That's how fine the line can be—all it took was a full morning of shopping to bring on symptoms. The soda and slice of pizza that the shoppers grab in the middle of the day may momentarily give them relief. It's not enough to fix the years and years of chronic dehydration; it only adds to it.

We know to fear dehydration in extreme circumstances. It's the specter that hangs over hikes through the desert and life rafts drifting in the ocean and emergencies that cut people off from resources. What we don't take seriously enough, because we're not aware of how serious it is, is the only slightly friendlier ghost of chronic dehydration that sits behind a two-way mirror, watching us, living with us, and causing trouble that we can't see. It's not so spooky at the beginning, though it can get us in the end. It's like that friend you've had for a very long time, with whom you've always gotten along just well enough, until one day he does something just jarring enough that you can't get over it.

Chronic dehydration is always riding your back, and it's been there for so long that you don't feel it anymore. If, over several months, you finally got properly hydrated, then let progress slip and went back to your old ways, you would feel that chronic dehydration return like a monkey on your back—and you wouldn't like carrying it around one bit.

We don't learn to hydrate. We learn instead, when we're young, that a cookie and a Dixie cup of apple juice are all we need to get through a whole afternoon at day care or preschool. While apple juice is good if it's organic and preservative-free, a few sips aren't enough to get a toddler through several hours of playtime—yet that's been a normal practice for decades. Throughout childhood, adolescence, and into adulthood, we learn and relearn similar lessons. When we have our own kids, we unknowingly teach and reteach them that it's okay to get by in life dehydrated. The difference when we *are* hydrated is astonishing. Like playing a game in the pool, carrying someone on your shoulders back and forth, from end to end, over and over, and then finally offloading the player after a winning slam dunk and feeling the weight lift away—that's what getting hydrated is like. If you're struggling with a chronic symptom or condition of any kind, whether it's been diagnosed properly or it's a mystery, getting hydrated could make a world of difference in your experience of that health issue.

Our eating and drinking habits that are part of our normal way of life here on earth are not pro–blood sugar stabilization, nor are they pro-repair and reversal of chronic dehydration. The fluid choices that people make are almost never adequate to truly hydrate. (Yes, I'm even talking to you exercise enthusiasts who drink a fancy electrolyte beverage after a long run—don't think that did the job. Many people who make exercise a big part of their lives are chronically dehydrated.) People's diets, overall, aren't hydrating enough. Add to that alcohol and random pharmaceuticals as well as the low-quality salt and preservatives that slip into so many foods, and it's a recipe for extreme dehydration every single day.

When you wake up in the morning, do you drink a liter of lemon water? Very few people do. It's an ideal protocol to protect you and keep you hydrated even when you're consuming your normal food and beverages throughout the day. That lemon water first thing could be enough to carry you. So could a celery juice or a smoothie—well, depending on what's in the smoothie. If it's a trendy recipe, chances are it's dehydrating, because it's filled with radical fat like tablespoons of coconut oil, nut butter, or whey protein powder and barely any fruit. Trendy smoothies aren't the only dehydrating morning routines. So are the traditional breakfast foods that people grow up on, like bacon, eggs, and toast with a glass of milk and maybe the processed, pasteurized, preservative-loaded orange juice of the old days. And how about coffee? So many people drink their morning cup

of coffee, and that's all they rely on before they head off to work. It may be lunchtime before they put anything else in their bodies.

For many of us, over time, our liver cells adapt to never getting proper hydration. Through a miraculous, unknown chemical function that I call the *camel effect*, our livers are able to keep the rest of our bodies hydrated in the long term. It's not perfect hydration; it's not ideal. It is, while it lasts, life-sustaining.

Even when it's bombarded by troublemakers, your liver takes in whatever little bits of high-quality fluid you randomly eat and drink, like the good sponge it is. It lives in wait for these moments when you do something good for yourself, even if it's by accident. Maybe six months ago, your aunt or grandmother offered you an apple, something you'd never eat otherwise—your liver took advantage. It took advantage of the romaine lettuce salad you ate last week at the block party and the navel orange that a friend shared with you while you were watching your kids' soccer practice. Your liver identifies molecules of living water from fruit, vegetables, and leafy greens as unique and scarce passersby in the bloodstream, grabbing on to them as if it's a child in an Easter egg hunt who's just found the eggs with the prizes inside.

Next, your liver stores these molecules of water for the droughts to come, this time like a child who stashes her or his Halloween candy and ekes it out for weeks. Your liver knows that it's the human condition that we don't often do a heck of a lot to hydrate the body properly. This goes back millennia—hydration isn't always an easy option. The resources aren't always there. And so, in the liver's wisdom, it compresses the precious bioactive water molecules, concentrating them. When you take in liquids from soda or coffee or black tea or other dehydrating sources, your liver releases some of the stored and highly concentrated bioactive water molecules so that they touch the inactive water's contaminated, over-filtered, or otherwise dead molecules, using the inactive molecules to expand the active, concentrated ones and pass along information, in the process transforming the inactive water into a vibrant, activated, living source. This transformed water can then do its good throughout your body, hydrating other organs such as your heart and brain as it travels through the rest of your bloodstream.

You've been relying on the camel effect for ages without knowing it. It's how you can go for so many years chronically dehydrated as so many people do. Once again, you have your liver to thank for your survival. What if the liver starts to falter? It does take a cleaner, better-working, more hydrated liver to maintain the ability to pass along concentrated bioactive water molecules to hydrate the blood. It needs to be a liver that's still upholding its ability to naturally detox and deal with the onslaught of typical troublemakers that are always visiting. If we're not looking out for ourselves, on the other hand, the miraculous camel effect chemical function slowly starts to disappear. If we've had a poor diet and poor hydration methods from a young age, it can disappear earlier in life. If we were lucky enough to be handed more fruits and vegetables and fewer dehydrating items when we were kids, the camel effect could last longer. Either way, at a certain point, when the liver gets sluggish, weakened, or otherwise compromised and pushed for too many years with too little hydration, its ability to adapt and protect us with this chemical function diminishes. The liver becomes so stagnant that poisons back up into the bloodstream and lymphatic system—and this, my friend, is an equation for what I call *dirty blood syndrome.*

Our blood is very complicated. So complicated that if we believe that we, as a society, know every mystery it contains, we're sadly mistaken. If we believe medical research and science have discovered all of the millions of chemical functions occurring within our blood, we're losing it. If we believe that the entire array of hormones that travel through our blood has been found, we're in great denial. And if we believe that the vast, universal circle of immune cells and beneficial microorganisms that are part of the inner workings of our blood has been found, discovered, and understood, then we're really just lost. Simply the truth that our blood is dirtied by scores of toxins would spin the heads of lab scientists—if only they knew what floats in our blood. It would take multiple blood panels to view just a fraction of what dirty blood has to offer science and research as a window into what causes human suffering. Our blood is a river you certainly wouldn't want to drink out of—unless you cleaned it up and made it truly safe.

When you're dehydrated, you have dirtier blood, bottom line. And you don't want dirty blood. Thick and filled with an abundance of toxins and other troublemakers, it leads to the symptoms and conditions described in this chapter, as well as to symptoms and conditions with dedicated chapters later in Parts II and III. It all depends on which type of dirty blood you have.

ENERGY ISSUES

We don't want to confuse energy issues with fatigue, whether chronic fatigue, adrenal fatigue, neurological fatigue, or even a case of mild fatigue, the unknown causes of which you can read about in my earlier books. The type of energy issue I'm talking about here is very common in people at the beginning stages of sluggish liver. These are people who used to have all the energy in the world and could go all day long. Then, as the liver started to become burdened and dehydrated, they began to experience mild dirty blood syndrome, and their energy started to flag. For those who were used to going at 100 miles per hour, with nothing stopping them from getting all of their tasks accomplished, this decrease in energy wouldn't be enough to stop them from going to the company baseball game or to send them to the doctor's office. It *would* be enough that they'd feel a lag at different points during the day, when they least expected it. It's one of the very first signs of a dysfunctional liver that's resulted in dirty blood pumping through the body. When the heart must pump harder to send blood through the body, it's a new experience that can feel draining.

Again, this isn't the fatigue of a highly active case of EBV causing ME/CFS, though it also doesn't mean someone *doesn't* have EBV hiding inside the liver, getting ready to make its move to the thyroid and create a case of Hashimoto's or a variety of mystery neurological symptoms. It's also not a metabolism problem. *Metabolism* is a term used all the time to cover up for what's not understood in the body, like undiscovered dirty blood syndrome. This energy issue is the type where someone's been skating by fairly well and is just starting to notice changes in stamina. In this case, changing the diet and cleaning up the liver and the blood can bring her or his energy back pretty darn quickly. Whatever diet you choose in this case, even if it's not the right type for someone with serious symptoms and conditions, the liver will give you a standing ovation of thanks for the improvement.

DARK UNDER-EYE CIRCLES

Dark circles under the eyes can start as early as childhood. A discerning parent will take a child to the doctor, asking what's causing them, and many pediatricians will say that it could be an allergy, perhaps an allergy to gluten. When adults notice their own dark under-eye circles, they'll also often ask why. Dark circles, they think, are normally reserved for mornings after late nights working or partying, hangovers, or maybe getting over the flu, so what's causing them if none of those are a factor? People will brush on concealer or visit a spa, throw some cucumbers on their eyes and wrap themselves in seaweed to address it—only it won't fix the problem.

It's ironic, because cucumbers and sea vegetables taken *internally* actually do contribute to healing. Sure, cucumber slices on the outside can get results for run-of-the-mill dark circles, like when someone is temporarily dehydrated from eating a toxic food or staying up too late on a stressful night or drinking too many martinis. Even sexual activity can bring on dark under-eye circles, and believe it or not, cucumbers applied on the eyes can actually bring some improvement. For the real, deep-seated reasons why people deal with chronic dark circles under the eyes, you need more than an external application of cucumber and seaweed—you need to drink cucumber juice for true hydration of the blood, lymph, and liver and start adding some Atlantic dulse to your diet to draw out toxic heavy metals and other poisons while providing yourself with critical, life-sustaining minerals.

Dark circles or even sunken eyes for weeks or months mean there's a hidden problem: a liver problem. It's true for children, too. Dark under-eye circles leading to a diagnosis of a gluten allergy or gut problem only edge toward what's really going on. In truth, this symptom has everything to do with a toxic, dehydrated liver creating toxic, dirty blood. Where the skin is thin under the eyes, it gets dark because the blood flowing through is lacking oxygen and filled with poisons, both from present-day exposure and from the troublemakers we inherit through our family lines.

As you'll read about in Chapter 28, "PANDAS, Jaundice, and Baby Liver," many children grow out of a sluggish liver. In that case, the dark circles disappear. Many people don't grow out of it, or they develop or redevelop a sluggish liver when they're older, at which point this symptom can affect adults. It's not a sign that your liver is failing you. It's a sign that your liver has struggled to stay in balance and protect the person it lives within, holding back as many toxins as it could, and at a certain point became so strained that it was forced to let some of them go.

If you're thinking, *Well, I don't have dark under-eye circles, so I must not have dirty blood syndrome*, not so fast. There are different levels and types of the toxins and other pesky presences that I call liver troublemakers. Some troublemakers can make dark circles appear; some can be released from the liver into the bloodstream without creating dark circles (and cause other problems instead). When the liver is sluggish, stagnant, troubled, and not performing to its full potential, it can release a whole cocktail of old and new troublemakers that can contribute to those smudges beneath the eyes. For example, pharmaceuticals are one of the troublemakers that can create dark circles. Even if you're not on them currently, medications you took years ago that your liver stored away at the time could be releasing into the bloodstream now. Toxic heavy metals can create a long-term shadow under the eye for children and adults, too, as can the family of various pesticides.

Gasoline and other petroleum exposure, solvents, and conventional household cleaners can bring that darkness or even an indentation beneath the eye.

So overall, dark under-eye circles mean we have some dirty blood on our hands. What determines how severe they are is hydration. Proper hydration on a daily basis can help clean up dirty blood and improve the liver just enough that the circles dissipate. Still, energy issues and under-eye circles aren't all that dirty blood can cause.

RAYNAUD'S SYNDROME

Raynaud's is a condition that many live with today. Its symptoms include discoloration of the skin, sometimes with tingles and numbness, most often in the extremities. It's a result of poisons from the liver backing up into the bloodstream—that is, dirty blood syndrome. Why doesn't everyone who's chronically dehydrated also have Raynaud's? Because the backlogged poisons in this case are a specific type of troublemaker: viral waste matter.

While other troublemakers such as mercury and additional toxic heavy metals can certainly contribute to the liver's struggle, as well as feed the virus so it can create more toxic waste, those presenting with Raynaud's do have a specific resident of the liver: the Epstein-Barr virus. Regardless of whether a physician has found and diagnosed EBV in a Raynaud's patient's blood work, the virus is in the body. While much of the EBV might have moved on to the thyroid or beyond, some of it has remained in the liver.

You can learn more about antiviral protocols as well as EBV's viral byproduct, viral corpses, neurotoxins, and dermatoxins in *Thyroid Healing*. When this waste matter, which contains traces of toxic heavy metals, escapes from the liver, it can hover and float close to the skin, changing the pigment in those areas and creating those dark splotches Raynaud's patients know too well. The thick, dirty blood and viral liver create the circulation issues of Raynaud's—when neurotoxins, dermatoxins, and other troublemakers back up from the liver into the bloodstream, they tend to gravitate to areas of lower circulation; that is, the fingers and toes. And the more poisons in the blood there, the less oxygen; hence the discoloration many experience. Tingles and numbness can come about from the rogue neurotoxins congregating in the blood.

If someone with Raynaud's is eating a diet that feeds the virus, the symptoms can become severe. While many Raynaud's patients hear that the phenomenon occurs as the result of an autoimmune disease that's causing the body to go haywire, they should hear the truth instead: it's a viral and liver problem creating a blood problem that can be cleaned up, not the body turning against itself, as the misguided autoimmune theory speculates.

GOUT

Dirty blood and gout go together like a scarecrow and a cornfield. A knife and a kitchen. A horse and a buggy. If you take away the scarecrow, you'll lose the corn quickly to the birds. Take the knife out of the kitchen and you'll be eating microwave dinners instead of preparing your own meals. Take the horse away from the buggy and you and your date will be stuck freezing in the middle of the street, your romantic jaunt through the cobblestone streets a no-go. What do I mean? Without dirty blood, you won't have gout.

Look at gout in its simplest terms, and it's a condition marked by swollen, painful joints, often in the feet and hands. With no antibodies showing up in blood tests to signal RA and no obvious signs of osteoarthritis, medical communities don't know where to go with the symptoms before them. Historically, gout has resulted in many different misdiagnoses. With the gout we identify today, many doctors say that crystals in the synovial fluid of the joints are causing the aggravation and inflammation. Some doctors see crystals as cause for an instant gout diagnosis. Others don't need to see crystals to decide by process of elimination that they're looking at a patient who has the condition.

What is gout, really? If everything were working right in the medical field, here's what you'd hear at the doctor's office: "Looks like you've got a liver condition. It appears that you have crystals in your joints formed from large accumulations of uric acid. Crystals tell us that the liver isn't filtering properly and the kidneys are paying the price. When the blood becomes thick and filled with an overflow of poisons from a dysfunctional liver for far too long, it carries a poisonous load—that is, it's dirty blood. As a result, waste can settle in different areas of your body. The joints are one such place, because as with Raynaud's syndrome, the joints in farther-reaching points of your body are naturally places of lower circulation. Your joint problem is really a liver problem."

So when someone gets a gout diagnosis, it should be a diagnosis of a liver condition. It's puzzling to think that crystals are viewed as the cause of gout when people exhibit the same gout symptoms without crystals present. That's because crystals aren't the cause of gout or the cause of gout's pain—you have to go deeper. While having an improperly working liver doesn't automatically translate to crystals, crystals do automatically translate to an improperly working liver. Crystals are just one component that happens to be found in a big batch of muck, and sometimes they're not there—though plenty of troublemakers still are. If researchers understood the sewage that can fill our blood and then looked for all the poisons that make it up, they'd be dismayed. Suddenly, they'd be saying, "Maybe it's not the crystals. Look at all this toxic sludge that we don't even look for in the lab: the oxidation from heavy metals, the petroleum from pharmaceuticals, the neurotoxins and other viral debris from a pathogen living inside the liver . . ." Understand that toxins and poisons have weight to them. When they flow to our extremities, they tend to sink and collect there because of their heavy nature. They don't make their way back in the bloodstream so easily, because a liver that's sluggish and dysfunctional results in blood "pull" back from the extremities that's weaker and slower than the blood "push" out to them from the heart.

If you don't have crystals in the joints, either urate ones or the calcium ones associated with pseudogout—and even if you do have crystals—here's what you're supposed to hear from your doctor: "This is viral inflammation of the joints. Viruses love to live inside our livers. They also produce a lot of toxic sludge, which gives the liver even more poisons to handle than it already has to in daily life. It means the liver can't hold on to as much as it would like, so many viruses find their way out of the liver, traveling to the joints and creating pain and inflammation. Even though antibodies aren't showing up in your blood work, what you're really experiencing is a form of RA, where the Epstein-Barr virus has been feeding in a liver filled with troublemakers until it finally escaped to your joints."

Many people who have been diagnosed with RA due to antibodies present in the blood also happen to have urate crystals; they're just ignored because of the antibodies. When they can't find an antibody, then they'll call the condition gout. It's a classic case of ignore-what-you-don't-see in medicine.

Another common symptom that accompanies gout causes confusion: swelling in the extremities. This is not only the joints themselves becoming inflamed; it's fluid retention around the hands, feet, knees, and even elbows. These areas can become painful, and it can occur with or without crystals present in the joints. After a doctor has tested a patient's heart and kidneys and found both to be functioning well enough, the swelling is considered mystery edema. What the patient should be getting is a diagnosis of poor lymphatic circulation due to a stagnant, dysfunctional, compromised liver, with lymphatic fluid retention putting pressure on the nerves in various areas of the body. Instead, if elevated enzymes don't show up on a liver test, then no alarm bells ring at the doctor's office. The liver condition stays completely under the radar, both for that doctor and for the broader reach of medical research and science.

You'll notice something else interesting about gout, which is that people with gout often have diabetes as well. No one knows why this correlation occurs. Well, the co-occurrence is not a coincidence. As you'll read about in Chapter 15, diabetes is more than a pancreas problem; the liver also plays a pertinent role. Medical communities, if they knew the truth about both gout and diabetes, would put two and two together, realizing that they're both liver problems and therefore interrelated. They'd have to figure out how viruses and toxins work, and how the blood becomes filled with these poisons; it would mean medicine would have to expand.

People with gout should refrain from eating heavy proteins and fats; the more protein and fat they eat, the more sluggish the liver gets and the worse their symptoms become. This has nothing to do with a food belief system; it's purely about what an individual with gout needs in order to heal. Reducing protein and fat in the diet gives gout (and pseudogout) sufferers relief, because it gives the liver a chance to recover and clean up the blood. If urate and calcium crystals were present, they'll reduce. Whether or not crystals were a problem, gout symptoms will fade. We must shift our thinking and see crystals only as one road sign that doctors happen to see out of many they can't. It's as though scientists are driving through a fog, and only one deer crossing sign is visible. If the fog lifted, they'd see all of the other road signs—slow, stop, speed limit, detour, one way, do not enter, dead end, merge, construction, blind curve, train crossing, evacuation route, and more—that would help them better navigate the way forward.

VARICOSE VEINS

When people have varicose veins or spider veins, you'll often hear them sarcastically thank their foremothers and forefathers. We remember relatives having these dark, visible blood vessels in the feet, ankles, legs (often in the calves), torso, or arms, and so we think of them as genetic.

That's not how it works. At the doctor's office or even the cosmetic surgeon's office, where people often go to get varicose veins removed, this is one more symptom that should instantly be diagnosed as a liver condition—and not a genetic one. It's only because liver troublemakers can be passed down from parent to child that you see this occurring across generations. Within the same family, you can have the same poisons residing in the liver and creating

dirty blood. As with the other symptoms and conditions in this chapter, you can have a compromised liver and dirty blood and not develop this issue. And as you'll read about in Chapter 36, "Liver Troublemakers," there are so many factors that can clog up a liver. It's the signature toxin cocktail you have that determines how it makes itself known.

What really happens when someone develops varicose or spider veins is that their blood has become chronically dehydrated and chronically thick over the years. You'll hear doctors and nurses report times they went to draw blood from a patient and it was so thick that when they removed the needle, the blood strung along with it like molasses or a length of yarn. That's the extreme of chronically thick blood. Even when this doesn't happen, it doesn't mean the blood's not thick.

Let's get something straight: We're not talking here, or anywhere in this chapter, about blood that's thick from an abundance of platelets. This isn't about whether the blood is thin or thick from platelets, whether platelets are causing extra clots, or whether a lack of platelets is causing wounds to bleed. We're not talking about platelet disorders. While they're serious and also deserve attention, they're a separate topic. Platelet issues mean there's a viral infection in the liver and spleen.

The thick blood we're talking about here is the type that's thick because it's become chronically dehydrated over the years at the same time the liver has filled with poisons that have backed up into the blood year after year. A higher-fat diet, where blood fats are always elevated in the bloodstream with no relief because someone eats three high-fat meals a day, often without realizing it, can also contribute to thick blood. This thick blood isn't easy on the vascular system, and so the body adjusts. It realizes that due to its viscosity, the blood is often moving more slowly than it should as it travels through arteries and veins and will eventually cause problems. Not that it's moving slowly all the time. There will be moments where our stress level reduces and we take better care of ourselves and get hydrated, whether we realize it or not. The blood will thin out for a time and flow smoothly. Then, when we get dehydrated again, more toxins will back up from the liver into the bloodstream and the blood will thicken again.

When the blood gets thick, our blood vessels tend to narrow slightly, because water is the natural expander of our veins. (One more reason to stay hydrated throughout life—it keeps veins from constricting.) Less water in the blood means the heart must work harder to bring up soupy, toxic, dehydrated blood from the lower extremities, and this increased suction pulls the walls of the veins inward, which makes the movement of blood slower. Slow-moving blood makes the heart work even harder, which in turn puts the brain on alert. To alleviate the heart's strain, the brain calls out for increased blood flow. In response, certain proteins, enzymes, and hormones that are undiscovered by medical research and science start cell production in order to broaden pathways for blood. This spurs the expansion of existing veins and the growth of new ones, in what's almost a mutation of your blood vessels. That's when you see those varicose and spider veins appear.

They're not a perfect solution, and ultimately, they don't solve the problem. What they do is serve as a warning flag for someone to change what she or he is doing and detox the liver in order to clean up the blood. When that happens, it can stop the growth of additional varicose and spider veins, and existing ones can even reduce over time.

INFLAMMATION

Inflammation can occur for two different reasons, and sometimes both at once. The first is injury. You fall on ice, you get hit playing sports, or some other accident occurs, and the body will react with inflammation. Invasion is the other reason the body can get inflamed, and in the case of chronic inflammation, the invader is a pathogen. No matter what else you're told out there, these are the two sole reasons for inflammation.

You'll frequently hear that chronic inflammation is the result of the body's immune system going after itself—that is, that it's an autoimmune response. That's because medical communities don't yet have the tools to detect just how often viruses such as EBV and HHV-6 and bacteria such as strep are present in the body. These invaders, which sometimes also cause injury by damaging tissue, are the real sources of your body's inflammatory responses. The body never attacks itself. Any antibodies present, even if they're labeled autoantibodies, are really there to attack a pathogen and attend to, repair, and heal tissue injured by that pathogen.

As you know well by now, the liver is a campground for various pathogens such as viruses and the poisonous materials that feed them. And of course, viruses will also release their own poisons such as neurotoxins, which go after the nerves and contribute to inflammation. The virus cells themselves, once escaped from the liver, can also attack different parts of the body. For example, as I detailed in *Thyroid Healing*, EBV will attack the thyroid, creating the thyroid inflammation known as Hashimoto's thyroiditis. Virus cells will also go after weak spots, which is how you can find yourself with an old injury that either won't heal or flares up for no apparent reason.

Say you bang your knee very hard, and it swells up—you'll grab a bag of ice to treat the inflammation. In the case of chronic inflammation, your body is also working on ways to bring it down over time. When you lend your hand to the effort by taking a natural approach and eating healthier foods and starting a supplement protocol, the body will respond in kind and you'll notice some results. Seeing inflammation come down as a result of natural foods and supplementation has been an epiphany for so many doctors in recent years. After witnessing some patients feel better with these changes, they'll write books, spreading the message like gospel. That's great. I commend them for taking initiative with new and back-to-basics approaches. What you need to know for your own health is that these celebrated approaches don't mean that the inflammation won't come back one day, nor do they mean that you'll get the best possible improvements. So far, these professionals' understanding of why a select group of their patients feels better only scratches the surface. It's the tip of the iceberg.

The real reason that people get relief in these cases is that picking healthier foods and supplementing with certain nutrients cleans up the liver and the blood. That gives less fuel to viruses and bacteria, and with pathogens faring less well, they can't cause as much inflammation. Pick any random diet that's even quasi-healthy and inflammation will reduce, because it keeps out some of pathogens' favorite fuels while also letting the liver unburden itself a bit so it can clean up the blood. The thicker and dirtier the blood, the better pathogens can fare and the more inflammation results; the cleaner the blood, the less inflammation you experience.

Going gluten-free is a popular part of many anti-inflammatory diets, following the belief that gluten is inherently inflammatory. The real

reason it helps is that taking out gluten starves any bacteria or viruses present—because gluten is one of their favorite foods. Medical communities are completely unaware of this, because they don't believe that pathogens "eat," yet they do. (You'll read more about pathogenic fuel in Chapter 36, "Liver Troublemakers.") For real relief that delves beneath the surface to the root of chronic inflammation, the Liver Rescue 3:6:9 in Chapter 38 and antiviral, antibacterial protocols in *Thyroid Healing* and *Medical Medium* are there for you.

INSOMNIA

There are many different causes of insomnia and troubled sleep, which is why I devoted five chapters to the secrets of sleep in my book *Thyroid Healing*. What's important for you to know here is that the majority of sleep disturbances and insomnia are from dirty blood syndrome. Even if your sleep issues have another cause, an unhappy, burdened, struggling, or weakened liver doesn't help.

A few different aspects of dirty blood syndrome affect sleep. For one, there are the poisons present in it. As the blood fills with runoff from toxic heavy metals oxidizing in your system, virus pollution (by which I mean its waste matter such as byproduct and neurotoxins), pesticides, and other chemicals from the troublemakers list, the brain gets saturated with it—and the brain is essential to a peaceful night's rest.

Then there's the liver itself. Like the fine-tuned machine that it is, when it's not firing on all cylinders or functioning at optimum level, it tends to shake, rumble, and roar. Or think of a horse you're riding that's agitated and angry, likely to spook. Either way, you won't get a smooth ride, and that includes in your sleeping hours: In the middle of every night, your liver wakes up, usually crankily, to start working for you, so that in the morning you can cleanse what it's collected through your urine or bowel movements. As your liver begins to fire up to perform this job, it can go into a subtle spasm because of all the toxic matter it has to deal with, both from within itself and from the dirty blood flowing back into it. That spasm can even squeeze some of the poisons it contains back into your blood in unpackaged form, making it dirtier. While it's not a spasm you can feel, the liver's bubble and squeak creates enough of a disturbance in the body that it can wake you up in the wee hours. Add in the brain disturbances from the toxic matter in the blood, some liver inflammation, some anxiety and hidden posttraumatic stress disorder (PTSD) from not sleeping well in the past, and maybe a partner snoring beside you or noises outside, and you'll get a good case of insomnia cooking. Tend to your liver, get hydrated, and take dirty blood syndrome out of the recipe and you'll have a fighting chance of sleep and a whole new relationship with going to bed.

A HEALING WELL

In some of the chapters to come, you'll read about other ways that dirty blood can affect your life. You'll see more about how with all they have coming at them, our livers are overflowing, and how in the process, they're losing their neutralization abilities.

In Ireland, there's a famous healing well. People have gone there for hundreds of years to get water—a highly active, living water in its most powerful form. It's extremely grounding water with a charge that neutralizes. If you were to dump trash into the well, the water is so potent that at first, the well would actually neutralize it. The more garbage and toxic chemicals you threw in, though, the more that neutralization ability would weaken—until it finally died. While there would still be water in the well, it would be dead in ways we couldn't even measure or decipher, because we couldn't measure or decipher its healing mystery in the first place.

That deadening is what we're trying to keep the river of your blood from doing, and that means supporting the healing, grounding, neutralizing wonders of your liver. Discovering how to save it from becoming poisoned means learning how to save yourself from dirty, polluted blood. It's one of your greatest lines of defense in life.

CHAPTER 11

Fatty Liver

As we go through life, we eat to survive. Challenging circumstances, which can range from traveling to having limited resources to living with excess stress and pressure to perform, can hold us back from eating the healthiest food. "I'll eat that doughnut," you may say, because you're on the run, trying to keep up with a demanding schedule and out of time to find another option. "I'll have that slice of pizza," you may decide, because it's easy; it's there in the moment. A bagel with cream cheese, a buttered croissant, ice cream as an after-dinner treat, chicken parmesan while out at a restaurant, a hot dog from a stand on the street, or barbecued ribs when your friend is paying. Buffalo chicken wings, shrimp fried rice, a piece of chocolate cake, maybe a fried egg or two, a slice of bacon: a little here, a little there, these are foods that get us by when life is harder and faster than we can keep up with.

Whether we know better or not, we eat like this to get by . . . and we eat like this for happiness. With all we're up against in today's world, it's impossible not to get wound up and emotional—so it's completely understandable that we choose the foods we do for comfort,

flavors that satisfy cravings, and even a sense of companionship.

Now, what if we're a little more conscious about food? What if we have a little less going on, a little more time to take care of ourselves? What if you're fortunate and have the resources to pursue other ways of eating? We may look to a trendy diet that seems incredibly healthy. We'll go less often for croissants and pizza and ice cream. We'll look for leaner cuts of meat and cut out grains and processed foods. Isn't this the answer? Not as much as we would think when it comes to avoiding fatty liver. Today's trendy diets are still not the choices your liver would make.

Our livers are focused on receiving a massive stream of blood, one that needs cleaning, processing, pampering, filtering, testing, measuring, weighing, decoding, and even interrogating so that the next 2,000 chemical functions that the liver performs can take place. And this is where your liver's most important concern comes into play: How thick is your blood? The thickness of your blood makes or breaks whether you develop a fatty (or pre-fatty) liver. What that thickness is harboring determines how fast you'll develop fatty liver.

LIVING AND BREATHING

Why is blood thickness the deal breaker? Why does it mean everything? Because the thicker the blood, the less oxygen can reside in it. The less oxygen in the blood that goes to the liver, the more trouble the liver has breathing. Yes, your liver breathes, and in order to respect that, we can picture the liver as a set of lungs, with the left lobe the left lung and the right lobe the right lung. Another way to envision the liver is as a sea urchin living in the depths of the ocean, extracting oxygen from the sea water. If the thickness of the blood holds a host of toxic particles, it will make the liver's breathing even harder. As a result, its life force will weaken. Think of yourself trying to breathe in an environment where the air is very dirty, smoky, or smoggy. Maybe as you walk down the street, someone in front of you is puffing on a cigarette, or maybe there's a forest fire near your home that's filling the air with ash—it will make it difficult to breathe. For people who are sensitive or asthmatic, air quality means everything. And a hot, humid day with an elevation of air pollution or a stuffy room at work with toxic scents in the air matters both to someone with sensitive lungs and to someone with no sensitivities. Now imagine your liver as your lungs and your blood crowded with pollutants—poor air quality is just like the strain that thick blood creates. When the blood has a high blood-fat ratio thickening it up, it's a concern.

High blood fat is not really on the radar of medical research and science—determining healthy ratios of blood fat is not a concern on anybody's agenda, whether researchers, doctors, dieticians, or nutritionists, and that's a serious oversight. There's no way to measure it accurately in today's world; you can't hop on a scale like you do to measure your weight or have your skin pinched with an instrument like you do to measure body-fat percentage. What I'm talking about is different from today's testing for triglycerides and cholesterol. You could go to your doctor's office for a full physical and have everything check out fine—the stress test, your weight, your heart rate and other vitals, the sound of your lungs, even a blood panel—all the while experiencing a high blood-fat ratio that never gets detected.

What physicians need at their disposal is a simple blood test that can be administered on the spot to determine blood-fat levels, like the kind used to measure blood-glucose levels in diabetics. It should be a routine part of any physical exam, so that a doctor can instantly say, "Whoa, what was your last meal? Your blood fat is off the charts. At this rate, you're going to develop fatty liver, gout, or heart disease in ten years, or even experience a heart attack."

Let's say it's Noah at the doctor for his physical. Ideally, the doctor would engage him in a dialogue: "So, Noah, what did you eat for dinner last night?"

"I ate out at a restaurant and ordered chicken with broccoli."

"What was yesterday's lunch?"

"A turkey club on gluten-free bread."

"And how about yesterday's breakfast?"

"I had two eggs with bacon and skipped the toast, because I decided to have a carb-free morning."

The doctor would lean forward. "Noah, that's great you skipped the toast. What we really need to be concerned with is how much fat is in your diet. A simple blood test is showing high fat in your bloodstream, and your recap of recent meals is indicating that it's consistently high. This will end up starving your liver of oxygen, setting the stage for illness and disease. You don't have to eat wheat, nor should you really, though you do need to consider bringing more fruit into your diet, along with other healthy carbohydrates and additional vegetables or leafy greens."

That's how the medical world should work on Planet Earth. Concern shouldn't always focus on sugar and carbs, to the point that vital foods such as fruit get eliminated from the diet. Sadly, blaming sugar as the cause of fatty liver is a huge mistake in the health industry right now. This mistake exists because sugar is never eaten on its own. It's always eaten with or very closely before or after fat, and nearly always an unhealthy fat at that, and that's what causes health issues. Fat's the problem. No one's sitting around eating gobs of standalone sugar. They're mixing it in coffee with cream. They're having it in cakes, cookies, and pastries. It's in the barbecue sauce that they use to coat their pulled pork. It's eaten as a treat such as a candy cane after a high-fat, festive meal. Not acknowledging that sugar is always consumed with fat is a prime example of both the conventional medical and alternative health industries operating with blinders on. They have tunnel vision that only allows sugar into view, and when a theory is seen from that limited perspective, it easily becomes law.

You can think of the roles of fat and sugar in fatty liver like this: Say you (sugar) were driving along with a friend (fat) when suddenly, she pulled in front of a bank, took out a gun, and ran inside. For a moment, you'd be paralyzed. Finally, you'd get your wits about you and hop in the driver's seat—just as your friend ran back out with a sack of cash and tossed it through an open window. When police arrived at the scene, they'd see you behind the wheel of the getaway car, and at the time of sentencing, you'd get blamed for the entire operation, as though your friend had never been there. You wouldn't want to be framed for a crime you neither masterminded nor committed any more than sugar should get the blame for causing fatty liver.

THICKER THAN WATER

Less oxygen makes such a big difference to the liver because the river of blood that enters the liver from the digestive system is already lower in oxygen to begin with. It's not possible to lock down a standard oxygen percentage of blood entering the liver, because it depends on what someone's eating, when they're eating, how long they've been on a certain diet, how many toxin obstacles they're up against, what time of day it is, and what day of the week. Any named standards are arbitrary.

Much of the rest of the blood entering through the hepatic portal vein is in need of filtering and processing, because it's full of toxins, pathogens, pharmaceuticals, minerals, vitamins, enzymes, amino acids, antioxidants, other phytochemicals and nutrients, fats, and more. For many people, the amount of toxins coming in is high, which makes the liver's job harder. Often, too, the ratio of nutrients is low, which is another strike against us. These two factors are manageable, however, if the blood is thin enough. Yet again, here's what pushes the liver over the edge: high blood fat.

Fat thickens the blood enough on its own, resulting in lower water content, at which point someone can become chronically dehydrated for many years. Imagine someone who barely drinks any water, aside from the water in a cup of coffee, a can of soda, an energy drink, wine, beer, or caffeinated tea. When someone's in this position of not drinking water or fresh juices, dehydration is even worse, which thickens the blood even more. This opens the door to strokes, heart attacks, kidney damage, high blood pressure, adrenal fatigue, and elevated cholesterol, as well as any central nervous system symptoms and conditions worsening along the way.

What does it mean for the central nervous system to worsen? Well, say you're dealing with ME/CFS, tingles and numbness, aches and pains, balance issues such as vertigo, restless leg syndrome, anxiety, or depression. These are all central nervous system–related symptoms, and they can worsen with lower oxygen levels and higher blood fat. What's even more important to understand is that every single autoimmune condition that someone may be labeled with can worsen with higher blood fat and lower oxygen levels. That's because the pathogens that are the real cause of autoimmune conditions, as well as the cause of many other diseases and health issues, can grow, proliferate, and expand with higher blood fat, causing the illnesses to worsen. Sure, you may experience symptom improvements on a high-fat, low-carb diet because you're subtracting gluten, dairy, and processed foods that feed pathogens. It's still not the answer to getting 100 percent better. Meanwhile, well-meaning doctors and other practitioners put autoimmune patients on a high-fat, low-carb diet in hopes that it will stop what they believe to be the body attacking itself, never realizing that the higher blood fat actually allows viruses and bacteria that are off their radar to prosper—meaning that someone's lupus, Hashimoto's, RA, and more worsen. In truth, most fatty livers have a pathogen living inside the liver, contributing to its sluggishness, and constant high blood fat does not help it. Blood fat cycling higher also diminishes oxygen levels even more, slowly aging and even killing the liver, which in turn quickly ages you.

As long as a seemingly new, trendy everyday diet consists of higher levels of fat as the main calorie source, it will burden the liver, possibly resulting in an undiagnosed pre-fatty or fatty liver condition—regardless of whether someone is exercising regularly and maintaining a healthy weight. Exercise and weight don't determine pre-fatty or fatty liver. Rather, it's about what the liver is up against in the river of blood running through it, and how hard your liver must work to protect your pancreas, heart, brain, and the rest of your body.

SACRIFICES FOR SURVIVAL

Our livers can sense what we eat. While you would think your stomach can, too, it can't. Your stomach doesn't have its own intelligence. It's just a pouch that gets its marching orders from your brain, which communicates through various nerves such as the vagus, as well as smaller nerves. Your stomach is an important tool, and it is well respected by your liver and pancreas— treated with more kindness by your liver than the kindness we pay our stomachs. Still, the stomach is not a very smart organ, nor is it supposed to be. If it were smart, it would punish us every time we ate foods we shouldn't eat. In a way, maybe that would be a good thing. It would warn us instantly with every unproductive food and reward us with every food that helps us. That wouldn't give us freedom, though, and the stomach's role is to grant us freedom. While the liver and pancreas can remain responsible, the stomach is supposed to give us leeway, because the world is so difficult. So many of us don't have many options in what we eat, whether because of an area of the country or world where we live or because of our resources. For that reason, the stomach doesn't punish us. It's there as a buffer to protect us, and the liver and pancreas care about it like a craftsman cares about her best set of tools in the workshop.

As fats enter the mouth, in whatever form of food or drink, the liver instantly starts to eject bile in order to be able to break down those fats as quickly as possible. For one, it wants to disperse the fats to make the passage of our blood easier for our vascular system. Secondly, it wants to thin out the blood before it gets to the liver. If the liver senses that the fat content of a meal is high, this bile production becomes extreme.

And if this happens often over time, the liver starts to weaken, unable to perform this job as well, and as a result, rogue, undispersed fats enter the liver continually. Because the liver will do anything to protect you and your pancreas, it starts taking on those fats. It's why the liver is the first part of the body to become fatty or heavy. Before a person develops any sort of weight problem that can be detected by outward looks or a number on the scale, that person's liver develops a "spare tire" or "muffin top."

The pancreas also suffers when the liver is in trouble like this. If your liver has any issues at all, you're going to be much more prone to pancreatitis as well as have a harder time recovering from it. Many people live with chronic pancreas problems, and I'm not just talking about diabetics. So many individuals live with chronic inflammatory pancreas issues that they may or may not even realize they have. For any pancreas issue whatsoever, the liver is really important to straightening it out so you can get better, heal, and regain full pancreas function.

Taking on fats due to a high blood-fat ratio for years, the liver weakens further, unable to disperse and eliminate fats as it should, and as that happens it becomes sluggish and starts to break down. Its ability to draw nutrients out of the blood becomes compromised, and many of these vital nutrients can end up trapped in the fat cells, inaccessible. Toxins, too, become harder for the liver to collect and process out, so many of them get lodged in the fat stored in and around the liver, along with those nutrients. The liver slowly becomes imprisoned by fat, developing into a pre-fatty and then a fatty liver. This fate can be avoided or reversed if we lower our fat intake, regardless of what dietary belief system we subscribe to, because lowering fat helps the liver get stronger and improve bile production. You get a second chance, with that better bile able to dissolve and break down fats to free you. Certain healing herbs and foods such as ginger can assist you with that. (More in Chapter 37.)

Otherwise, with the blood thick from high fat levels, bile production weakened, and fats in the blood unable to disperse, the intrusion of fat pouring through the hepatic portal vein especially (as well as from the hepatic artery, since the liver can't filter out all the excess fat that comes through the portal vein, so it comes back later) is equivalent to an avalanche in the Alps, with hundreds of skiers caught on the slopes—like the chemical functions that your liver performs being caught in the path of too much fat. As the snow cascades, some skiers will crawl out and ski away from danger while others will be helpless, frozen forever—which is to say that the liver will fight for some of its most important chemical functions to stay intact, propelling out whatever chemicals it can to save you. It's sort of like how if you were skiing with a child when the avalanche came, you'd do anything you could to push the child toward safety before you sacrificed yourself and got buried by snow. One of your liver's sacrifices can be weight gain.

CHAPTER 12

Weight Gain

If you were to ask a thousand health and fitness professionals why someone was overweight, the majority would answer "slow metabolism," with the close runners-up being "eats too much," "eats too many carbs," and "doesn't exercise enough." They're the answers you've heard before, whether from doctors, trainers, family, friends, headlines, or the nightly news. And yet, if you're the one struggling with your weight, you know that it's not a simple formula.

It's merely the stereotype that when people are overweight, it's because they love food, overindulging in fried items, sweets, and other treats while spending too much time on the couch. This isn't based on an accurate perception of what those who deal with mystery weight gain are really up against. It's often not a straightforward matter of expending more calories than you consume—you've likely tried tracking calories and found it both crazy-making and ineffectual. It's probably felt awful to think that you were born with an inadequate metabolism while your neighbor or coworker or best friend hit the jackpot. There's a tremendous amount of noncompassion and downright cruelty in how people view those who are overweight or obese, and in how they view themselves.

It's time for the world to understand what mystery weight gain really is, and the first step is understanding what it isn't: not about eating too many carbs or being lazy or lacking self-control; not caused by hypothyroidism or polycystic ovarian syndrome (PCOS) (though both of these conditions can be a sign of future weight problems); and not a result of a slow metabolism—because there's no such thing as a fast or slow metabolism.

This last one may come as a shock, since we're conditioned to believe in metabolism as a well-understood medical fact. We've grown up hearing the word used as though it's a rock-solid law of the universe, when the truth is that "metabolism" is nothing more than the antiquated discovery that the body is a living organism that assimilates food and uses it for energy. Telling people that a slow metabolism is the reason they have trouble losing or keeping off weight isn't a real answer; it usually leads to despair, making people feel like they were born with faulty bodies and they're stuck that way for life. The reality is that many of the mechanics of how the body gains and loses weight remain medical mysteries, and metabolism is merely a convenient label. There's so much more to know.

THE LIVER'S STARRING ROLE

What is weight gain really about? You won't be surprised by now to hear that most of the time—an overwhelming amount of the time—weight gain is really about the liver. While two other factors, the thyroid and the adrenals, can often be involved, it's important to remember that they both lead back to the liver. Let's look at how that works.

The Thyroid–Liver Link

It's trendy right now to blame weight gain on the thyroid. Yet as I revealed in detail in *Thyroid Healing*, a thyroid problem does not cause weight gain. There are thousands of people in the U.S. alone, never mind globally, who have a thyroid disorder and still maintain what we'd call an average weight. It's true that many others with thyroid disorders do gain weight, whether long before a diagnosis, at the time of diagnosis, or later on. That correlation should not be mistaken for causation. Whether someone has a hypothyroid or Hashimoto's thyroiditis, or even if the thyroid was killed off or removed, the gland is not to blame.

Health-care professionals started linking the thyroid with weight trouble because the thyroid is believed to be the body's metabolism regulator. Notice that word "believed"? Again, metabolism is only a theory that's been repeated so often it sounds like fact. How the thyroid truly works is also not fully understood by medical research and science. So you've got the metabolism myth to begin with, and then it's combined with the mysteries of the thyroid—that's not an equation that somehow leads to a conclusive answer. Two unknowns don't make a known.

Here's why you'll see a correlation between thyroid issues and weight gain: because thyroid issues are viral over 95 percent of the time, and chronic viral infection weakens and burdens the liver—in part because the virus that causes thyroid problems nests in the liver on its way to the thyroid. When the liver gets damaged by viral activity and overloaded with its waste matter, it can't filter as it's meant to, which leads to eventual weight gain (we'll examine how in more depth in a few pages). Body temperature fluctuations, brain fog, weight coming on in the middle of the body: while we're led to believe they're thyroid-caused, the truth is they have *liver* stamped all over them. If you've dealt with a thyroid condition and a weight problem side by side, it's because they're both symptoms of the same underlying viral issue. *It's not the thyroid itself causing weight gain.* (You'll find much more on this topic in *Thyroid Healing*.)

The Adrenal–Liver Link

The adrenal glands: they're getting a lot more attention than they did just a few years ago. In some ways, that's great. It means patients' struggles are being taken more seriously and medical communities are more driven than ever to acknowledge the interconnectedness of the human body. Compassionate practitioners should be applauded for searching far and wide for ideas that they think can help their patients.

Here's where we need to be careful: taking another part of the anatomy, the adrenals, that's not yet fully understood by medical research and science and using the leeway of that mystery to throw as much as possible under its umbrella. Fatigue? Difficulty focusing? Depression? Anxiety? Insomnia? Call it all adrenal, goes some current thinking. Because the adrenal glands are still being explored, it seems just as plausible as not to attribute a health issue to them. Weight gain is yet one more item being thrown under the umbrella of the adrenal label. Adrenal fatigue, elevated cortisol, high cholesterol, hormonal imbalance—they're all being blamed for slowing down someone's metabolism so that she or he holds on to a "spare tire" regardless of exercise. This theory is not accurate. This is another situation where there is a real correlation going on, only it's not the direct causation it appears to be. And again, it's certainly not a slowing down of the metabolism, since metabolism really doesn't explain weight gain or loss.

In truth, it's the level of excess adrenaline we're faced with that sets off a chain reaction that can lead to weight gain. That reaction begins with the stress and overstimulation of our nonstop lives. As you'll read more about in Chapter 19, "Adrenal Problems," your liver initiates a remarkable shielding process when your precious adrenal glands pump out high levels of adrenaline. In order to shield you from excess adrenaline's corrosive effects, the liver sponges up the adrenaline—and goes a step further by enlisting old, stored hormones as bait and trap to defuse the new ones. A bonded hormone compound results, and if the liver isn't in tiptop shape, it can't flush it all out. Instead, it must store it—and as you'll read about in the next section, when the liver has too much to store, the result is usually weight gain.

LIVER STORAGE: THE MISSING PIECE

What weight gain really comes down to is how fast or slowly your liver functions. That's not to say that this is blaming your body for being "faulty." It's not about genetically inheriting a liver that's either lazy or more vigorous. It's

about what we've come back to over and over in this book: what your liver is up against.

When someone can eat all the cookies he wants and not gain an ounce, it's not because he has a fast metabolism. It's because he has a liver that hasn't yet hit its fat-storing or poison-storing limitation and therefore functions at a faster pace. That doesn't mean his liver isn't overburdened or overstressed. You could be thin and still have a liver illness developing or a liver complication that's causing symptoms such as high blood pressure, acne, or jaundice. Weight is about the troublemaker storage department of the liver—for the person who can eat what she wants and not gain weight, it hasn't been compromised yet.

Compromised fat storage doesn't automatically mean that diet is the issue. While for a given person, eating a lot of high-fat foods can certainly be a factor, there are several others that should be considered, too. Anything that overburdens the liver can be a factor. This includes toxic heavy metals, DDT and other pesticides, herbicides, fungicides, solvents, plastics, industrial chemicals, and other toxins—if any of these have built up in the liver, they're taking up valuable storage space, which can become a problem if they build up to a certain point. (See Chapter 36 for a list of liver troublemakers.)

There's also viral and bacterial damage. One virus that should be infamous for disrupting the liver's functioning is Epstein-Barr, the virus that causes thyroid issues, fibromyalgia, RA, lupus, Lyme disease, ME/CFS, sarcoidosis, cystic fibrosis, Ehlers-Danlos syndrome, and much more. EBV has a nesting period in the liver, during which time it can drill into the tissue and scar it, making it sluggish and damaging some of its storage capabilities. EBV also throws off poisons, excreting waste in the form of byproduct, neurotoxins, dermatoxins, and viral corpses that give it more to process out and, when the liver is too overloaded for that processing, more debris to store within itself to protect you.

Another factor is the excess adrenaline and cortisol situation we'll look at in Chapter 19, "Adrenal Problems." After the liver has swooped in and saved the day with the old hormones that bond with and neutralize the new ones—a process still undiscovered—so much of the bonded hormone compound can accumulate in the liver that the organ runs out of space in its usual storage banks.

Finally, there's the damage that unchecked adrenaline can cause to the liver. Sometimes, in times of prolonged or high stress, or when the adrenals are overcompensating for something wrong elsewhere, such as low thyroid hormones, the adrenals can flood the body with so much adrenaline that it can't all be neutralized. This excess, active adrenaline is harsh on the liver—it can actually have an almost pickling effect, especially if someone is also eating a lot of salt, consuming plenty of vinegar such as from salad dressing, and drinking a little alcohol, perhaps a glass of wine at night. Being compromised with adrenaline slows down our livers and gives them yet more to try to store.

Ideally, the liver would be in robust enough shape to process fats, toxins, and hormones with ease, neutralizing and getting rid of the toxins altogether while only holding on to high-quality fats and hormones that could be useful to your body later. The reality is that for most people, the liver simply has too much to do. As a river of blood rushes into the liver, its assembly line of liver lobule workers scramble to process and package all the good, bad, and ugly. If there's too much bad and ugly, those workers get too tired and overwhelmed to deal with everything coming at them, and the liver's next-best option for shielding you is to store the excess. Trying to find space for all of it, though—at the same time the liver is moving at only a sluggish pace—becomes a challenge.

Oftentimes the liver will need to stash excess fat cells, hormones and hormone compounds, poisons, and toxic waste matter in the same compartments—wherever there's room, even within the storage bins meant for nutrients, if necessary. Storing goodness and garbage together like this is not the liver's normal course of business. It's what it's forced to do in dire straits in order to adapt and protect you: to prevent fat from getting through and gathering in your arteries and your heart, to prevent cholesterol from building, to prevent insulin resistance that can lead to diabetes from occurring, and so much more. Pushed to its limits, the liver grows weaker and more sluggish over time. Its protective processes break down.

GAINING WEIGHT WITH AGE

What happens in the liver that allows for weight gain as we age? So many people go through so much of their lives eating what they like, whatever that may be, following a philosophy of moderation, breaking that philosophy over and over again, and still maintaining a normal, healthy weight. Then, eventually, the inevitable happens for all except a rare few: a thickening waistline, more pounds on the scale, and the sinking feeling that their bodies have let them down.

For many, liver problems will build quietly in the background for decades before the liver gets to such a sluggish point that its fat storage capability becomes dysfunctional. It's why people will say that they maintained a steady weight for 10, 20, 30, 40, or 50 years and then suddenly started gaining weight for no apparent reason.

Often, trainers will insist that it's because the metabolism started slowing with age, and that the answer is to eat a better diet and exercise more to increase the metabolism. Yes, people can often get results from diet and exercise. It's important for you to know that it's not because these factors raise the metabolism. Rather, eating more unprocessed foods and moving the body both help clean the liver, detoxing it and bringing it more oxygen. Parts of the liver get rejuvenated from exercising and eating better, and that's what helps these people drop pounds. It's not the metabolism being "fixed" from diet and exercise; again, it has nothing to do with metabolism.

With the person whose outward appearances are fine, the liver can be on the edge of sluggishness as fat deposits start to accumulate in it, taking shape and form. Eventually, people often get to that point where there's a sudden shift, weight starts to come on even though they're not doing anything differently, and we have the beginning of someone telling them, "You have a slow metabolism." This is the point that over 50 percent of those who struggle with their weight have reached: when exercising vigorously and watching what they eat doesn't stop the number on the scale from going up.

In these cases of mystery weight problems, the liver has become so sluggish that it needs extra special healing support. Excess fat cells, pathogenic waste, excess adrenaline, and/or toxins have oversaturated the liver. When it's in this state, the liver can't process fat as well as it's meant to, so fat cells begin to collect in it at a more rapid rate. The liver becomes so congested internally that fat builds around the outside of it, with pre-fatty and then fatty liver developing. Fat cells then begin to accumulate in the intestinal tract, and eventually, the heart

and arteries get saturated. A raised A1C level can occur, along with a diagnosis of prediabetes. Weight around the waist begins to cling.

That's the fat cell side of weight gain. If everyone walked around with their livers in their hands, we'd see just how many people suffer from pre-fatty or fatty livers. Instead, we judge based on outward appearance, and that means that thinner people often feel justified calling someone "fat," with no idea that if we went by inward appearance, their livers would get the "fat" label, too—they're just not exhibiting its effects on the outside yet.

When someone is called "fat" because they're heavy on the outside, or when they think of themselves as fat, most of the time, fat is only part of what's making them heavier than they'd like to be. There's another side of weight gain, particularly mystery weight gain, and that's fluid retention. If you're carrying around 60 extra pounds of weight despite your best efforts, there's a good chance that only 40 pounds of it is body fat and the other 20 pounds is fluid that your body's holding. This undiagnosed lymphedema is a result of your lymphatic system being forced to act as the filter your liver's meant to be. The liver is intended to be the filter for macro waste matter, while the lymphatic system is supposed to process out the micro. When the liver gets strained, though, more waste slips by it. The resulting sludge that's passed off to the lymphatic system is thicker than what it's meant to handle, so lymphatic vessels and lymph ducts get clogged. Lymph fluid can't flow as it normally would, resulting in the lymphatic system trying to push lymph around the blockages. Pockets of lymph fluid start to collect, which translates to fluid retention. Simply knowing this is one of the keys to moving forward.

MYSTERY SOLVED

What about the 80- or 90-year-olds who are still thin for no obvious reason? What's the difference for those rare few? Rumor has it that it's because they have good genes or robust metabolisms—and rumor has it wrong. When someone is able to keep her or his weight down naturally for an entire lifetime, it's because the liver never got pushed over the edge. That person's liver never got maxed out with poisons, viruses, toxic heavy metals, pathogens of various strains and mutations, plastics, drugs, pesticides, herbicides, fungicides, solvents and other toxic chemicals, dioxins, and extra volumes of fat. That person's bile production stayed strong, with active, vital bile salts teeming with enzymatic life. Whatever fats and unauthorized pathogens and poisons the liver had to deal with over time weren't enough to tip the scale.

Take a look at a family with a few generations who've struggled with their weight and then a family that's stayed thin through generations, and yes, it can seem like genes are the explanation. It can seem like that second family won the genetic lottery! While genes play many important roles in our lives, though, they aren't the answer here. Truth is, a different key inheritance is in play: toxins in the liver. For those who never struggle with their weight, the poisons they inherited through their bloodline were at lower levels than for the rest of us. Maybe a grandmother didn't subscribe to using DDT like the other 99 percent of people on the block. Maybe a father didn't work in a factory. Livers in the family were less saturated, and as a result, offspring came into the world less burdened and less likely to deal with weight gain. It never had to do with genes. (For much more on the gene blame game and the metabolism myth, see *Thyroid Healing*.)

There are plenty of cases of siblings, those with the most similar DNA in a family, with drastically different weight experiences to demonstrate that weight is not all about genes. One sibling's liver could be extremely high in toxic heavy metals and carrying a higher family load, while the other's viral load is dormant and doesn't hold as many toxic heavy metals, translating to weight gain for one and not the other. We can't forget that everybody is different.

Weight gain should never come with a sense of doom and destiny attached, nor should it come with judgment. The focus on starving yourself, working out like crazy, or cursing your family line—these are all part of the past for you now. Connecting to the truth that much extra weight is actually extra fluid can be incredibly freeing. It means that weight loss is not a grueling matter of burning calories. It's about releasing the dam so the weight can flow away. Let's also remember that those extra fat cells someone's carrying around usually aren't the result of a fast food, couch potato lifestyle. It could be that someone exercises every day and eats measured portions of only the foods said to be healthiest, and yet body fat accumulates, because EBV or any number of other liver troublemakers have hampered her or his liver.

The next time you notice someone who's overweight or look at yourself in the mirror with disappointment, see what it's like to erase the stigma and pay true witness. Don't immediately think of the treadmill; exercise your compassion instead. Remind yourself that extra weight is no one's fault, and weight is not fate. There's a path forward, and it comes from knowing the truth: that healing the liver—and addressing the factors that burden it in the first place, such as a viral load, adrenal strain, and toxic exposure—are the true keys to weight loss.

CHAPTER 13

Mystery Hunger

Like weight gain, mystery hunger is one of those health issues that is often treated unkindly. If you're dealing with nagging hunger that no amount of food can fill, rest assured that no matter how others treat you or what you may think of yourself, there's nothing wrong with who you are as a person. It's not gluttony. It's not a character flaw or a moral failing. It's not your fault. There's a very real explanation for why mystery hunger can plague somebody.

Compassionate practitioners who have taken up the cause of constant, unusual, and problematic hunger have brought different theories to the table. One is that it's a psychological overeating disorder. Another theory is that their hunger "shutoff switch" is malfunctioning due to a brain or stomach disorder or condition. A third theory is that excess hunger is hormonal; when a woman is pregnant, ovulating, premenstrual, menstruating, menopausal, or coming off menopause and she feels famished or an impulse to binge-eat, it will often be blamed on hormones. Lately another theory that's gotten a lot of attention is hyperthyroidism; many people are told that an overactive thyroid is causing them to have a heightened metabolic rate, which means they burn calories faster than normal, which in turn makes them hungrier than normal. There's also the theory that the extra weight someone's carrying around is the very source of their mystery hunger, which is so disheartening. Boredom is put out there as a theory. So are SAD, depression, and diabetes—which no one realizes are related to the liver. And finally, we have the theory that the discomfort that acid reflux causes can prompt someone to want to eat all the time.

Make no mistake: these remain theories—unproven possibilities floated out into the world in the hopes of offering patients the feeling of having an answer, even though they aren't truly answers. Of all of the theories above, the oldest one in the book is that it's psychological and "all in your head." It's also one of the most painful diagnoses to receive; it can make you feel like you're at odds with your own mind. Food isn't one of those elements we can remove from our lives entirely, so the challenge of simply eating less and ignoring the persistent tug in the gut asking for more can feel insurmountable. Now, let's not discount eating disorders. It's true that some of us overeat to soothe difficult emotions, and that food and trauma and addiction can get wrapped up in one another. This isn't the whole picture, though. It leaves out a critical physiological need that plays a big role in triggering the impulse to overeat in the first place. It's the same physiological need that causes mystery hunger when food addiction isn't involved: a starving liver.

CRITICAL CLEAN CARBOHYDRATES

How can a liver be starving if someone's eating all the time? Because a starving liver is not a liver that's hungry for fat calories. It's a liver that's run out of glucose and glycogen reserves, so it's crying out for replenishment in the form of *critical clean carbohydrates*. You can remember that as CCC, or the three Cs, as an easy way to connect with what your body wants.

Think of a woman who's pregnant and always ready for her next meal. Her hunger will often get a hormonal label or—and this is at least better than hormone blame—people will explain her hunger as the need to eat for two. The truth is that overwhelming hunger during pregnancy is because a pregnant woman's liver needs an abundance of natural sugars to build up more glucose and glycogen stores in order to protect and feed her baby's liver while it's in the process of developing. A baby's liver depends greatly on her or his mother's liver condition, and the mother's liver plays a critical role in delivering carefully prepared, highly absorbable nutrients to her baby's liver, which will then identify and absorb the nutrients, taking them in for liver cell growth. (For more on babies' and children's livers, see Chapter 28.) It's the liver's cry for glucose to feed her baby that drives that woman to bring snacks wherever she goes.

It's not only pregnant women who need natural sugar to feed their livers; we all need CCC. So many people are dealing with low glucose and glycogen reserves, causing our livers and even our nervous systems to go hungry and pass along that hunger to us. When our reserves are low, our heart, kidneys, reproductive system, and spleen are hindered, too, though it's the liver and nervous system that hold the hunger—mostly the liver. (As far as the nervous system goes, in times of crisis, your brain needs glucose, so it calls out for the liver to release glucose to help protect and soothe it.)

LIVER STRESSORS

How do we run out of the liver's glucose and its stored version, glycogen, in the first place? An overabundance of stress to the liver. One frequent stressor is pathogenic activity—that is, a virus and/or bacteria in the liver feeding on its storage of poisons such as toxic heavy metals, byproduct and sludge from other pathogens, plastics, and petroleum from drugs. As the virus feeds, it leaves behind waste products, creating an even larger landfill deep within the liver, which gives the liver a greater struggle to fuel itself with what it needs to function: glucose.

The Epstein-Barr virus is one very common pathogen that takes up residence in the liver, and it also happens to cause hyperthyroidism—which explains why hyperthyroidism and hunger often go hand in hand. It's not a metabolism issue that causes that all-the-time hunger associated with hyperthyroidism; it's the liver's glucose deficiency from battling EBV. Many people with hypothyroidism struggle with mystery hunger, too, due to the same viral cause.

(It's worth noting that the weight loss that can go along with hyperthyroidism isn't from an overproduction of thyroid hormones affecting metabolic rate, which is the current medical theory. Weight loss really occurs because certain varieties of EBV that cause hyperthyroidism release poisons that are allergenic to the body, prompting a constant flow of adrenaline that acts like an amphetamine and causes some people's bodies to shed pounds. More people with a hyperthyroid actually struggle with weight gain than loss, a fact that confuses medical communities. And almost everyone who starts off underweight with either a diagnosis of an accelerated metabolism on its own or a diagnosis of hyperthyroidism with accelerated metabolism ends up gaining weight later in life. Someone may remain thin for 10, 20, 30, or more years, and then finally around age 50, the burden that the liver was carrying for all those years catches up with it. Someone will be told, "Your metabolism slowed down with age," when the reality is that the liver became clogged—and can get unclogged if you learn to work with it.)

When someone experiences mystery hunger and is also overweight, it's often a sign that the liver is in a pre-fatty or fatty state. In this case, the extra fat cells accumulated in and around the organ create the liver stress, hindering its capacity for glucose storage. For a refresher on pre-fatty and fatty liver, revisit Chapter 11.

If someone is underweight or at a normal weight and constantly hungry, there's a good chance that excess adrenaline is contributing to it. Rushes of adrenaline, whether from demanding schedules, emotional challenges, or going hours without eating, saturate the liver and hinder its ability to build up glucose reserves, essentially starving the liver lobules that are working hard and in need of fuel. That last one, skipping meals, is especially important, because it's the most within our control. Going for half the day without eating is not a way to prove your worth and conquer hunger; it's a way to make yourself hungrier in both the moment and the long term. When you don't eat often enough, your blood sugar drops, and without glucose reserves your adrenals pump out excess adrenaline to compensate. Your liver is forced to soak up the excess adrenaline, and by the time you finally eat, your liver is too saturated to hold on to the glucose it needs. Even if you fill your belly, you may never feel full, or if you do in the moment, the hunger is going to nag again soon. This is also the explanation for why adrenaline rushes of other kinds can contribute to mystery hunger. You may be eating regularly, and yet if you're constantly experiencing fight-or-flight, adrenaline is filling the liver, and the organ's not getting a chance to refuel with glucose from your meals.

It's common that people going through an emotional crisis like the loss of a loved one or a breakup will stop eating and find food is the last thing on their minds as adrenaline consumes them in their pain, sorrow, and suffering. I've seen this happen many times over the decades, and you probably have, too. It's heartbreaking. As time passes and life moves forward, the situation will often flip, and an insatiable hunger will take over for a period of time, because the liver is begging for food after being nearly starved.

Someone can experience all three liver stressors that contribute to mystery hunger at once: pathogenic activity, a pre-fatty or fatty liver, and excess adrenaline. In that case, the liver is even more sorely in need of glucose reserves. So those are some initial steps to address mystery hunger: lowering a viral or bacterial load, caring for the adrenals (see the previous books in the Medical Medium series for more on both of these), and helping the liver shed excess fat (see Chapter 38, "Liver Rescue 3:6:9" and Chapter 40, "Liver Rescue Meditations"), whether you think you have a weight issue or not. Then there's the critical piece of giving our livers the glucose they need.

GLUCOSE OBSTACLES

We're fooled into thinking that we get more glucose into our bodies than we do. After all, aren't we constantly hearing that in today's society, we eat too much sugar and too many carbs? A slice of apple pie, honey-roasted peanuts, a BLT made with juicy, ripe tomato and whole-grain bread—aren't we constantly giving our liver sources of its precious simple sugar, glucose? The truth is that the sugars we eat can only help us if they're uninhibited; for our livers to benefit, the glucose we ingest needs to be free of tagalong fats that hinder its absorption. When we eat radical fat with sugar, then as hungry as the liver is, it can't replenish its glucose reserves because the fat disengages the liver's ability to separate the sugar.

Pork ribs smothered with marmalade barbecue sauce is a prime example of a food combination that helps explain a starving liver. As much sugar as there is in that sauce, none of it is going to help out your liver, not even the high-quality glucose coming from the oranges in the marmalade, because the pork fat blocks its absorption. Your liver's responsibility to protect your pancreas (and brain and heart) takes priority, and your liver's work goes instead into breaking down the radical fat and even taking some of it on if needed to lower your blood-fat levels. The same goes for a ham and cheese sandwich: because of the fat levels in the ham and the cheese, the lactose (milk sugar partially composed of glucose) concentrated in the cheese isn't accessible to refill the liver's glucose and glycogen reserves. The bread carbohydrates' glucose building blocks can't benefit the liver either because of what's in between those slices of bread. With apple pie, depending on the recipe, it's the butter or lard or shortening or egg in the crust that blocks the apples' precious sugars from replenishing the liver. With honey-roasted peanuts, it's the high fat content of the peanuts and the oil used to roast them that stop the vital sugars of the honey from refilling the liver's glucose reserves. With the BLT, it's the fat in the mayonnaise and the bacon that interferes with the precious sugars in the tomato. These are missed opportunities for the liver to get a boost from the sources of glucose in our snacks and meals. If it's here or there or only happening for a short time, it's no big deal. If it's year after year and decade after decade, it becomes a very big deal. The cunningness and edge that the liver needs to sort, separate, organize, and catalogue all of the elements it needs for your survival get interrupted by the repeated fat-sugar combination.

It's not solely eating fat and sugar at the same time that can be an issue. Eating fats continually throughout the day can also get in the way of glucose absorption, because many fats stay in the bloodstream for a while. Even if you have, say, a chicken Caesar salad at noon and then wait until two o'clock to eat an apple, the salad's leftover fats will still be in your bloodstream, and the apple's natural sugars aren't going to be able to offer your liver as much help as if you ate it with no radical fats in the bloodstream. Typically, the fat from pork products takes about 12 to 16 hours to disperse after eating, other animal products' fats take 3 to 6 hours, and plant fats take 1 to 3 hours. This is the unknown reason—unknown even to the experts who design diets—why high-fat, high-protein diets are starting to incorporate more plant fats. What doctors observe is that patients experience better health results when some of their protein sources come from avocados, nuts, seeds, and coconut. They don't realize it's because these plant fats disperse after an hour or three, allowing more vital sugars, like from a mid-afternoon apple, to get to the liver. (Apples, by the way, are vital members of the CCC family and some of your best allies. They have thousands of years of built-in information coded within them, so they rise above nearly anything else you're eating to do at least part of their job.)

Alcohol is the ultimate glucose fake-out. Once your liver gets a taste of alcohol, it fights desperately to use the alcohol's sugars to fill its glucose and glycogen reserves. At the same time, your liver must absorb the alcohol to protect you, which fights the liver's ability both to extract the sugar and to function. Remember those liver lobule elves from Part I? The size of a large grain of sand, these elves have no tolerance for alcohol; the adulterated, methylated, homeopathic sugar of alcohol intoxicates them in an instant. Still, the sugar is a lure. Like a mirage on the horizon promising replenishment, every sip of alcohol dangles potent sugar in front of the elves, and so they keep crying out for more even though they won't really be able to use it.

Knowing this can help decode alcohol cravings. The person who avoids eating carbs yet relies on nightly wine is drawn to that wine because it's the liver's shot at grabbing glucose. Since the alcohol prevents the liver from absorbing the sugar, the glucose reserves never actually get refilled, and so the liver sends that craving again the next day. Alcohol addiction is often only partially addiction to the alcohol itself; it can also be a very real sign of a liver starving for glucose.

ANSWERING THE CALL

Aside from taking care of underlying liver issues, the best approach to saying good-bye to constant hunger is to feed your liver—and yourself. Eat often (every one and a half to two hours) and eat well, with the goal of replenishing your glucose and glycogen reserves. Be mindful that alcohol won't count as glucose replenishment. Use the fat-digestion timetable above to plan some hours in the day when fat won't hinder glucose absorption, and during that period, pick some foods from Chapter 37 or snacks from Chapter 39 to give your liver exactly what it's craving. Holding off on fats until later in the day, as in the Liver Rescue Morning in Chapter 38, is one technique that can be a big help.

And remember: Your hunger is nothing to conquer. It's not a shortcoming. It's a call for help from your liver—and now you know exactly how to answer that call and feel satisfied again.

CHAPTER 14

Aging

Fear of aging—and what aging can do to the body—drives so much in our society. Anti-aging trends abound: skin lotions and potions and creams, tonics, exercise programs, supplements, injections, and cosmetic surgery. Diet programs and superfoods get labeled "age-reversing," whether they really help protect you or not. Hormone replacement is heralded as a fountain of youth (even though, as I revealed in *Medical Medium*, it only ages you faster). Even strategies to think and act more youthful catch our attention. We're constantly trying to beat the clock and look younger, feel younger—to stop Father Time.

There's nothing new about a desire to avoid the pitfalls of aging. There's nothing wrong with it, either. Of course we're just like the generations before us, going back to long, long ago—of course we want to hold on to our health and hold on to our very selves as we get older. The answer is in not getting distracted by the false promises of every anti-aging craze. The answer is in knowing what really ages us.

So what does determine the aging process of our bodies? We know that each time the planet revolves around the sun, we get a year older. We think genes can play a role. We believe stress can age us rapidly. There are many truths and many theories, because many factors do play a role in how fast we age. Still, even with all the different experiences and exposures we go through, there's one foundational factor that plays the largest role—it's the one that can either age us more quickly or slow down our aging. It's the source that holds the secrets, the old secrets we believe exist in the cosmos or hidden somewhere on earth and yet are really hidden with *us*.

Humankind's magic time machine to yesteryear? It's not some fanciful invention of the future. The fountain of youth? It's not a made-up piece of history. Time machine, fountain of youth, whichever you prefer to call it, we each have one already; it's an ancient part of who we are. More real than you can know, it's been sitting patiently within you since before you were born, ready for action. It's a wellspring of renewed life, a holy place of rejuvenation. It holds the answers, the power, the truth; it holds youth. It's the origin of longevity and the age reversal process. Your liver: it's everything when it comes to preserving yourself.

Handled wrong, it can backfire. Handled with ignorance, handled with unknowing and recklessness, it can be forced into survival mode. It won't cheat you. It won't stab you in the back. It won't forsake you. It won't tear your heart out and stomp on it. It won't *purposely* age you or make you look older. It won't turn away because it's weak and has no loyalty. The liver will only turn away to take what's left of itself after long-term sluggishness or even abuse and, in desperation, direct its resources to protecting other aspects of your physical self and keeping you alive. Skin becoming saggy or discolored and losing its elasticity is a common complaint, and like other symptoms of early aging, it's a sign of a liver slowly losing its various chemical functions. Aging faster and looking weathered happen for a very good reason—to save you from a much worse fate. Your liver, if it gets to this point of realizing with its highly intelligent chemical function database that it's not being given what it needs to keep itself healthy and keep you young, will put its last reserves into protecting your brain, heart, and pancreas with all its might.

How we care for our livers determines our health, aging process, and much of our well-being mentally, physically, and even emotionally as we get older. People care for their health with many different methods, though they often don't think of them as liver-specific. They go to the spa to get a massage and a full-body seaweed wrap; they go on dietary cleanses and take vitamins and other supplements; they visit their doctor for checkups—some of this just happening to care for the liver in bits and pieces along the way. These little snippets of accidental, indirect attention do help our livers hold on to some health value, some health stock, as we get older. Yet it's a crapshoot, a tease, as if someone dangled a carrot in front of

your liver, and only once in a great while did it get to catch that carrot and grab just a little bit of beta-carotene for survival. Brief respites are like telling the organ: "Now you have it, now you don't"; "Here you go. Now I'll take that back"; "This could be yours, but nope, only a little"; "Is this what you need? Oops, sorry, you didn't get it fast enough"; "Would this really help you? No way, not today. Sorry." And the game goes on.

THE FIGHT TO KEEP YOU YOUNG

Did you ever have that teenage experience of being handed the keys to your first car, backing out of the driveway with the windows rolled down, and feeling unstoppable as you took to the road? When we give our livers unintentional, minimal favors, though they leave it wanting more, they are still blessings. They're fleeting moments of freedom and rejuvenation that give us the keys to the youth car. Fleeting they are, though. Without liver awareness, we're that invincible young teen who seems to know it all—until a fender bender puts an end to the joyride. With any luck, that's where it stops: with a small accident, a small burden or impediment to the liver, a wake-up call to the owner that this vehicle needs better looking after. Otherwise, left neglected and uncared for long term, left to get dirty and rusted and broken, that car isn't a youth car at all anymore; it's a banged-up jalopy limping along on the road and spewing exhaust.

If we don't want to age before our time, we don't want the liver taking all the hits. We don't want it to get so bruised by life that it can't carry us on all the adventures we picture for ourselves. We want it to get more than a hint of liberation that's soon followed by a crash; we want to eliminate the crashes altogether and make freedom the default. Because that—caring for the liver, rather than accidentally toying with it—is the true secret of looking and staying young.

Once tapped into, our livers hold special chemical functions for keeping us young. Some of these functions, of course, exist around the ability to detoxify. Getting rid of junk is crucial to keeping your liver fit for duty. The most profound anti-aging function is your liver's ability to take an antioxidant it either has stored or is using fresh from the most important source that exists, fruit; bond it with amino acids it's been storing; and then send these new, improved phytochemical compounds into your sea of blood on a targeted mission: to stop healthy cells from dying. This isn't the same as when antioxidants directly from foods offer benefits such as preventing oxidation by cleaning free radicals from the body. Those antioxidants are indeed critical for anti-aging; from their food sources, they're instilled with a broad mission of repairing, supporting, and correcting tissue throughout the organs and body. Antioxidants that have been upgraded by the liver take it to the next level. When the liver alters certain antioxidants, it coats them and codes them with special information, infusing them with a recipe of knowledge that goes beyond tissue support; it stops cell death. This antioxidant upgrade process stops us from dying. It's true armor, not the illusion of protection and strength that radical fats give us.

When we're hurting the liver, on the other hand, it's dying slowly over time from the battles and wars, from lifestyle exposures, and from elements in our environment over which we have no control. The liver ages before the rest of you out of protection, so you don't have to struggle as early as it does. Along the way, it fights to keep you young. Then at a certain point, if you don't know how to support it, its profound chemical function of delivering

upgraded, amino acid–enhanced antioxidants gets depleted or weakened, especially since you're not replenishing its reserves with proper foods. Its precious time-reversing strength and ability dwindles as it runs on low battery, and it's forced instead to direct its energy, for as long as it can, to the chemical functions that go into keeping you alive.

DNA INDICATORS

With aging, we're quick to think genes. "What condition is your DNA in?" is where today's trend lies.

We always see what's wrong before we're aware of what's making it wrong. Instead of identifying the true source of why our DNA can diminish at all, medical research and science look at flawed DNA and put the cart before the horse. They point to the DNA itself as the issue and blame us, our very essence, as the source. If you want to be enlightened about aging, you need to look beyond genes. They're an indicator, not the answer. They're a sign of something happening, not the cause. An altered gene is not the instigator; it's just a measuring stick in a pond showing that it's drying up.

The truth is that DNA has nothing to do with aging. The condition of our DNA is not proof of a flawed family line; it's a warning about the state of our livers. When DNA weakens, wears down, frays, or becomes injured—which science mistakes for mutation—it's a signal that the liver is losing its strength to keep us young. The very chemical function that our livers possess to keep our cells from dying is the same antioxidant chemical compound that keeps our DNA from becoming weakened or frayed. When we do anything to support our DNA, we are without realizing it supporting our liver, giving it those snippets of rejuvenation. Our DNA will show improvement, in truth, because we supported the liver.

If someone looks good, strong, and young for her or his age and isn't exhibiting symptoms of illness or other health complaints, instead of saying, "Hey, you've got good genes," we should say, "Hey, you've got a good, solid liver. That thing's a cleaning machine. You must not have been exposed to too many toxins in your life."

THE KEY YOU ALREADY HOLD

Longevity enthusiasts need to be careful not to look in the wrong places for anti-aging answers. That's not a comment on their intelligence. You could be one of the smartest people on the planet and you could still lose your car keys and wander your house, looking in all the wrong spots. Once you got in the car, you could still take a mistaken turn and travel down the wrong avenue. No smart person is immune

to making mistakes, which is how the most intelligent people out there end up pursuing the latest spins on genetic technology without realizing they're not even looking in the right part of the house to find the anti-aging key.

In truth, everything we do that helps our livers also slows down and can even reverse the aging process. People have stumbled across ways to do this without realizing that the liver is the key. Exercising and adding more fruit, leafy greens, and vegetables to a fat-overburdened diet, as well as taking time off to go on retreat and seek spiritual connections that bring down our adrenaline—these happen to care for the liver, and that addresses aging.

There's so much more we can do when we see the liver for its true role in keeping us out of harm's way and when we learn to harness the hidden power of antioxidants and amino acids and glucose and every other liver rescuer you'll read about in this book. We don't need to leave our lives behind to find that fountain of youth. With the knowledge you hold in your hands, you can drink from it any day you choose.

"Even if there are moments when you feel you cannot persevere, these words will persevere for you. They're here for you to grab on to; they're the hands that reach out to pull you up."

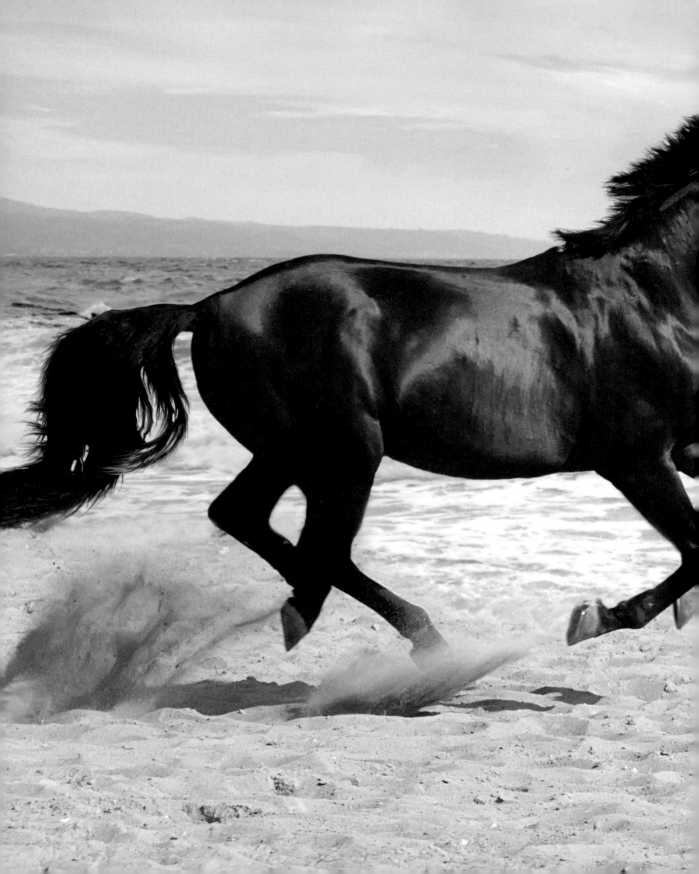

PART III

THE CALL TO BATTLE

MORE SYMPTOMS & CONDITIONS ENLIGHTENED

CHAPTER 15

Diabetes and Blood Sugar Imbalance

When you think diabetes, you may think, *Been there, done that*. We're taught that diabetes and blood sugar are all about insulin, so they're all about the pancreas. In the case of type 1 and 1.5, we're taught that it's autoimmune, with the body attacking the pancreas. What relationship could the liver have with an illness that medical research and science already have sewn up? How does diabetes end up in a book about the liver? Maybe this chapter is just misplaced.

Or is it? When it comes down to it, though it may seem like the medical establishment already knows everything about blood sugar, in reality it hasn't even scratched the surface—there are causes unknown to medical communities of how diabetes comes to be.

Insulin production does have a lot to do with the pancreas, and the pancreas is undoubtedly part of diabetes. That's why the chapter "Type 2 Diabetes and Hypoglycemia" in my first book, *Medical Medium*, took a close look at the gland. At the same time, that chapter also looked beyond the pancreas to the adrenals and what we'll explore in much more detail here, the liver—because in diabetes, the pancreas is not the only thing that's wrong. (Take note that the body never attacks the pancreas. More on types 1 and 1.5 diabetes in a moment.)

It's never enough to stop with the obvious. That's like a plumber coming to plug a leak temporarily—which isn't to say we aren't thankful for the momentary fix. Without the plumber knowing which valve to shut off or which weakness to patch, the water gushing out of the pipe would ruin the house. Same goes for modern medicine: without the know-how of monitoring blood sugar and administering insulin and medication, we'd be in serious trouble. Still, despite these excellent methods for managing diabetes, medical research and science have not yet found the source of the problem. Like the plumber's valve shutoff or pipe patch, today's measures to control diabetes only form a stopgap until the real issue—in the plumber's case, perhaps a rusted spot or a weakness in manufacturing—is discovered. So if we want the truth about our health, we need to look for the underlying *whys* and *hows*. Why does an A1C level rise? How do we develop insulin resistance? Why is sugar considered the enemy? How can we reverse the true cause of diabetes?

GUESSING GAMES

The scapegoats of our time, which I call *escape-goats* because they give the medical establishment an easy out (picture a hole in the barn door allowing goats to get away), are bad diet and no exercise. Cookies, cakes, fast food, too many hours on the couch—we're told by the best experts that all we need to do is exercise more and reduce our intake of sweets and fried, processed, and preservative-laden foods, and we'll fix the problem. That obscures the apparent randomness that medical research and science first observed with diabetes—a randomness that drove them to believe originally that it had no identifiable cause. Take two people of the same age, have them eat what they like and never exercise; one may become diabetic, the other may not. Over time, experts got smarter and observed that for those with diabetes, changing diet and exercise regimens did result in improvement of the condition.

That didn't account for *cause*, though; they needed a third escape-goat. To explain the fact that so many who don't take care of themselves never develop diabetes, they theorized that a genetic weakness of the pancreas must predispose certain people to diabetes. Adding gene blame to the diet-and-exercise theory was the only way for medical communities to feel comfortable with the mystery of who develops diabetes in the first place. It fostered an entitlement in the medical industry so its members could live in their own skin without looking further for answers.

Now, it's true that diet and exercise play a role in preventing prediabetes and type 2 diabetes. That's not the whole picture, though, and while genes play a vital role in our lives, they are not responsible for diabetes (type 1 *or* type 2) or blood sugar imbalances. There are some issues with simply observing a group of people and noting who gets diabetes as a basis for understanding its cause. For example, just because someone's blood tests don't show diabetes doesn't mean she or he isn't *pre*-prediabetic at a level not yet detectable or diagnosable by medical research and science. That person will show up in the study results as nondiabetic when the reality is that she or he is in fact on track to developing diabetes way down the road.

This brings up an important point. The way that medical research and science view type 2 diabetes today, there are two stages: prediabetes and diabetes itself. While medical communities realize there are some type 2 diabetics who require less, if any, insulin, and some who require more insulin, prediabetes and type 2 diabetes remain the major distinctions. What's off the radar of the medical world is that before prediabetes develops, there are pre-prediabetes, pre-pre-prediabetes, and even pre-pre-pre-prediabetes. Hopefully research and science will discover how to detect these very early stages of type 2 diabetes and name them (perhaps as stage 1 prediabetes, stage 2 prediabetes, and so on), because for the sake of intervention, it's critical to realize they exist. The testing for these will need to center around the liver; as you'll soon see, the liver is integral to the development of type 2 diabetes.

What about type 1 diabetes? While liver care is still essential for those with type 1 diabetes, this one occurs from injury to the pancreas. That injury can come from a bout of food poisoning, a viral infection, a bacterial infection, a toxin, or even a physical blow to the gland. It is not autoimmune. *It does not come from the body attacking the pancreas*, only from outside forces hurting the pancreas. Someone can eat out at a restaurant, for example, pick up a pathogen or parasite that damages the pancreas, and come down with type 1 diabetes. Pancreatitis can develop from an accident. Or a stomach virus can travel to the gland and hurt it, damaging its insulin-production abilities.

The newer term out there is type 1.5 diabetes, also known as *latent autoimmune diabetes in adults* (LADA). Its true cause is the same as type 1's, this time with the pancreas injury coming later in life than with juvenile diabetes. Again, this is not truly autoimmune—it's just that the term is convenient wrapping paper that the medical establishment has used to keep type 1.5 diabetes/LADA packaged up in a box. No form of diabetes comes from the body attacking the pancreas.

While a doctor can detect a cyst or tumor on the pancreas, the damage to the pancreas we're talking about here is not visible with today's MRIs, CT scans, PET scans, and ultrasounds. Some pancreatic scar tissue isn't even visible to a surgeon's eye on the operating table. Is the pancreas injured at the top, bottom, left side, right side, middle? They wouldn't be able to tell. It's as if doctors are driving in a blizzard with no visibility, and since the upper echelons of the medical world don't want you to know where its faults lie, it's presented to you like it's a clear day. One of the faults you're kept from hearing about is that medical research and science know virtually nothing about the root of types 1 and 1.5 diabetes. To cover up this lack of knowledge, development, understanding, and accomplishment when it comes to the pancreas, they point to the old autoimmune theory as law.

The viruses that no one realizes can chronically injure the pancreas, causing types 1 and 1.5 diabetes, are those in the herpetic family. That doesn't mean you'll get a diagnosis of a herpetic family virus or that it will show up in a blood test; there are many undiscovered viral strains that can go unseen and undiagnosed. Slowly, one of these viruses can attack the pancreas, causing it to become dysfunctional over time. It's why many type 1 and 1.5 diabetics experience more problems as they get older: because the virus, undetected by medical tests, has never been stopped.

When it's a blow to the pancreas that injures it, the gland can develop scar tissue over time. Once-healthy tissue around it can become less viable and lose life, microadhesions can grow, and the state of the pancreas can worsen, bringing on either type 1 or type 1.5 diabetes. Medical research and science are still generations from uncovering this truth or pinpointing where in the pancreas each individual diabetic's issue lies. It's just boxed up with the autoimmune wrapping paper and a pretty bow and set before you like it's a gift.

Noting the existence of type 1.5 diabetes, even though it's mislabeled as autoimmune, is progress for medical communities. It's still not all the way there. If medical research and science were truly picking up on all the subtle levels of distinction among cases of diabetes, they would identify diabetes types 1.1 through 1.9, too. For that matter, the medical world would realize that in addition to type 2 diabetes, there are types 2.1 through 2.9. On top of that, everyone is unique, and there are subtle twists that make every individual's case of diabetes slightly different in some way. There's so much more for the world to learn about the pancreas and liver issues that lead to diabetic conditions.

Even studying a group of individuals who are all doing exactly the same thing isn't going to reveal what leads certain people to develop diabetes. There are dozens of reasons that researchers don't realize are such big factors for why different people following the same diet-and-exercise plan will have different health outcomes. One person, for example, may have had certain toxic exposures while someone else inherited heavy metals or has a greater pathogenic load. The degree of stress in another person's life, if diet and exercise aren't being employed as supports, could accelerate a case of prediabetes. Where someone has worked or lived, the water she or he has been drinking throughout her life—all of this makes a difference, and yet these factors are not accounted for in studies, so the variability in who does or doesn't develop diabetes is chalked up to genetics. This genetic diversion only prevents progress. While it may seem like advancement, it's not leading toward the truth; every seeming development is, in fact, building a barricade from the truth, preventing you and even medicine from reaching the answers about why people develop diabetes and how they can get better.

Even still, these additional factors don't give us the root answer. It is obvious that the kinds of foods we eat make or break our healing in many ways, and that they make or break prevention. Yet following a trendy diet isn't a guaranteed treatment or preventative, unless the foods in that diet are geared to help the underlying problem—and how can a health professional craft such a program without true knowledge of what really causes diabetes? Letting go of foods such as doughnuts and pastries *is* going to help your health. Beyond taking out junk foods and other clearly poisonous concoctions, though, diets remain guessing games, like shaking out a rug in the wind. There's nothing inherently wrong with following a diet that's trending; a lot of people can get results with guessing games.

And then sometimes the wind can blow the other way. The game can bring all that dust and dirt that you're trying to send away right back into your face, even landing in your eyes and blinding you from seeing the truth.

In other words, someone's A1C level can improve on a trendy diet. The eating plan can seem to get type 2 diabetes under control. Maybe you end up requiring less insulin or medication, or maybe your prediabetes or type 2 diabetes miraculously disappears for a while. Your stress is down, the wind is blowing the right way; it all feels very rewarding. Trouble is, it's unpredictable. Many people will see their improvements plateau at a certain point and then even diminish. That's because there's way more to the story of your health, your body, your organs, and your blood sugar than avoiding sugar and other carbohydrates. The reason this chapter belongs in this book is because the origin of that story goes back to your liver, continues with your liver, is all about your liver. Even when your symptoms are at bay, even when it seems like your low-carb, low-sugar diet is making everything better, even if you keep your diet the same, your liver is still likely getting worse—which means diabetes could still be waiting for you with the next change in the wind. Here, now, it's finally time to give the liver the spotlight it deserves.

YOUR HERO, THE LIVER

Yes, it's important to avoid unproductive carbohydrates, refined sugars, and processed foods. Doctors advise you to get rid of these with good reason. If you don't, you'll get more insulin resistance and unstable blood sugar readings. Your A1C will be out of normal range. Your fasting sugars won't be right and neither will your nonfasting ones; you'll be instructed by your doctor to drastically lower or even remove altogether carbs and sugar from your diet.

Here's the first spot of trouble: this advice will be indiscriminating. Natural sugars and other healthy carbs from foods such as fruit, honey, winter squash, and potatoes will be counted as ones you don't want in your life, when the truth is that they're CCC; they contain some of the exact healing elements you most need. Here's the second spot of trouble: you'll also be told to keep fats in your diet. Not only that; many health professionals will advise to add even more fats to the diet—often using the label "high protein," when the reality is that high protein translates to high fat.

This combination of limiting carbs and upping fats is a trapdoor for diabetics. Not being able to reach for a healthy sugar that the body desperately needs while falling victim to the protein law and increasing fats in the bloodstream, even if they're from healthy sources like nuts or seeds, leaves so many people with health that will eventually worsen. It's especially sobering when you consider that a high-fat diet is how prediabetes and type 2 diabetes develop in the first place.

That's right; diabetes doesn't appear from sugar, carbs, and no exercise. It begins as a liver problem in a very early stage: a sluggish, stagnant, or pre-fatty liver undetectable by medical testing. Remember: one critical job of your liver is to save your pancreas—to protect this delicate flower like a guard so you don't get diabetes.

The liver's glucose storage is a huge piece of preventing diabetes. As you read about in Chapter 3, our livers take glucose from the food we eat and store some of it fresh and at the ready. It stores the rest of the extra glucose as glycogen, a pasty, thick, dense carbohydrate that turns back into glucose when the liver activates it with

precious concentrated water molecules and a chemical compound it produces to bring glycogen back to life. The liver stores this precious glucose and glycogen for a number of critical reasons, including some of the organ's undiscovered chemical functions. One function that's very important is making sure we don't get diabetes. The variability in who does or doesn't develop diabetes has nothing to do with genes. It has greatly to do with whether your liver has enough storage of glucose and glycogen.

Your liver knows that on Planet Earth, you're not always going to have access to food. It has an understanding built into its cells that since the beginning of humankind, we've experienced times when we must miss meals. There has never been a guarantee that we'll have convenient access to nourishment. It may be a week of not being able to find food or, in modern times, a day when we subsist on coffee until breaking for our first meal at two or three in the afternoon. Even with perfect, healing foods at our fingertips, sometimes we choose not to eat, and the liver knows this. Within the very nature of the liver, from long before we were born, is the knowledge of how to release stored glycogen and convert it into accessible sugar to be released into our bloodstream to stabilize our blood sugar when we haven't eaten. This means everything, and it matters to everyone, from those who have diabetes to those developing it to those who don't have it and want to keep it that way.

If the liver weakens because of high-fat foods, pathogenic activity, toxic heavy metals, or other poisons, it can't store glucose and glycogen like it used to, plus it's forced to use up any reserves as fuel to deal with the overload of both troublemakers and responsibilities as it tries to keep so many other critical functions in the body going. Imbalance of blood sugar begins with your liver losing its sugar supply. Beaten down and out of balance, your liver's reserves will drop until it doesn't have enough glucose and glycogen to protect your pancreas anymore. Usually, the pancreas is very stable, able to keep up a steady, balanced, minute-to-minute release of insulin as needed, because the liver's release of glucose and glycogen storage keeps blood sugar balanced. Without the liver offering glucose between meals to keep the blood stable, the pancreas feels the pressure and loses its stability, forced to fluctuate to highs and lows in its insulin production. Those highs happen when the pancreas sends out insulin to seek out every morsel of sugar it can to push it into cells of the body. Elevated fats in the bloodstream make this job much harder if not impossible. As a result, the pancreas weakens, insulin production lessens, and insulin resistance hits a crisis point. Blood sugar will become unstable. That's when hypoglycemia can occur, or when your doctor will observe A1C levels off the charts and label you with *prediabetes*, and you'll be on your way to developing full-blown type 2 diabetes.

FATE COMES DOWN TO FAT

Sugar isn't the real culprit with diabetes; the culprit is fat. Sugar simply reveals the problem, like a messenger. Take the sugar away—put someone on a high-fat, low-carb diet—and the problem will *seem* to minimize or even go away. Blood sugar will *seem* to stabilize. Will it really stabilize? On paper, yes. Internally, no. Eliminating sugars merely hides a sick liver. And if you're not fixing a sick liver, then you're not fixing the root of the problem so you won't be able to prevent a blood sugar condition from worsening down the road. Any natural diet or supplement regimen that seems to show results for prediabetics or type 2 diabetics only does so indirectly by taking away

the messenger, sugar, and unknowingly helping out the liver with some vegetables, nutrients, and practices like exercise.

We're not meant to be punished by diabetes. We're not meant to live in fear of developing this seemingly mysterious disease. If we can't stick with a strict diet and exercise every day, we're not meant to be struck down. Instead, if you develop diabetes, you're meant to know the core cause and work on that. Then you have more room to make mistakes and not be perfect, because you know what really matters with diabetes and other blood sugar issues.

Know this: if the ratio of fat in a diet is high, regardless of how award-winning, trendy, or convincing that diet is, any blood sugar improvements you see on it will be an illusion. A sluggish, stagnant liver will continue to worsen over time from a high-fat diet. Even as blood sugar *readings* are stabilizing, the real blood sugar issues will continue to build silently. It simply won't be evident because there's no messenger (sugar) shouting in your face that danger is near—even though the danger hasn't passed. The minute you play with your diet, indulging in a cookie, a dinner roll, a ham and cheese sandwich, or your favorite ice cream, things will get out of control. Your blood sugar numbers will start to change. Your A1C will lose control. Insulin resistance won't be masked anymore; it will start to show itself again. Your doctor will say it's because you succumbed to eating sugar or other carbohydrates; what the doctor doesn't know is that your type 2 diabetes, prediabetes, insulin resistance, hyperglycemia, or hypoglycemia were there all along under the radar, waiting and wreaking havoc.

As you saw in the earlier chapter "Mystery Hunger," when your blood is dominated by fat sources in your diet, it starves your liver of glucose, never allowing it to restore its reserves.

Not only that, it also inhibits sugar from doing its job in your body altogether. Now, blood filled with dietary fat—don't confuse this with someone being overweight and harboring deposits of fat in the body. We're talking here about blood fat, and there's a difference; you could have high blood fat and be physically thin. When the blood is filled with fat, it by default blocks sugar from having direct access to the organs, glands, and nervous system, including the brain. Fat in the blood makes it very difficult for the hormone insulin to attach to sugar and then speak to tissue cells to open up and receive that sugar so it can perform its critical, sustaining role as fuel to keep us alive.

We sense our cells' sugar deprivation—that in order to function, our bodies need sugar—and that surfaces as cravings. All too often, we turn to unproductive sugar in answer. We eat cheese because we're told it's protein, when really it's a concentrated fat-sugar combination that doesn't advance our health, because the fat content won't let the sugar do its job. We cave for birthday cake because our bodies are so hungry for sugar—and again, it is rogue sugar that clashes instantly with the fat inside of the cake. If you get antsy on that high-fat, low-carb diet and reach for a bagel with cream cheese in the morning, followed by a sugary iced drink after lunch and then a glass of wine after dinner, glucose levels and insulin resistance will become more and more problematic. You'll think it's because fat was your ally and that this introduction of sugar is the real problem. In reality, the problem was there all along from the high fat levels in your bloodstream as a result of everything else you were eating; the sugar simply revealed it. The indulgence foods made it more and more obvious that a high-fat diet was not sustaining. Not that I'm advocating any of the above as health foods. Refined and processed flours and sugars are not ideal—items such as white flour, corn syrup, table sugar, and agave syrup aren't going to help your health.

TRUE BLOOD SUGAR SUPPORT

In a healthier trend, we've been told to eat green apples and berries because they're low-glycemic and safe. Experts have observed you can eat them on a high-fat trendy diet, though it doesn't mean either fruit is respected. They're merely tolerated—allowed in with mixed feelings, even fear. Truth is, fruit is so forgiving that the lower sugar content of these fruits won't clash with fats; they're natural, healthy sugars that a diabetic on a high-fat diet can get away with. Thank goodness people are letting these God-given gifts into their lives. Still, calling these fruits "safe" is missing the point entirely. We should be allowed more than a Granny Smith and a handful of raspberries. We should be able to opt for *all* fruits in our diets, even when we're diabetic. In the end, it's these natural sugars that will truly heal and reverse a liver condition so you don't have type 2 diabetes (or prediabetes, hypoglycemia, hyperglycemia, or insulin resistance) anymore.

High fat interferes with a full recovery. Even when it's a diet that's diverse in its fat content, bringing in lots of coconut, avocado, nuts, seeds, and leaner meats, plus including plenty of vegetables—a diet that many experts think is like striking oil when it comes to your health—it still results in too much fat in the bloodstream. While it is an upgrade and a healthier diet, it still hides blood sugar issues that are continuing to build in the background. It still hurts the liver.

Ultimately, the liver truly, desperately needs to recover for someone to put type 2 diabetes and related blood sugar issues behind them.

Isn't it ironic that what the liver really needs, high-quality glucose, is what the popular diets of today keep us away from by limiting or eliminating healthy carbohydrates? It's not possible to completely reverse prediabetes or type 2 diabetes—long term, for good—if the liver doesn't get to restore its sugar storage bins. The only way to do that is to consume less fat and bring in natural sugars and other healthy carbohydrates—that is, CCC.

Types 1 and 1.5 diabetes can also be improved and even healed in rare cases, though it's going to take a lot of diligence, effort, understanding, and extra pampering of the liver and pancreas. Foods matter for types 1 and 1.5 diabetes just as they do for type 2 diabetes. To protect the liver with these conditions, too, fat should be the concern rather than sugar; blood fat shouldn't be high. When a viral pathogen is slowly causing injury to the pancreas over time, it's also important to stay away from foods that feed viruses, keep them alive, and allow them to continue to do damage. And yet, the best experts in the field and the literature you find out there won't identify what viruses eat, that they even eat at all, and that they can injure the pancreas, causing types 1 and 1.5 diabetes, or injure the liver, causing type 2 diabetes. These sources are still in denial. The enduring truth that will be there waiting for them when they're ready is that viruses can fuel themselves on the foods we eat, and that can either advance a virus's cause or hinder it, depending on what we put in our bodies. That's one reason why Part IV of this book offers dietary direction, so you can look out for the foods that feed viruses while bringing in the ones that repel them. If you're already on a diet you feel is working, you can gain even more control over your type 1 or 1.5 diabetes by avoiding the virus-feeding foods from Chapter 36, "Liver Troublemakers."

No matter which blood sugar condition you have, when you lower your dietary fat intake—which means lowering your protein intake; you should think of fat and protein as one and the same in order to truly understand what you eat—you're healing your liver. You're not hiding anything the way a high-protein, low-sugar diet does. You're fixing the real problem. If you're an animal protein lover, keep your meats lean and eat fewer servings. If you're plant-based, keep your consumption of nuts, seeds, coconut, and oils down. And regardless of your diet, try to refrain from eggs and dairy altogether if possible. By lowering the fat in the bloodstream and allowing for more foods that can help with the actual problem, we get out of the vicious cycle that happens to every diabetic and nondiabetic who cuts out carbs: cravings to the point of breakdown, reaching for forbidden foods when our cells cry out for relief, suffering the health consequences of high fat plus sugar, and starting all over again. Fruit-bashing trends teach us complete fear and hysteria, so when a sugar craving comes, we're backed into a corner. Instead of choosing fruit, we often reach out for the old, familiar, unproductive choices we were eating before becoming ill.

It's unavoidable that we need glucose to survive and thrive. When blood fat is high, it means that the body won't be able to properly use the sugar in the unproductive foods we binge on, so the sugar will have nowhere to go and will start causing problems. The key act of lowering your radical fats helps restore your liver and protect it. It's still okay to bring in some healthier fats, so long as your bloodstream isn't saturated by fat. (We all know the term *saturated fat*. That's not what I'm talking about here. When I say a bloodstream saturated by fat, I mean fat, whether saturated or unsaturated, healthy or unhealthy, bad or good, dominating the bloodstream.)

Lowering fats means you can allow healthy sugars and carbohydrates back into your diet without causing blood sugar instability and insulin resistance. Instead of limiting yourself to a few slices of apple and a pint of berries, if you're reducing your fats, you can successfully bring in potatoes, sweet potatoes, winter squash, bananas, and all other fruits. This protects you from the irresistible impulse to binge on a bad carb when glucose reserves get extremely low. When blood fat is low, and when we choose proper, natural sugars, they benefit anyone with any health challenge, diabetics included, in untold ways.

Vegetables are still critical. Leafy greens such as lettuce, arugula, and spinach; herbs such as parsley and celery; tomatoes and cucumbers (technically fruits); and our other veggie favorites are needed in the diet, in part to provide mineral salts—the right kind of sodium, which plays a role in binding to natural sugars. Medical research and science have not yet discovered this process of mineral salts helping to drive glucose into our cells more efficiently, with the least possible resistance, and yet it's vital. It explains why people love green smoothies so much and why snacking on celery or leafy greens alongside fruit is an ideal choice for regulating blood sugar.

As important as vegetables are, we still need that winter squash, sweet potato, potato, and fruit for the calories. Melon on its own is a fantastic choice. Diabetics are often told to stay away from melon when the reality is that all melons, including watermelons, make an incredible food for diabetics because they hold natural sodium combined with natural sugar. (Remember to eat melon on an empty stomach to avoid a stomachache from this predigested food getting held up in your gut by slower-digesting foods.) If you like green smoothies and you make them with mostly greens and just a touch of fruit, you'll get hungry because your body's calling out for calories, and you'll think you need a yogurt or almond butter or boiled egg (all of them fat sources) to sustain yourself. Let more of your calories derive from natural, healthy carbs and sugar than from fat, and improvements will come—help is on the way.

One of the reasons that exercise is so helpful for controlling diabetes and prediabetes is because it burns up fat calories and improves circulation, bringing more oxygen into the blood and driving that oxygen into the liver. As you've learned, the more fat in the bloodstream, the less oxygen. Walking, running, biking, working out, playing sports—these help use up fat calories that would otherwise be tough to use efficiently. Animal protein sources, for example, bring with them fat calories that are more difficult for the body to use from the get-go than fat calories from sources such as coconut or avocado. (It's a good reason to reduce animal proteins from, say, three servings a day to one and then to sub in some easier-to-use fat calories.) Exercise gives the body a way to use up those fat calories, no matter the origin. What makes an even bigger difference is if someone is exercising while also eating a diet lower in fat. Circulation and oxygenation of blood improve more, resulting in faster and stronger liver health improvement, which can in turn help correct a prediabetic or type 2 diabetic condition and provide a critical foundation to help improve and even sometimes heal types 1 and 1.5 diabetes—something that's been said to be impossible in both the conventional and alternative medical worlds. It *is* possible in rare cases, when you know what you're doing.

THE HEART OF THE MATTER

The medical buzz today is that if you have diabetes, you have a higher risk of developing heart disease. That's because along the way, practicing physicians discovered that they were often prescribing medications for the heart alongside those for diabetes. Without understanding the true connection, they attributed this co-occurrence to the same elements as diabetes itself: no exercise, poor diet, and the looming theory used to explain any disease that doesn't make sense—genes.

The truth is that glucose fuels the heart. This muscular organ, when it doesn't get enough glucose—because the liver has run out of glucose and glycogen storage—can atrophy or enlarge. So there's your connection: the liver's sugar storage. You've already seen how this factors into diabetes. In order to protect your heart, too, your liver must have ample glucose ready to send into your blood to deliver straight to your heart, nourishing it just like the other muscles in your body. If we're on a high-fat diet, the heart struggles to receive these critical sugars. We think of protein building muscle when the reality is that we build muscles by using them and then fueling them with quality carbohydrates and sugars—and by our livers keeping our blood clean so that the carbohydrates and sugars aren't mixed with the toxins and other troublemakers of dirty blood, and our muscles receive them in their purest form.

Our hearts rely critically on sugars, so when we lack glucose and glycogen storage in the liver's banks for far too long, the heart doesn't get the sugars it needs on a daily basis, making it more prone to heart disease in some shape or form. A sick liver with no remaining glucose and glycogen reserves and a bloodstream constantly filled with fats for years—they're how

both diabetes and heart disease can develop; that's the connection. Heal your liver and restore its reserves, and you help take care of both.

THE ADRENAL ELEMENT

No discussion of diabetes is complete without addressing adrenaline. Your adrenals have the built-in protection mechanism of releasing adrenaline for your body to use as a noncaloric sugar replacement when your liver runs out of glucose and glycogen reserves. You don't want to rely on this fallback. You always want to have enough sugar in your liver, or in your bloodstream, so that your adrenals don't need to save you.

Trouble is, we don't realize we're relying on our adrenals to save us. We're basically trained to run our livers down in life and to skip meals or snacks in the name of fulfilling other obligations like school, work, and caring for our families. We have no idea that our livers lose their reserves and that adrenaline becomes our glucose replacement that ends up hurting the pancreas. If running on adrenaline like this keeps going on and on, through high school and then college and well beyond, then the liver spends all those years sponging up adrenaline while the pancreas is also scorched by it, compromising both the liver and pancreas further.

For many women, it's around age 30 (and for many men, it's usually around age 40) that the adrenals reach a weak point, unable to fill in for glucose as well anymore. With the liver's storage banks of glucose and glycogen used up, too, the stage is set for hypoglycemia, hyperglycemia, or diabetes.

To prevent or reverse this, take your healing measures one step beyond lowering fat, increasing healthy carbohydrates and natural sugars, and getting more oxygenating exercise—and add grazing to your life. By eating a nourishing snack or meal every one and a half to two hours, you prevent the blood sugar dips that force your adrenals to fill in for low glucose. In turn, you save your adrenals, liver, and pancreas, and you put yourself on the true path to healing.

CHAPTER 16

Mystery High Blood Pressure

Millions of Americans—and many more globally—have no identifiable heart, vascular, or kidney problems and yet hear that they have high blood pressure. Sitting in the doctor's office and being handed that label of *hypertension* seems more conclusive than it really is. Despite the big word, you're still left in the dark. Much of the time, when a doctor diagnoses a hypertensive issue, what's truly causing the high blood pressure remains a mystery to medical research and science. As with type 2 diabetes, the mystery of who gets it is often explained away as lifestyle, passed off as a need to exercise more and eat "right," and if that doesn't work, to go on medication. If only medical communities knew that this isn't the whole story. High blood pressure often has more to do with the liver than the cardiovascular system.

HIDDEN FACTORS OF HYPERTENSION

Have you ever used a straw in a glass of water? You sip, the suction pulls up the contents of your glass to your mouth with ease, and you swallow. Cola, with its syrupy nature, takes just a touch more effort to draw up the straw. What happens if you're drinking a milkshake? Sipping its contents through the straw becomes harder; it takes more suction. And what about if you try to draw up jelly through a straw? You'll find it's very difficult.

Your heart draws blood directly from your liver. When the liver is in good working order, it's like sipping water through a straw. When the liver is stagnant, sluggish, hot, fatty, or toxic, it becomes a clogged, dirty filter. As a result it becomes inflamed and constricted, so it can't process blood well, nor can blood travel through the liver as easily as it should. It makes the blood dirtier and thicker with debris and increases the suction needed for the heart to pump up blood from the liver. As someone's liver becomes more and more congested due to liver-unfriendly food choices while she or he is also chronically dehydrated, as we all are, the heart can be forced to use 10 or even 50 times its normal power to draw blood through the body. It goes from sucking water through a straw to drawing up cola to a milkshake to jelly. The result of all this increased suction is increased pressure—that is, high blood pressure. Mystery hypertension is born.

In order to save the heart from the strain of hypertension, medical communities should be looking to the liver to understand these mechanics of how a burdened liver leads to a burdened cardiovascular system. If they did, they would find that the liver is playing a role here even when the traditional liver tests we looked at in Chapter 9, "Liver Enzyme Guess Tests," don't indicate an issue, and they'd conclude that this variety of high blood pressure should be diagnosed as *liver hypertension*. They'd discover that even when a blocked artery is clearly diagnosed, that itself started with the liver, one way or another. This would empower patients to go to the source and clean up their livers to get relief. It would empower patients who weren't yet suffering to take care of the liver to begin with to avoid ever risking the possibility of developing high blood pressure.

I know that taking care of anything or anyone—whether a pet guinea pig or our own needs or another person's—isn't easy. Most of us live our lives hanging by a thread, just doing what we can to survive and get through the day. Taking care of your liver and high blood pressure may not be at the top of the list. At those moments when you have a bit more of a grip and a spare morsel of mental space, at least now you know what to do. Without that knowledge, you don't even have the opportunity to avoid or truly fix the problem.

Yes, poor diet and no exercise can lead to high blood pressure—because they can negatively affect the liver. As always, though, we need to be aware that "good" and "poor" diets are not necessarily what we've been led to believe. In the case of mystery hypertension, it's a high-fat, high-salt, high-vinegar diet that you need to avoid. Notice I didn't mention sugar. While it's popular for a diet to leave out sugar, it actually plays no role in liver hypertension. Besides

alcohol, an obvious liver troublemaker, it's really too much fat, salt, and vinegar you need to look out for—which may be surprising, given that so many diets rely on them. Most people are on a high-fat diet, many without realizing that the majority of their calories come from fat, and have no idea that for years, the excess fat they've been consuming has been making their blood thicker and pastier while also congesting and dehydrating the liver, with fat cells accumulating inside and around the organ. With salt, when we overdo it with the wrong types, especially in combination with a lot of radical fats in the diet, fat in the bloodstream is forced to encapsulate it, which creates denatured, dehydrated fat cells that are harder for the liver to send out and away to exit the body; the denatured fat cells end up clinging to the liver. (Natural mineral salts from whole-food sources, on the other hand, especially those in celery, are actually very good for the liver and blood pressure balancing, lowering it when it's high and raising it when it's low.) Further, people don't realize that vinegar can actually contribute to a sluggish and stagnant liver almost as much as alcohol. (See Chapter 34, "Liver Myths Debunked," Chapter 35, "The High-Fat Trend," and Chapter 36, "Liver Troublemakers," for more on fat, salt, and vinegar.)

Then there are the people who eat what truly is a healthy diet. They stay lower fat, and the fats they do eat are high quality. They don't eat much salt or vinegar or drink much alcohol. They exercise. How to explain mystery hypertension then? As we examined in Chapter 8, "Sluggish Liver," a sluggish, stagnant liver can have another source: toxins. Whether heavy metals, pathogens such as EBV, viral waste matter, plastics, DDT, chlorine, fluoride, or any number of other poisons, the buildup can clog the liver, too, having the same effect of forcing the heart to pump harder and, in turn, raising blood pressure. If you think you couldn't have been exposed to any of these, ask yourself if you've ever had a fluoride treatment at the dentist's office. Even just one in your lifetime? Where did the fluoride go when it entered your mouth? Did it all disappear? It went straight to your liver, and this byproduct of aluminum manufacturing has been there for however many decades it's been since your fluoride treatment. With DDT, you may think that if your family isn't from a rural area, you couldn't have inherited this pesticide through your family line; chances are, you still did.

It's not one or the other, "lifestyle" or toxins. Someone can have a little bit of everything going on: inactivity, eating poorly, toxins inside the liver—plus a couple of extra factors. Across the board, dehydration is important to address. Most people in the U.S. alone are chronically dehydrated, which thickens the blood, contributing to the heart's strain bringing it up from the liver.

Finally, we need to consider stress. You may hear that hypertension is caused by stress constricting blood vessels throughout the body. In truth, bouts of stress are just the sprinkles on the cupcake of high blood pressure. It takes a lot more to make the batter that bakes into the cupcake itself. There are people under very little stress who are living with hypertension on a daily basis. Then there are people under enormous stress who haven't developed hypertension, because they don't have a liver issue yet. It doesn't mean a person who doesn't have hypertension won't develop it over time; chances are, she or he will eventually experience a liver problem that leads to high blood pressure.

The real relationship between stress and high blood pressure has to do with adrenaline and the liver. The liver is the seat of courage—our day-in, day-out bravery stems from it—which

also means the liver pays the price with every daily battle we face. When we're pushed past our limits, our adrenals pump out stress-based adrenaline, which, as you keep reading about, the liver must sponge up in order to protect the body from damage—and a liver saturated in adrenaline makes it hard for blood to smoothly process through and find its way back to the heart.

Now, your adrenal glands produce different blends of adrenaline for different situations. There's a big difference between your liver soaking up everyday adrenaline blends from going about your life, such as taking a brisk walk or dreaming, and the blends for times of confrontation, attack, fear, anger, and loss of trust. That's why it takes a brave liver to soak up this adrenaline for intense times. Whether from someone cutting you off on the turnpike, a disagreement at work, or a family emergency, your liver must bear the surge; it's like a fiery flood that can injure the liver lobule elves if they're not in top working order to neutralize it, and that injury makes it more difficult for blood to travel through, raising blood pressure in the process. The liver does it, though in the same sacrificial spirit as a father taking a bullet for his daughter: whatever it takes.

SOLVING THE EQUATION

Each person's exact equation of these different hypertension factors is unique. What they all add up to is that to bring your blood pressure back to healthy levels, liver care is essential. If you're not taking care of your liver, you can't truly take care of your heart and vascular system. You could be checking all the boxes that you've heard of before, like exercising, staying away from chocolate cake, taking heart-healthy supplements, and eating a low-carb, high-protein diet with lots of vegetables, and you'll at least be better off than if you weren't working out and trying to eat as healthily as you know how. Still, the common recommendations out there don't fully address the real source of heart health: the liver. Even if you're all muscle and don't have a scrap of visible body fat, it doesn't automatically mean you're protecting your heart. The heart attacks of today come whether you're healthy, doing cardio, or lifting weights or not. There's no discrimination in that regard. Thick blood and a weakened, sick liver are what are responsible for the heart attack epidemic. Care for your liver, on the other hand, and at the same time you protect yourself from vascular and heart disease.

CHAPTER 17

Mystery High Cholesterol

When it comes to cholesterol, like blood pressure, we often think it's all about the heart and vascular system. We know the terms *HDL* (high-density lipoproteins), *LDL* (low-density lipoproteins), *VLDL* (very-low-density lipoproteins), though there are even more varieties of proteins, triglycerides, and lipoproteins that medical research and science have not yet discovered. We picture hardening of the arteries and plaque inside the heart valves, and rightfully so.

How does it start? It can't form on its own, out of thin air. You don't wake up one morning with elevated cholesterol because the cholesterol fairy visited you in the night and, instead of replacing a tooth with a quarter, replaced your peace of mind with a prescription for statin medication. High bad cholesterol or even low good cholesterol must come from somewhere.

Medical research and science account for the mystery by saying that in addition to the high-cholesterol foods we choose, our bodies create this troublesome cholesterol. It's a simple explanation to appease us. And sure, eating fewer fried foods, oils, and cheeseburgers is going to make your life better and improve your cholesterol readings. At the same time, mystery high cholesterol is bigger, badder, and more straightforward than medical communities realize.

THE LIVER'S ROLE IN CHOLESTEROL

Elevated cholesterol conditions have everything to do with the liver, the master of balancing, regulating, storing, organizing, and more. You're well aware by now that no matter how masterful, while looking after us in our every sleeping and waking moment and not getting restored along the way, our livers get beaten down. One casualty is cholesterol regulation. The liver's extraordinary chemical function of producing what's called good (HDL) cholesterol starts to wane. As the organ becomes overburdened by fat, whether from beneficial or taxing, unhealthy sources, it can't keep its production lines open for good cholesterol anymore. Nor can it manage what's called bad (LDL) cholesterol.

Imagine you're driving all day and all night long on a road trip, until you can barely drive anymore. Desperate, you start to look for a diner that's still open. At 3 A.M., as you pull into the parking lot of one you finally find, you see lights shutting off inside. You sit in the car, exhausted and depleted, then decide it's still worth a try. At the door, a waitress is posting the CLOSED sign with a note underneath: "Opening late tomorrow. Time TBD."

You knock just in case, and she opens the door. "Sorry, the kitchen is shut down for the night."

As you look behind her, you see employees inside, cleaning up and organizing for the next day. "People are still working. Is there *anything* you can get me?"

Like the diner's night crew sweeping floors, gathering garbage, wiping windows, making sure there's enough butter for tomorrow, and cleaning up the vomit in the bathroom of some college kid who came in drunk, your liver has its hands full with regulating and containing bad cholesterols that will otherwise begin to saturate the bloodstream and vascular system. It's consumed with cleaning and storing and reorganizing in its desperate need to protect you. For years and even decades, it fights like this to control bad cholesterol. It never gets a pat on its back, with us saying, "Hey good job, liver, my friend." It never gets a salute or accolade or medal of achievement. It gets stuck with us not understanding its limits and pushed past our own limits in life, showing up at the door and asking it to do even more. Your liver is like the waitress taking pity on you during your long journey, going to get you a buttered dinner roll after operations are shut down for the night.

When we choose foods that have the makings of good cholesterol, the liver stores away those components, knowing it will most likely face a stretch of rainy days when we're choosing high-fat foods that tax it, weaken it, and break down its core good cholesterol chemical functions, allowing bad cholesterol to rise throughout the body. When we consume bad cholesterol, our livers first try to neutralize it,

though not eliminate it altogether, because that bad cholesterol in the bloodstream isn't causing harm as long as it's free-floating; it's not the maker of heart disease. The liver likes it out there as a warning flare or a message written on the wall inside an ancient pyramid that we may someday stop misinterpreting and instead decode in its true meaning: "HELP." The liver does have a responsibility to try to manage an overabundance of bad cholesterol, so while it leaves plenty in the bloodstream, it also corrals some, storing it up in imprisoning containment units in the hopes that it will one day get the chance to detox it out of the body by releasing it through the bloodstream, kidneys, or intestinal tract.

We all have our dreams and aspirations, and so does the liver. The liver's dream is to keep us safe. It knows this dream may not come true. Still, it soldiers on. If the liver becomes heavily burdened by an onslaught of toxins, viruses, and/or bacteria, it can't release the small, fatty deposits of bad cholesterol that it has stored up inside for safe release out of your body. The dream dies. Instead, these cholesterol deposits join with any other fat cell deposits in and around the liver. These are fat deposits that come from a diet high in fat—again, whether good *or* bad fats. If you're saying, "High-fat diet? That's not me," switch "high-fat" to "high-protein," and you may have an awakening. Regardless of what your trainer says, regardless of how seemingly healthy the diet, high protein translates to high fat, which will slowly lead to a pre-fatty and then a fatty liver (which can easily go undiagnosed), and then high cholesterol.

Weight doesn't determine cholesterol levels; a sluggish, pre-fatty, or fatty liver does. This is another instance where you could be in good shape and taking care of yourself physically, while eating what seems to be a good diet, and still have elevated bad cholesterol or good cholesterol that's too low. Someone who's thin can get a high cholesterol reading. If she or he has a pre-fatty liver with a boatload of toxins and pathogens that have been building in it over time, regardless of that person's weight, the liver will reach a point where it can't store cholesterol and other fat, good or bad, anymore, and it can't produce good cholesterol in the first place. This will keep the excess bad cholesterol floating through the bloodstream, un-neutralized and unorganized, with nowhere to go. Eventually, it will end up lining places like the heart and arteries, causing the problems we associate with high cholesterol.

This doesn't mean that medication such as a statin is the solution. While a statin has the ability to make bad cholesterol reduce or even disappear on blood test readings, your cholesterol has only been manipulated; you still have a problematic liver condition. Statins are the ultimate creators of a now-you-see-it-now-you-don't, smoke-and-mirrors effect—only it won't have you ooh-ing and aah-ing. Think about one of the principles of magic: nothing ever really disappears. So when a statin seems to make your bad cholesterol go away, it doesn't really vanish. Where does it go? The medication forces the cholesterol to start rapidly sticking to the heart and vascular walls. It was better off free-floating as a warning sign that a liver issue that could lead to cardiovascular issues was developing.

Even the liver knows that bad cholesterol, if it can't be contained, is better left free-floating than stuck to the heart and arteries. Elevated blood cholesterol itself is not the recipe for strokes and heart attacks that medical communities believe it to be. In reality, the recipe is elevated blood fats from a diet high in radical fats—a high-protein diet with a lack of omega-3 fatty acids and antioxidants alongside too many omega-6 fatty acids and their distorted,

dysfunctional cousins (that is, fatty acids that have been mixed with the wrong ingredients, overheated, and mutated by cooking techniques such as frying). These fats and fatty acids bind to the walls of the cardiovascular system and build up and up and up because meanwhile, the liver weakens over time and loses bile strength and production levels that would otherwise disperse fats. Higher fat levels in the bloodstream don't allow room for proper blood flow, so when someone gets a small, common viral or bacterial infection in the blood, there's not enough space in the blood vessels for these infections to play out naturally. As a result, blood clots can form or larger infections can develop from the lack of oxygen, and those infections can flow onward—in some cases, toward the brain. Statins take free-floating cholesterols that wouldn't normally bind to the walls of the cardiovascular system and force them to mix with radical fat, combining to create plaque there, bringing you closer to heart disease.

FOR THE BETTER

Long before detectable signs of plaque or hardening arteries form, the liver condition that eventually causes them begins. This means that you can stop a cholesterol problem long before it starts; protecting yourself against high cholesterol means learning to look after yourself and your liver. You don't want to be knocking on your liver's door after closing, asking it to open its production line. You want to be proactive, learning how to pace yourself along the way, so you can be in this life for the long haul. If your doctor has already identified a cholesterol or plaque issue, fear not—it's so reversible, it's not even funny. Incorporating the right foods and tending to your liver with the other techniques from Part IV can change these issues for the better.

CHAPTER 18

Mystery Heart Palpitations

There are different ways to describe heart palpitations and other arrhythmias. There's ectopic heartbeat, for instance: a mystery skip or jump feeling in the chest that appears when all seems well with the heart. There's atrial fibrillation. There are even muscle spasms in the chest that resemble sensations of the heart acting irregular.

When someone exhibits serious arrhythmia, a good cardiologist will usually find the answer. Then there are the mystery palpitations and fibrillations that have no apparent rhyme or reason. If you're experiencing strange feelings around your heart and a cardiologist gives you the all-clear, saying your heart itself checks out fine, with no sign of deterioration or degeneration in the tricuspid, mitral, aortic, or pulmonary valves; no sign of a leak anywhere; ventricles looking good; no presentation of endocarditis or other random, mystery inflammation that's often called autoimmune; and no obvious signs of heart disease or heart enlargement, then your issue will often be categorized as heart palpitations or ectopic heartbeat that are hormonal in nature. Translation: it's a mystery to medical science. (The hormone blame in this area started because these heart palpitations seemed to affect women in greater number than men, and because their onset was often around menopause.) With some rhythmic issues of the heart, the best guess is that it's some sort of electrical issue rather than hormonal. Nowadays, the thyroid is another easy source of blame. If someone has been diagnosed with Hashimoto's thyroiditis and also experiences heart palpitations, that thyroiditis becomes the instant escape-goat.

GUMMING UP THE WORKS

There was a day when heart rate irregularities that obvious cardiovascular problems couldn't explain were brand new to our society—and it wasn't that long ago. Don't get me wrong; heart attacks, heart disease, and other general heart problems have been around for a long time. While they're more prevalent now than ever before, they didn't start recently. People had plenty of heart attacks back in the 1800s, 1700s, and even further back. What's new is the *mystery* heart palpitation. Not until the 1940s did millions of people in their 40s and 50s begin to experience these unexplainable discomforts in the chest.

There's a reason it happened to a certain age group at a certain point in time. It's when a viral condition that they'd carried with them since childhood in the late 1800s and/or early 1900s finally surfaced, after just the right amount of incubation time and the right types of triggers. Before the late 1800s, the virus had been docile; then it strengthened into a less kind force at the precise time these people were coming of age. It was the beginning of the modern-day viral explosion. The virus was Epstein-Barr, and it's still with us today. Now its strains and mutations are more accelerated than ever before. It affects women (and men) in their child and teen years all the way up the ladder of ages. You can read more about Epstein-Barr's history and still-active presence in our lives in *Thyroid Healing*.

Specifically, the virus's effect on the liver has contributed to mystery heart palpitations all these years. Another component has been DDT. Back when the viral explosion was beginning, DDT was also taking hold—and taking a toll on the liver. We don't think of ourselves as exposed to DDT anymore. Yet the reality is that we can inherit it through the bloodline from parents, grandparents, and so forth; plus old DDT still lives in our environment, and its new, accelerated pesticide cousins are in use today. Then there's the rise of pharmaceuticals and petroleum byproducts, which had reached new heights by the 1940s and since then have become an even greater presence in our lives—and livers. These are all pieces of the puzzle that contributed to the creation of mystery heart palpitations and all the other elements that we're still dealing with today. Again, it's not these components themselves directly causing heart palpitations; it's the fact that they take up residence in the liver.

When mystery heart palpitations first hit the scene, there was pandemonium. It wasn't just one or two cases trickling in to any given doctor's office; people were filing in at record numbers. Many years ago, I met a 90-year-old retired country doctor. For fun, we would talk shop, and he would tell me stories of his medical practice back in the day. One was the story of heart palpitations, what he described as a crazy phenomenon that had started when he was still practicing in the 1940s. He'd never seen anything like it before, and neither had his colleagues; they were all confused. He said it was as if someone were playing a joke on all the doctors. At first, everybody thought there was something in the water. Since he was drinking the same water as those in his town, though, that theory didn't make sense to him. Over time, the new advancements in hormone replacement became popular. He remembered the day when hormones became the blame for everything, and he didn't buy into that, either. He knew it was a big pharmaceutical campaign to rally for a new, profitable treatment. This doctor knew in his heart and soul that palpitations weren't a symptom of perimenopause, menopause, or postmenopause—because women had never exhibited symptoms of the "change of life" before. (More on menopause in my first book, *Medical Medium*.) In the remaining years of his practice, he never found out the answer to what causes mystery heart palpitations.

I couldn't help telling him what I'd learned from Spirit: that they had to do with the liver. The man's eyes lit up. Out of all the organs, the liver had always interested him the most. I talked about pesticides, such as early DDT.

"Oh, I remember that," he said, then spouted out a recollection of how DDT was *everywhere*, part of normal everyday vocabulary. I told him that DDT had ended up in people's livers, and he said, "It's most likely in mine."

"Why do you say that?" I asked.

"I used it in my garden for many years."

When I was finished explaining the liver troublemakers of pesticides, the viral explosion, pharmaceuticals, toxic heavy metals, and petroleum byproducts, and how that all translates to heart palpitations, he pronounced, "By golly, I think you're right!"

By golly, indeed. The mystery heart palpitations that started in this doctor's heyday and continue today are caused by a jelly-like substance produced by your liver when it's occupied by certain troublemakers. Usually, the liver doesn't get overloaded enough to produce this sticky gunk until someone has passed the age of 30, though it can still happen at younger ages. This unique substance isn't usually dangerous. It doesn't hurt you directly; it doesn't normally cause heart attacks or strokes. What it does is gum up the works.

At first, the liver holds on to it to protect you. Before even that, the byproduct isn't sticky. It's just a buildup from a virus, EBV, feeding off its favorite fuels in the liver—those usual suspects of old pharmaceuticals, petrochemicals, plastics, solvents, old DDT storage bins that we all have, toxic heavy metals, and so much more. When we never give the liver the opportunity to cleanse properly, such as with Liver Rescue 3:6:9 in Chapter 38, then rather than getting thinned out and dispersed, the buildup continues to build up and starts to get sticky. This is when the liver will still keep it contained. One of its strongest drives is to not release anything toxic into the bloodstream.

A liver in good working order will normally produce a chemical compound to help dissolve this sticky buildup. The compound is very astringent and bitter; you might have even tasted it before, because it can come up into the stomach with bile that creeps up there. This compound only works as a degreasing agent when it touches oxygen in the blood; the compound is like a match, and oxygen is like the matchbox it needs to get lit. Since high fat levels in the bloodstream drive down oxygen levels, it has a harder time finding that oxygen when the blood is full of fat—it would be like if you were trying to light a match and someone were holding your arm so that the matchbox was just out of reach. Without that spark, you couldn't light your candle, just as without oxygen the liver's special chemical compound can't become a degreasing agent that breaks up byproduct stickiness.

The liver can't perform miracles when we unknowingly hand it problems. We usually can't help contracting viruses or being exposed to pesticides. It's not our fault that we don't get an education on how to take care of ourselves for the long haul. How many times over the years have I heard that not even medical school teaches how to care for yourself? Too many times to count. So we hand our livers impossible jobs without realizing it, and one of them is to contain this buildup, among other junk.

This jelly-like byproduct I'm talking about here is a specific type. It's not the normal garbage that your liver is trying to store away if it can't detox it. It takes the right toxins (the ones we discussed above) and the right virus (EBV) to form this particular substance. And you don't need to exhibit one sign of liver disease at the doctor's office in order for this gunk to give you heart palpitations. You don't need to show one sign of heart disease. If you were to find yourself at the movie theater feeling a jump in your heart for the very first time, and you decided not to ignore it and went instead to get it checked out, there's a good chance that even with all the tests, nothing would show up.

To understand how the buildup of this substance leads to heart palpitations, imagine big, wet snowflakes. On a day when the temperature is hovering at 32 degrees Fahrenheit, the snowflakes drifting down from the sky will melt almost as soon as they land on the grass and sidewalks; they won't stick. If the conditions are right, on the other hand, and the temperature drops, the snowflakes will start to build up, creating a layer of snowfall. If the temperature rises again, the snow will disappear over time.

When your liver can't contain its jelly-like buildup after a certain point, the substance leaves the liver through the bloodstream, overrides the chemical compound meant to dissolve it if the liver were in better shape, and finds its way to the heart, where it sticks inside valve entryways. It's not a heart or valve disease; rather, with the right conditions, these little bits of "jelly" act like big snowflakes piling up on one another (on a microscopic level too small to observe if you could suddenly see inside your body). As the substance builds up, it can make the heart valves stick slightly, sending the heart into a slight, nondangerous spasm—resulting in that uncomfortable feeling in the chest.

The "right conditions" to cause this sticking, like temperatures dropping and causing snow to stick, include a diet high in fat, an overload of troublemakers, and the resulting thick blood. Fattier blood equals thick blood equals dirty blood. Fatty, thick, dirty blood holds less oxygen, and you want higher oxygen in your blood because it acts together with your liver's specialized chemical compound as a degreasing and dispersing agent for this jelly. The fine bits of jelly buildup in the liver that get released are supposed to be dispersed before they get a chance to stick to heart valves.

Note that the oxygen saturation tests out there these days can easily show that you

have adequate oxygen in your blood even when you don't, because they test on a macro level. What about a micro level? We don't yet have tests that pick up on that smaller scale, because medical research and science don't realize there is one. When they discover this nuance, they'll be able to develop tests that help determine if someone has enough oxygen in the blood to disperse an item such as this jelly.

Don't confuse jelly buildup with plaque. Plaque in the arteries, smaller blood vessels, and valves is the beginning of heart disease. What we're talking about here is a whole different substance, one that changes with the most minute shift in the blood's oxygen level—though you can have both heart disease and this unrelated, sticky residue at the same time. The oxygen level shift here is a much smaller difference than that between 98 percent and 99 percent; rounding up to the nearest percentage point is not precise enough for this kind of pinpointing. For true precision, we need to go out to over 100 decimal places. Here's what that looks like: 98.99999999999999999999999999999 99999999999999999999999999999999 99999999999999999999999999999999 999999999999

When it comes to the oxygen saturation of your blood, there's a world of difference between the figure above and 99 percent.

So oxygenation of blood (or rather, lack thereof) is one big piece of the puzzle when it comes to this substance gumming up your heart valves. At the same time, you need enough viral activity in your liver that's feeding off toxins and then releasing them for the other conditions to be just right.

Flutters, a jump in the heart, a skipped-beat feeling, a fish-jumping-out-of-the-chest feeling, a popping sensation that goes up to the throat, and more: there are many different forms that palpitations can take. Mystery atrial fibrillation has a lot to do with this jelly. When blood oxygen levels are very low, viral activity is high, and the liver is very toxic—even when the organ is not exhibiting disease—the jelly can become very thick and build up to the point that it causes this irregular heart rate on a fairly regular basis. Not every case of mystery arrhythmia is caused solely by the jelly. A rarer cause is when someone has a high level of toxic heavy metals such as mercury in the brain, meaning that electrical brain signals end up hitting those metal pockets and ricocheting down the vagus and other heart-related nerves, causing spasms or mystery symptoms that are neurological.

FREE FLOWING

How to avoid an out-of-rhythm heart? Think of the conventional medical approach to arrhythmia: a prescription blood thinner. That should tell you something about what medical communities have observed makes a difference. Now, wouldn't you rather go to the source and thin your blood naturally? I've seen so many people get rid of mystery heart palpitations, ectopic heartbeats, and other arrhythmias by cleaning up the liver and lowering the amount of fat they eat. If you suffer from heart palpitations and you're looking to a trendy high-fat diet to be your answer, you really need to find another avenue. Lowering the fat in your diet not only thins your blood; it allows the liver to safely release what's been holding it back.

CHAPTER 19

Adrenal Problems

Medical research and science are unaware that our adrenal glands actually produce 56 different adrenaline blends geared to a number of different functions. Some of those blends are mild, namely the ones for actions such as talking on the phone, dropping off your child at school, checking the mail, putting together a list of what you need at the store, and doing the laundry. There's a world of difference between the liver soaking up that everyday kind of adrenaline versus the more normally publicized kind our adrenals produce in times of high stress, exertion, alarm, and sorrow.

When it is this second type of adrenaline, our livers take special pains to protect us, since our adrenals must produce a strong brew of adrenaline to get us through betrayal, jealousy, hurt, pain, fear, attack, loss, confrontation, being stabbed in the back, having our trust broken, not being heard, and adrenaline-rush activities such as skydiving, bungee jumping, and extreme cleansing. Even someone making a wayward comment in the workplace because they didn't think first can get our blood boiling and give us the shakes because of the adrenaline surge it triggers when our brain registers a threat. The liver is there to clean up afterward. It's a natural process that gets us through life's ups and downs.

With information, demands, and feedback coming at us faster than ever, we have a lot of surges of this caustic adrenaline nowadays, sometimes more—a lot more—than is ideal. The adrenals must work that much harder, and so must the liver. Each one of our livers deserves a bravery medal for taking on the job of adrenaline management.

EXTREME CLEANSE EFFECTS

With any type of cleanse, detox, or diet we try, regardless of how popular or celebrated it is in the health world, we need to pay serious consideration to possible side effects that may not be helpful—and may even be harmful. Liver cleanses are a prime example: they need to be liver-friendly. That sounds strange to say, doesn't it? When you're doing a liver cleanse, wouldn't you automatically think it's liver-friendly? You'd think that someone labeling it with "liver" would instantly mean it's safe for the organ. Well, not necessarily. And there's much more to it than that. When you're administering a cleanse or trying one yourself, you not only need to look out for the liver and its needs; you also need to be mindful of another critical part of the body: the adrenal glands. The Liver Rescue 3:6:9 in Chapter 38 does both.

I remember once watching a friend pull weeds out of his garden. As I sat nearby, he told me that with so many responsibilities and commitments that month, he hadn't had a chance to tend to his plot. The weeds had gotten away from him. He kneeled there, uprooting the unwanted growth, getting closer and closer to his prized pepper plants. In the fertilized soil around them, the weeds appeared especially thick and strong. My friend gripped a massive thistle.

"Are you sure you want to pull that one out?" I asked. "What if you snip it at the base instead so you don't disrupt the peppers? Aren't they the ones that win you prizes at the farmers' market every year?"

"Yes," my friend replied, "I've won three years in a row. But I need to get this thistle out, or it will starve the peppers of nutrients."

So he tugged, then he pulled, then he yanked as I sat cringing. It seemed he was trying to be as careful as he could at first, though he quickly became obsessed; madness took him over. Finally, he put all his weight into it and uprooted the thistle with a heave—only that wasn't all he uprooted. Along with the thistle, three pepper plants were now sideways in the garden bed, their roots exposed to the air, with clumps of dirt everywhere. Immediately, as a medic would tend to an injured body on the battlefield, my friend tended to his special plants. Carefully, he replanted them and did everything he could to make up for his mistake, watering them with care, feeding them with his own mystery concoctions of nutrients as well as new ones he'd never tried before. Despite all his extra measures, in his heart he knew he'd made the wrong decision in fixating on the thistle. The hit his plants had taken was just too much.

The pepper plants took a full month to reestablish themselves, and they never truly recovered. While the peppers did turn red eventually, and he was able to bring them into the kitchen and use them in salads, they never reached the prized size he needed; they were too stunted to bring to the farmers' market competition. People asked him what had happened, and he told them he'd had to leave town to attend to some business. The next time I saw him, he said, "I should have just cut the thistle to the base, added rich compost around the peppers, and kept with the program. I'd have had the peppers I wanted and maybe even better."

When we're trying to cleanse poisons out of the liver and we cleanse too hard, trying to get rid of everything at once, we disrupt and uproot too much. Many of the cleanses out there create a storm inside the liver—and they also tap into our emotional center, creating a mission-based madness that drives us to feverishly cleanse the liver to the extreme. In the process, what we should think of as our prized peppers—located in the back, one on each side, above the kidneys—take a hit.

That's right; the adrenal glands are much like peppers in that they generate serious heat. Have you ever been outside in the cold without a jacket? You start wiggling your fingers or jogging in place, and it helps because this gets your adrenals to work. When you move your muscles, these heat-making glands send adrenaline into your system to get you nice and warm. It's a misconception that it's the increased circulation alone that warms you up when you move. Really, it's the adrenaline (1) revving up your heart to pump faster so that (2) blood carries that extra adrenaline through your blood at a higher rate that has the warming effect. There are some hot pepper plants nowadays, and they generate a lot of heat units; we need to be careful we don't use them in the wrong way and burn ourselves. We've also got to worry about those two peppers in the back, the adrenals. We need to be gentle with them.

With a misguided cleanse, not only does the liver take on more stress; the adrenals take a hit, too. To begin with, they're usually stressed and weakened already. People with health problems normally have adrenals that have become slightly compromised and aren't functioning at their best. Many deal with recurring bouts of adrenal fatigue or ongoing, chronic adrenal fatigue. When you cleanse the liver, the adrenals have a responsibility to uphold that no one knows about: to match the toxic material released from the liver with enough adrenaline to create a rush that acts as a flushing mechanism. That is, for every one part of poison that your liver detoxes, your adrenals must send out two parts adrenaline. It's a more liver-friendly brew of adrenaline than many, though it still has an impact on your liver. Medical research and science can't yet measure the amount of toxins released by the liver at any given time, especially during a cleanse, nor are they even aware of this poison-adrenaline relationship.

When it happens as it should, the least amount of adrenaline needed is used, because the toxins are released properly and evenly, without setting off alarm bells in the body. When the liver is forced to cleanse in a way it's not supposed to, on the other hand, as poisons flood the bloodstream, bells and whistles sound throughout the body as if the town dam has broken or as if it's a three-alarm fire.

The liver itself sends out a warning, too. Imagine that you've been tasked with removing boulders from the top of a hill. Your foreman forces you to take on one that's too heavy, and your first instinct is to hold it back, since it's so hard to maneuver. Unable to keep that up for long, you feel it getting away from you. The boulder starts rolling down the hill, off path, directly toward a coworker at the base. What do you do? You scream to your work friend, "Move out of the way!" That's what your liver does, too: when it's forced to release poisons in too-high quantities at a too-rapid pace, it sends out chemical compounds to alert the central nervous system that a rogue detox is about to occur.

The nervous system instantly alerts the adrenals to save the day by releasing adrenaline to protect the body in that moment. In this case, the adrenaline acts as a steroid compound to stop the body from reacting to any poisons as quickly as possible. It's still released in the two parts adrenaline to one part poison ratio—which adds up to a lot of two parts adrenaline if it's a lot of one part poison. In many cases, this adrenaline surge can make someone feel euphoric. A cleansing high occurs, and for those who have strong nervous systems and healthier livers and adrenals, the euphoric high can last for days and even weeks, preventing them from feeling the lows.

In many cases, when someone is on a trendy, extreme diet and starts to feel sick, she or he will be told it's a healing reaction. While it's true that we can have natural detox reactions in the right circumstances, if it's a harsh cleanse, then that reaction is not a healing one; it's a sign of too many poisons flooding the system at once. Not only that: when the liver is releasing large, unauthorized levels of poisons due to someone following trendy advice that's not geared to support the body in the right way, the adrenals will keep pouring out that two parts adrenaline to match the toxins. For someone with weakened adrenals, this is extra work that the glands don't need. The opposite of euphoria can occur, with lots of lows as the liver ends up absorbing back most of the poisons. For someone with a sensitive nervous system, it's not beneficial, either: the adrenaline itself, though it's there to stop damage, will start doing damage to the central nervous system over time. You may even experience symptoms such as the shakes, some light tremors, aches and pains, or dizziness.

(This adrenaline–nervous system relationship is one that medical research and science have only detected on a surface level. For example, for people who have Parkinson's disease, doctors don't recommend the use of epinephrine autoinjectors unless a shot is truly critical to saving a life, because they've observed that Parkinson's worsens with use of epinephrine. Well, that's because Parkinson's is neurological, and epinephrine [another word for adrenaline] is hard on the nervous system. The adrenaline–nervous system relationship is also why people with any nervous system symptom or condition, or just sensitive nerves, don't fare well under pressure or stress. Their nerves are so sensitized to adrenaline that they can't keep a "stiff upper lip.")

When experiencing a cleanse, you want it balanced. You're going to feel some highs, you're going to feel some lows, and you want it all moderate and within reason. Everyone has different health issues. Each person may react a little differently to a cleanse. What no one wants is a radical cleanse that has you utterly sick and ill, worse off in the end than when you started. I've seen this happen in the healing world out there for decades. As your body recovers for weeks and weeks afterward, it may feel like the extreme cleanse brought about healing. What's really happening is that you're healing from going too deep in the cleanse. You lose track of the fact that you're just trying to get back to

where you were before the cleanse—and so do a lot of the experts and health professionals who advocate these extreme cleanses.

One thing you want from any cleanse is a quick recovery. When the liver is forced to cleanse at a rapid rate, the adrenal glands can weaken faster, making it more difficult for someone to recover from a cleanse. The weaker the adrenals were to begin with, the longer the recovery takes. With adrenaline rushing through your system to address the toxins that have been pushed out of the liver, loss of sleep can occur, too, which can stress the adrenals even more. During an extreme cleanse, people often don't sleep as much as usual because they're wired on adrenaline. Afterward, they'll often sleep more than ever because their adrenals need to recover.

We have to protect our peppers—that is, our adrenal glands. No two are the same, not even inside the same person. While it's easy to assume that they're identical, and they may look the same when observed, the truth is that on a micro level, in size and shape, each is unique. Just like peppers, where two fruits on the same vine can have different curves and shades and heat and number of seeds, two adrenal glands are always a little different. I've seen thousands of adrenals over the decades, and in any given person no two are equal in strength. One of our adrenals is always weaker than the other—or, if you prefer the glass as half full, one is always stronger. I say this because it's important to know that when doing cleanses—and with any cleanse, the liver will be involved—the weaker adrenal is going to have to work even harder to produce the amount of adrenaline called for by the amount of poison being released. In fact, with anything we do in life, that weaker adrenal gland is going to have to work a little harder. It's that much more important, then, to take care of the pair. In addition to the healing information in Part IV of this book, you'll find more on how to do that in the chapter "Adrenal Fatigue" in *Medical Medium*.

ADRENALINE NEUTRALIZATION

Let's look more closely at the adrenaline-liver relationship in our everyday lives when we aren't going through cleanses. Whenever there's excess adrenaline in the bloodstream, the liver must try to absorb and neutralize the hormone, and that's both a miraculous process and a big job: sometimes too big a job if we're not careful.

Though *stress* is usually considered a bad word, a certain amount of it is actually good. It keeps us motivated and moving forward and engaged with what I call our *purpose-plus*. As I mentioned at the beginning of this chapter, a certain amount of adrenaline, too, is healthy and natural. (For critical information on using stress to your advantage, see *Life-Changing Foods*.) It's an overabundance of stress as well as overstimulation, dangerous cleanses, adrenaline-rush activities, and going too long between meals, that trigger our adrenals to squeeze out continual spurts of excess adrenaline, which are toxic and corrosive to the nervous system and the rest of the body if left unchecked. (The adrenals also release cortisol, which is like the good kid tagging along with the bad kid, adrenaline. When adrenaline is neutralized and behaves, cortisol evens out and becomes more reasonable and useful. If cortisol is hanging out with adrenaline on the night before Halloween, chances are cortisol is going to follow its lead and throw around eggs and toilet paper rolls.) Let's always remember that the toxic, corrosive nature of unchecked excess adrenaline is not because our bodies are out to get us. Without adrenaline's lifesaving functions, we wouldn't be here. It's what we're up against in this demanding world, not a flaw of our bodies, that's responsible for the floods of adrenaline we face.

Immune cells such as lymphocytes, monocytes, basophils, and neutrophils throughout the entire body are counting on the liver when adrenaline comes rushing out of the adrenal glands. These components of the immune system are nervous, and they run and hide because they don't want to be scorched. They know they're at risk of getting injured and hindered by adrenaline, so they're relying on the liver to take the hit. The liver's immune system must be the strongest and smartest in the body, with highly intelligent white blood cells protected by a filmy shield produced by a chemical function of the liver that is undiscovered by medical research and science and that uses an amino acid, a unique mineral salt, and a liver cell protein to help the immune cells withstand being scorched by adrenaline to a degree.

A liver in good working order can indeed protect the spleen and the entire immune system. In response to adrenaline surges, the liver—gracious, courageous savior of the body—acts as a sponge. Adrenaline enters in virtually any possible way, flowing into the liver through the hepatic portal vein and the hepatic artery, getting absorbed through pores all around the liver, as well as entering from adjacent lymphatic vessels. It doesn't have manners. It doesn't knock on the door; it breaks it down. The liver absorbs the surplus hormone to prevent damage elsewhere. It's a sacrifice, since adrenaline doesn't help out liver lobule elves. Excess adrenaline that your liver soaks up is also enemy to your liver's personalized immune system. An alarm bell rings (different from the alarm when the liver releases too many poisons at once) to alert your body that your liver's immune system is compromised and that many tasks need to be taken care of immediately, like liver immune cells running to protect important assets as a mother would run to a baby in a flood. The elves start *hup-two*-ing, and a miraculous chemical function starts to take action, producing a natural solvent-like agent that works to protect us.

The building blocks of this chemical compound are old, nonuseful hormones that the liver has collected, neutralized, and altered over time. These are normal hormones the body produced in the past, such as sex hormones and stress hormones, that lived out their original purpose, as well as hormones that we get from troublemaker foods such as eggs and dairy. Whenever the liver finds these rogue hormones in the bloodstream, its plasma-producing cells trap them, defuse them, and break them down to prepare them for their new, critical responsibility.

The next time we have an adrenal spike, they have a chance to live out that responsibility: when the alarm bell rings, the liver plasma cells activate and set free the old hormones, setting off the chemical reaction that transforms them into that solvent-like agent. Say you're experiencing a lot of fear or stress; falling in love; falling out of love; or going through anger, betrayal, hurt, sorrow, worry, or life's ups and downs, whether good or bad. Your adrenal glands are going to react by spurting out lots of cortisol and adrenaline to support you with fight-or-flight stamina. The body knows that the price you'll pay for that support is the damage too much of these hormones can do on a physical, mental, or even soul level. If rogue adrenaline touches a precious white blood cell from the liver's immune system, it will injure it. If rogue adrenaline touches the brain or intestinal lining, it will damage them. If it gets into the bones,

it can cause them to become fragile and thin. Alopecia—caused by the adrenals becoming weakened, getting out of balance in their hormone production, and underproducing a specific hormone—can worsen as adrenaline spikes weaken the glands further. Adrenaline spikes can exacerbate existing depression or bring it on in the first place. It can also fuel pathogens inside the liver, including viruses such as EBV, shingles, and HHV-6. There's one agent that can stop all this, the balance built in to the body to prevent damage: the new chemical compound formed from old, reconstructed hormones.

Once released, this agent's job is to be both bait and trap for the fresh, excess cortisol and adrenaline. These new, rogue hormones sense familiarity in the old ones and gravitate toward them with the idea that they'll be stronger together. If you don't think a hormone can think for itself, think again. Within biochemicals such as hormones is immeasurable data that cannot be decoded by the science or computers of today and will never be. If the human race survives the hatred, greed, and jealousy that propels it into wars and other acts of destruction and we're still around a thousand years from now, they still won't have it decoded. The amount of information inside a hormone is so vast that it's like its own universe. Some of that information directs hormones to be guided by the energy of the body and plugged in to the energy of the human soul. It's why hormones are so tied up in emotions—and one reason why adrenaline is released when your soul is scared.

When the new and old hormones bump up against each other, the old hormones' gluey quality grabs on to the new hormones like a sticky floor. Less quick and agile now, the new hormones become stuck; those old hormones bind onto them like nothing else can. It's a case of like fighting like, as when people cleanse their faces with oil or use mushrooms to heal a fungal problem. When these like hormones bind into each other—the fresh, excess stress hormones from episodes of raw, intense emotions or other extreme experiences binding with the old, stored hormones that have been remade—a miraculous chemical reaction occurs. They become one.

Together, these hormones are quite the pair. The fresh adrenaline and cortisol spark life into the old hormones, while the old hormones spark death into the fresh ones, dying down the information of fear, chaos, loss, betrayal, hurt, sorrow, and pressure. The end result is that the old hormones defuse the new ones. They're the roller coaster ride stoppers. They're the brick wall. Bonded together, a balance occurs. The liver now detects the excess adrenaline and cortisol as being within an acceptable neutral zone, no longer dangerous and therefore ready to be excreted or flushed out to the kidneys— if the liver is working very well and at the top of its game.

As you know by now, this isn't always the case. When the liver gets overloaded for any of the various reasons described in this book, its capacity to neutralize adrenaline and cortisol diminishes. Its ability to be the protective parent wanes. In an in-between state, the liver is still able to process some of the old hormone, and then it's forced to store the rest. If the liver is more beaten down, then it will store nearly all of the bonded hormone compound in special compartments within itself. That storage is in the hopes that someday the liver will catch a break and get a chance to release the compound for elimination from your body. When the liver doesn't catch that break, the bonded hormone compound becomes another stagnant waste item taking up space inside the organ. As you read about in Chapter 12, when the liver has

too much to store, the result is usually weight gain. When weakened, the liver can also lose its ability to perform its hormone neutralization responsibility. It will still help out as much as it can, though it won't be perfect, leaving some of the adrenaline free to do its caustic damage to the liver and beyond.

So many people who experience a time of betrayal, jealousy, hurt, pain, sorrow, negligence, irresponsible or narcissistic treatment, or another adrenal release will experience a bout of adrenal fatigue afterward. Or the digestive system will get sensitive as the liver weakens in the moment, busy soaking up adrenaline—not to mention that any un-neutralized adrenaline that gets by is extremely corrosive to the intestinal linings and stomach. Because of the fuel that unchecked adrenaline is to pathogens, it's not uncommon to be listless and fatigued, and experience malaise—to have a small bout of low-grade mono from awakened EBV or a low-grade shingles outbreak or even small eczema flare—after a tough situation such as the loss of a loved one, a broken heart, or a bad breakup with a friend or partner. The liver's immune system that usually keeps viruses such as EBV contained weakens in those moments of adrenal stress.

During an extreme cleanse, the liver is faced with a choice amid a storm of competing alarm bells: release old, stored-up hormones to go and bind onto all the excess adrenaline and neutralize it so it won't do its caustic damage, or don't, because the brain signaled the adrenals to release that adrenaline for a reason, to shield the body from the poisons forced out of the liver. The adrenaline is there as an intentional shock to the system, like a shot from an epinephrine autoinjector delivered after a bee sting, there to act as an anti-inflammatory to stop the body's reaction to the venom. The liver, ever the mama bear, knows what's most important in this case, to let the adrenaline do its job, and so it makes that critical move of holding back the stored hormones that would defuse the adrenaline. Doing so, the liver must take the hit of a lifetime when the adrenaline eventually comes flooding into the liver at full strength through the bloodstream. It's one reason why you can't always trust a liver cleanse to be liver-friendly. If it's a man-made cleanse derived from myths and theories and it has poisons dumping out of your liver by the bucketful, causing twice that amount of adrenaline to be pumped out to match it, then your liver is absorbing the full hit of active adrenaline along with the poisons that have left the liver, and that's very liver-unfriendly indeed.

It would be easy to think that a diet high in fat provides a buffer in the bloodstream from toxic adrenaline. Quite the contrary. Instead, fat suspends the adrenaline, keeping it in the body long term. Unable to be sponged up, defused, stored, or eliminated through the urine as it usually is, this fat-suspended adrenaline holds on to the information that went along with its release. That means a fatty liver or sluggish liver, which translates to extra fat in the bloodstream, also keeps heightened emotions active, like the moment at the office when you found out that you'd been left out of a critical meeting. It's a secret to why we sometimes find ourselves unable to let go of certain grievances. Clean up the liver and let go of the fat, and the liver can finally process the adrenaline to shield you from reliving the experience over and over again.

STRONGER FOR IT

Our adrenal glands and livers are incredibly resilient when we do the right thing. If you're not aware of how your adrenals and liver coexist, then you can make more mistakes and step on more land mines. The adrenals especially are extremely forgiving. Realizing how they function during cleanses and hard times is how we discover ways to take a little better care of them. Sometimes just a little attention, a little understanding, can go a long way.

It's when people don't understand how the adrenals work that they get on a slippery slope of trouble. What holds so many back is that the attempted insights into the adrenals out there don't make sense, because these glands are barely understood in the first place. You can only be stronger for the information here. The knowledge alone of the liver's role in supporting the adrenals can strengthen the glands.

When you take it a step further and look out for your liver with the different measures in this book, you look out for your adrenals and save them from stress. It's not about living in a bubble and avoiding every conflict or difficult emotion. You have a fundamental right to go through those challenges. You also have a fundamental right to access the wisdom they offer and to walk away better for them, not weaker. Our bodies know how to do this—if we can only witness and work with their true needs.

CHAPTER 20

Chemical and Food Sensitivities

Chemical sensitivities are incredibly frustrating for the people who deal with them. Part of that is physical suffering. The other large part is encountering an unsympathetic world. The average person who's never had to deal with a sensitivity will view someone with sensitivities as the ultimate hypochondriac or just think they're stark crazy. Unless there's a visible allergic reaction, like someone with a peanut allergy being rushed to the hospital after turning blue from a closed throat that's blocking airways, it's hard for an observer who hasn't been there to identify. (A peanut allergy is really a toxin sensitivity, by the way.) Anaphylactic shock, asthma attacks, hives—these reactions only describe one segment of the population. Chemical sensitivity sufferers' reactions are very often invisible to the outside eye, making it challenging for these people to find advocates. Instead, they're often told that they're making up their sensitivities or looking for attention, or that it's a psychological problem. They may be treated with an eye roll or a sigh or teasing. They may even be told they're attracting or manifesting the issue.

What we really need to do is find compassion. The people who deal with chemical sensitivities know how real they are. They're very, very

difficult. When the sensitivities are moderate to extreme, individuals will often confine themselves to home because it feels like the only safe place. Some are in a catch-22 because the house or apartment where they live sets off their sensitivities, too, whether because of a lingering carpet cleaning fragrance, outgassing construction materials, or another chemical presence in the home. Since the outside world has its own threats, often unpredictable ones, these people feel they have nowhere safe to go.

A DIFFERENT WORLD

Chemical sensitivities tend to vary from person to person and also from time to time for the same person. It's almost as if these sensitivities move and shift, and the condition alters. Out of nowhere, you may need to change soaps. One minute you're sensitive to perfume, the next it's hairspray, and if you've never been sensitive to your own all-natural shampoo, next thing you know, you could be. The inconsistency and unpredictability are part of the difficulty.

You may be one of those people who finds your sensitivity manageable. You've learned, for example, to avoid plug-in air fresheners when you can, and you get by. That's a mild sensitivity. Then there's the person who has to avoid multiple items. Conventional hairsprays, colognes, perfumes, candles, fragranced detergents, fabric softener, cleaning solutions, and, yes, air fresheners (which many people can't tolerate and rightfully so, because they're extremely toxic) become the enemy—just a whiff is debilitating. The hypervigilance required makes it so much more difficult to operate. Where are you going? To the house of a friend who uses conventional toxic cleaners, a plug-in air freshener, and chemically treated potpourri? How are you going to function? There's an activator around every corner. Even Christmas trees are sprayed with a concoction to keep them green as long as possible. Even *fake* Christmas trees are treated with nanotechnology solutions that can set someone off.

Those who are chemically sensitive are forced to become experts, and always to be mindful. What they view through their eyes is an entirely different world from what someone else may see. Anyone with chemical (or food) sensitivities has had to leave behind their rose-colored glasses. They must dedicate an immense amount of energy and time to reading labels, finding out what's truly in every product they come across, and researching ingredients' origins. They must be cautious about new carpets and furniture as well as home projects that involve paint, caulk, lubricant, or sealant. They must call ahead to hotels with special requests for hypoallergenic rooms, still with no guarantee that upon opening that hotel room door they won't be blasted with scent. Some chemical sensitivity sufferers are better educated than engineers and even chemists. While a chemist may be at the highest level in her area of expertise, she may also be wearing clothes saturated with multiple synthetic laundry chemicals, use air fresheners leaching out oils with unknown effects on humans, and hop in her car that was just detailed and wiped down with chemicals to make the leather shine and outfitted with its own dangling air freshener. Then that weekend she may decide to paint her house with high-VOC paint and later pour gasoline into her lawn mower, spill some on her hands, then mow the lawn and breathe in the exhaust. The chemically sensitive person is actually better versed in all the harmful exposures to which the chemist has just subjected herself. If someone mentioned the exposures to the chemist, she may say, "What doesn't kill you makes you stronger." That may make sense in other areas of life. Not in this one.

Those who are newly chemically sensitive have a very tough time of it. First, there's the process of becoming aware that something's wrong. It can create a tremendous amount of confusion. Headaches for the first time in your life, a funny taste in your mouth or a tingly tongue in certain settings, getting tired easily while walking through a department store and breathing in thousands of synthetic chemicals, or starting to feel a tight chest in the workplace from fragrances in the air day in and day out—these aren't fun symptoms to develop. Newbies have a difficult challenge, both with finding a doctor who doesn't say, "It's all in your head," or want to shove you in the Lyme disease trap, and with finding support from family and friends, who may be bewildered or become sick of it all quite fast since everything was fine before. Your bodily reactions aren't easy, and neither are the reactions you get from others. "Why can't you be like everybody else in the world who's living life, putting on makeup and perfume (or cologne and aftershave), going to the salon, breathing in car exhaust, and shopping at the mall with no complaints?" For anyone who's navigating a fresh sensitivity, this new reality can feel very limiting.

Then we have the people who are already experts. They discovered their sensitivities years ago, they know what they can and can't handle, they know what boundaries they can push—and still, it's unpredictable. They can go through times of feeling better and handling more and then waves of being able to tolerate less. It's a game of chance.

We can't confuse chemical sensitivities with reactions to obviously harmful chemicals. We're not talking here about highly regulated chemicals like those known to visibly burn the skin. We're talking about substances you can't see, hear, or feel—ones that many people can't even smell. How does someone develop a sensitivity to the invisible? What occurs? It all stems from the liver—and that's one truth that not even chemically sensitive people know yet.

All sufferers have their guesses about why it happened to them; they often have a landmark. Some people believe it all started the day they got sprayed by a pesticide while walking through a condominium park. Some people think it started the day they ate a certain food. Some say it was the day they had their house painted. Yes, these experiences can be triggers, and the realization that something's wrong can occur at these times—they aren't the whole story, though. What about the other person who got sprayed walking through the condo park that day and not only was he fine, he went to the hardware store, purchased his own pesticides, sprayed them on his own lawn, and didn't develop a chemical sensitivity? Maybe it could happen down the road for him, though not yet. That wasn't his landmark. For the person who did develop a sensitivity, it was about what was going on internally. The timing of that day in the

park was random. The sensitivity was going to happen anyway—it had already begun.

CHEMICAL SENSITIVITY SECRETS

It all starts with the liver, the big sponge of the body whose job it is to collect, catalogue, and keep in check thousands of troublemakers, both from the outside world and created within your body, in order to shield you. It's natural for the body to create toxic substances—for example, when you experience fear, the adrenals pump out that form of adrenaline that helps with survival in the moment and yet is so potent that the liver must clean it up as soon as it's done its job in order to protect the rest of your body from its caustic nature. We also eat foods with ingredients that are hard on the liver, whether toxic grease or invisible toxic chemicals. On cruise ships, the food is sprayed down with chemical agents to preserve it, and our livers must contend with that. Any type of drugs we ingest or shots we receive, going all the way back to antibiotics taken in childhood, give the liver more to process and contain. Pathogens, including EBV, find their way inside the liver, make a home, and create a mess all on their own, releasing waste matter such as dermatoxins, neurotoxins, and byproduct.

With all these troublemakers and more, your liver is in a constant ratio game. How much is coming in through the air you breathe and the germs you're exposed to and the rogue viral toxins that have escaped back into the bloodstream and the foods, drinks, and medicines you ingest? How much can the liver afford to let go for elimination from your body, released when you go to the bathroom, without overloading your system? That ratio of what's going into the liver versus what can go out is forever in play.

For many people, there aren't a lot of toxins leaving. The liver is sluggish, the colon is already dirty, and yet more poisons keep coming in from toxic food sources, fresh paint, a visit to a store filled with scented candles, an air freshener plugged into a dentist's waiting room wall, a delivery truck spewing exhaust as it idles in your driveway, the carpet cleaning in your office over the weekend, the fire-retardant chemicals sprayed on new clothes you just bought. The liver can't let go as fast as the poisons enter. Then a trigger finally pushes the liver over the edge. It could be a visit to the dentist's office to get a mercury filling drilled out, which outgasses mercury into your system (for more on this, see *Medical Medium*). It could be that walk through the condo park, getting hit with toxic weed killer. When the body has reached this too-toxic place—over time—and the liver has grown too sluggish to keep it all in check—again, over time—chemical sensitivity starts. The final triggers aren't the cause; they're the liver's last straw.

A sensitive central nervous system is behind chemical sensitivities. Toxins that the liver can't neutralize or contain overload the nervous system to the point that it eventually becomes sensitive or even allergic to certain poisons. This can take the form of funny feelings in the mouth, the sense that you can't breathe deeply or "right," blurry eyes, chronic headaches or migraines, fatigue, tingles and numbness, insomnia, dizziness, anxiety, depression, and more. Some of these symptoms can happen independently, for example as a result of EBV neurotoxins going after the nervous system. Chemical sensitivity can also cause all of it. If the liver weren't already overloaded and the scale weren't tipped so much—and if a given person didn't have an active EBV infection or another major problem—then a chemical sensitivity

wouldn't develop from one bad encounter. The switch would not be flipped.

Often, neurotoxins and dermatoxins from EBV *combined* with certain toxins stored inside the liver create chemical sensitivities. For a person who has EBV without the right kind of toxic heavy metals or pesticides in the liver, a chemical sensitivity may not develop. While she or he may deal with a sensitive central nervous system from the virus, that individual won't have the chemical sensitivity component. Neurotoxins and dermatoxins excreted by EBV that's consuming the right kind of poisons in the liver, on the other hand, weaken the nervous system further. They give someone extra eye sensitivities (including light sensitivity), brain fog, dizziness, tingles on the tongue, and numbness in the hands. People will think it's the chemicals they just breathed in—the incense in a store or air freshener in a bathroom or cloud of hairspray at the salon—directly causing this. In reality, the virus system has already fed off enough poisons in the liver to make them sensitive, so when there's an outside stimulus like a synthetic fragrance, the nervous system reacts instantly.

This unknown combination of factors happening beneath the surface really confuses medical research and science when they try to figure out the causes of chemical sensitivities. Doctors and other practitioners need to keep an open mind and learn that in most chemical sensitivity patients, the central nervous system is weakened and a viral infection could be playing a very large part in that. Not every chemically sensitive person is dealing with an active viral infection. Many have been sprayed or injured by certain chemicals and the body has developed a hyperawareness, causing the hypersensitivity sensations.

All of the above is why two different people can have two wildly different outcomes from the same exposure. It all depends on where someone is in her or his life in that moment—how much burden is on the liver, how limited the liver has become in eliminating poisons, what kind of viral activity is present, and how sensitive the person has become without knowing it. Many people can have a chemical sensitivity for a long time before they realize what's going on. When a sensitivity makes itself known, an emotional component kicks in that makes the physical suffering harder. *What could trigger it next? Is it getting better? Worse? Am I dying?* Many people can't put a finger on what that final push into sensitivity was, and that mystery makes it tough, too. Fear heightens, and a form of obsessive-compulsive disorder (OCD) develops from what they go through.

Freedom comes from knowing that it's not a single or silent trigger that turns your life upside down overnight. It's a slow build, which means it can be deconstructed. Healing from chemical sensitivities is about patience and understanding. It takes two focuses: caring for the liver and caring for the nervous system. I'm not blind to the fact that chemically sensitive people have difficulty detoxing. Many can't even take a single supplement in order to try to soothe the nervous system or detox the liver, because they're so sensitive. If this is you, don't think you're stuck. Food is the answer in this case—take care of your liver and nervous system carefully with food.

FOOD SENSITIVITY SECRETS

If you're someone with a lot of food reactions, I know what a difficult time you have of it. Every day, it must seem, a food you used to be okay with gives you a funny new sensation. Many people are told this is mold-related when the

reality is that yet again, it's a viral issue heightening chemical sensitivities: that is, an abundance of EBV neurotoxins taking chemical sensitivities to a new level. In some cases, it's because the food itself is viral fuel. If it's a troublemaker food, it can feed EBV, creating more neurotoxins that inflame the digestive tract.

People with a hypersensitive central nervous system also tend to have hypersensitive intestinal linings. One reason is that their adrenaline tends to get released more often, because their senses are heightened as they scan their every surrounding for triggers. When you walk into a store that you think could affect you, you can get nervous—rightfully so, given your past exposures and reactions—and that nervousness can trigger the adrenals to jump in and defend you, with a mild fight-or-flight occurring. Same if you're concerned about superbugs and you walk into a hospital to visit a friend. You're going to go in there with heightened anxiety, which is going to get the adrenals releasing adrenaline. Over time, this increased amount of adrenaline oversaturates the liver, as you've read about, and can also saturate the intestinal linings, giving them a mild scorching. The thousands and thousands of nerves in the intestinal linings can become inflamed and exposed, with nerve receptors irritated.

Eating different foods, you may experience discomfort as they rub the intestinal linings, touching all these sensitive nerves. It's easy to have a fearful response when this happens. Someone may say, "I can't eat lettuce—I react—but eggs are okay." The irony is that lettuce actually helps to massage intestinal linings, loosening debris and other pockets of waste matter so they can be eliminated and not provide viral fuel, while eggs feed pathogens such as EBV, resulting in more neurotoxins, eventually creating more chemical and food sensitivities.

Eggs feel good going down because they travel down the middle of the intestinal tract, turning into smooth, liquefied glue. Lettuce, on the other hand, starves EBV. Part of its magic lies in brushing the intestinal linings, yet with irritated nerve receptors there, it can easily feel like you're having a reaction to it. Ultimately, lettuce soothes nerves; the milky substance in its core has an overall tranquilizing, sedative effect.

Apples are another food that people commonly worry they can no longer eat. In truth, apple sensitivities trace back to someone biting into an apple covered with wax and pesticides that hadn't been washed off first. When that happens, the tongue will instantly pick up on the chemicals, and sensitive trigeminal and vagus nerves, which connect with the mouth, will trigger a reaction that may include itchiness, tingles, numbness, or a burning sensation. Chemically sensitive people who've experienced this often have to stay away from apples for a little while and then may find that if their nerves calm down, they can try an organic apple, peeled if needed, without having a reaction.

It can seem like a vicious cycle, where you're sometimes reacting to the very foods you know should offer relief. If that's the case for you, go slowly with bringing in special foods from Chapter 37 and use your energy to focus on avoiding as many of the liver troublemakers from Chapter 36 as you can, particularly the troublemaking foods in that list, to see progress. Turn to the chapter on hidden PTSD in *Medical Medium* if you need moral support. Above all, remember that you can still heal. Nobody with a chemical or food sensitivity is barred from feeling better someday. When you tend to your liver and nervous system, there is hope.

YOU'RE NOT THE PROBLEM

If your nervous system is very sensitive, you may still react to certain exposures after you heal. You'll still have to follow certain boundaries and rules that you decide for yourself. Walking into a linen store, for example, you may still get a headache or feel wiped out from the chemicals used to treat the fabric. What will improve is your bounce-back time—and getting back to normal faster makes all the difference.

Here's the thing: You have a right to react to a world that's toxic. You're not the problem; the toxic chemicals and constant stressors are. Sensitivity is a value—you're the canary in the coal mine. Even if your sensitivities go away completely with liver and nervous system care, they've left you with a gift: a heightened awareness of the perils of our world so that you can better protect yourself and your family for the future.

CHAPTER 21

Methylation Problems

If you've ever heard that you have a gene mutation that's responsible for methylation issues, it must have felt like an instant judgment that you have a faulty, destructive, unsupportive element of both your body and who you are. You might have been prescribed certain vitamins and other supplements meant to support the ability to methylate properly, though that likely didn't take away the feeling of defeat. When there's something making you feel unwell, that's hard enough to bear on its own. Add to that the gloom of being told you were born with an unfixable gene issue, or that a gene mutation problem mysteriously developed along the way, and that makes matters much worse—especially since this isn't true.

Methylation dysfunction isn't a gene problem. It's not a methylenetetrahydrofolate reductase (MTHFR) gene mutation; a gene mutation cannot cause a methylation compromise, breakdown, or disorder. A methylation issue is much bigger and different from popular recent beliefs in the alternative and conventional medicine worlds. Here, we're going to explore the truth of what causes a methylation problem and what causes a misreading on a gene test.

WHAT METHYLATION MEANS

First, what does methylation really mean? It's the body's ability to receive, absorb, and assimilate key, critical nutrients that we get through healthy foods as well as from water we drink, water that touches our skin, sun exposure, and fresh, clean air. When we take in a phytochemical, vitamin, mineral, or other nutrient, our body alters its chemical structure to fit perfectly to what we need most. It's a process that breaks down, alters, and makes nutrients more bioactive so they can benefit us in a more profound way.

Mainly, methylation is a miraculous role that your liver plays—day in and day out, during both your waking and sleeping hours. Your liver does it with the help of your ileum, a small piece of digestive real estate at the end of your small intestine, just before the colon. In order to convert nutrients for your body's best use, your liver and ileum work with each other, play with each other, rely on each other, communicate with each other, and back each other up. When one is hurting, the other will try to help.

Hepatic portal vessels draw critical nutrients from the ileum to the liver, with capillaries coming off the ileum and flowing into the portal system so they can end up in the liver's good hands. When the ileum is not functioning well, most any nutrients coming into the portal vessels from the ileum are diminished, and the liver is left to cope.

TESTING: NOT WHAT IT SEEMS

When an MTHFR mutation test comes back positive for an MTHFR gene mutation, a patient ends up with a diagnosis of a gene mutation, commonly of C677T or A1298C. It seems to make all the sense in the world that a gene mutation test would tell you if you have a gene mutation. Here's the thing: it's not actually a gene mutation. The gene is not injured or mutated or altered, even though we're told that's what the test determined. Not only is the testing process itself fallible; it doesn't accurately measure for a mutated gene. Just because science is able to view DNA under a microscope doesn't mean that's what they're doing here. (And when they do look at genes in other circumstances, it doesn't mean that they understand everything about them.)

All "gene mutation" tests are just testing for the presence of inflammation—not what's causing it, not what it really means, only its markers. What can be a positive aspect of testing is if it identifies that you have elevated homocysteine levels and an issue around methylation. If you've ever had a homocysteine test, you'll notice that in your blood work, it's listed under inflammation. It's good to uncover inflammation and methylation issues if they're happening. People with chemical sensitivities have methylation problems, too, and that can trigger a positive on a gene mutation test and/or show up as elevated homocysteine levels.

At the same time, this positive side of gene mutation testing is not enough to override the negative aspect, which is the damage that can occur to someone's mind and body when told she or he has faulty genes. You would think that the faulty gene answer gives people relief, because it's presented as an answer. Truth is, it doesn't give relief because it's not an answer. It's a deception and a detour into the world of medical bureaucracy to avoid finding the real truth of why chronic illness is elevating rapidly on a global scale. Be prepared to see everywhere—in ads, commercials, studies, reports, articles, books—that genes are responsible for everything. It's an endless campaign.

If you've received an MTHFR gene mutation diagnosis, you need to let go of the gene mutation part and hold on to the methylation issue part and focus on resolving the true cause of that in order to improve your health. Know the truth of why testing even showed a gene mutation: that it picked up on markers of inflammation, not a mutation itself.

HOW RIGHT GOES WRONG

How does a methylation problem occur, and what happens when it does? As we touched on, one of your liver's over 2,000 functions is the ability to change and convert nutrients to more usable, available, bioidentical forms so you can get the most out of what you're eating to survive. For example, if you eat a spinach salad, those spinach leaves are filled with various B vitamins. Those B vitamins can be helpful in their natural, original state. At the same time, your liver is aware of your body's needs in the moment. So if you're depleted because of, for example, elevated adrenaline from intense stress or an illness developing somewhere within your body, your liver will find and enhance the specific B vitamin you need out of the many that spinach gracefully offers. While medical research and science know about the basic existence of methylation, no one knows that in the methylation process, your liver takes "superfoods" to a whole new level, with your ileum playing a great role much of the time, creating supervitamins and other supernutrients from regular nutrients. This incredible chemical process that's accomplished by your body, not a science lab, makes nutrition so much more viable and easier for the rest of your body to use than it would be otherwise.

Another remarkable aspect of this process is that ahead of time, before you ever ate the spinach salad, your liver documented the need for that particular B vitamin. When the vitamin came, the liver could put it right to use. At the same time, your liver looks out for those nutrients it knows you'll need on the rainy days and dry spells of adrenaline rushes, sickness, and other challenges, such as getting exposed to pesticides, fresh paint, or other troublemakers. As you eat your salad, your liver is storing up other B vitamins (as well as other nutrients in the spinach) that it knows will come in handy one day. What it collects is all very specific to you and your needs—someone else's liver will store a different balance of nutrients from what your liver stores for you. Your liver continues to rely on you to make nutrients available to it on an ongoing basis. So if you're not eating spinach salads and other nourishing foods, where's the liver going to get the nuts and bolts it relies on to make methylated supercompounds to store and then deliver through the bloodstream to areas of your body that are in desperate need?

One vitamin that's critical to your body's ability to methylate many other nutrients is vitamin B_{12}. In truth, the body relies on B_{12} for tens of thousands of daily functions. It's like flour for a pastry chef—without it, none of the items in the bakery case could be made, least of all the prized wedding cake. The liver relies on this B vitamin and stores large quantities of it, delving into it continually as part of regular organ function. It also relies on B_{12} for a function the liver can perform when it's out of stock of essentials: the ability to produce trace amounts of certain nutrients and chemical compounds on its own. Your master chef, the liver, can only do this when it has its key ingredient, B_{12}, in enough supply to send it out to your brain, the rest of your nervous system, your heart, and other places in your body that desperately need it.

You may remember from Part I that under ideal circumstances, vitamin B_{12} is one of those nutrients that will travel from the ileum to the liver. Even before that, the B_{12} methylation process will happen in the ileum. The liver relies on that manufacture and methylation of B_{12}. When the liver is running low on all of the nutrients it needs, even B_{12}, the precious glue that holds it all together, the liver will excrete a chemical compound into your bile to travel through the intestinal tract and deliver a message down to your ileum. If all is as it should be, here at your ileum is a goldmine of B_{12}. In fact, it's better than a mine; it's actually a B_{12} production center. Rare microorganisms called *elevated biotics* (which you get from eating fresh, raw, organic, unwashed or lightly washed produce like cucumbers and leafy greens straight from the garden or farm) live only here in your ileum, and they're also responsible for producing the ultimate methylated form of B_{12} that absorbs into the channels of your body and finds its way back to your liver when called for, through capillaries that lead to the portal vessel system.

This B_{12} is the liver's number-one most important mortar to hold together all the bricks that build the castle of your health. When there's enough of it, the liver stores ample amounts to send into the bloodstream as an assistant to almost every vitamin, mineral, and other nutrient that it releases to aid your body in any way. It's the B_{12} that makes everything go right—the catalyst, the magic carpet, the royalty that blesses us with vitality. That medical research and science have discovered it is a triumph. That's where the progress stopped. It's like discovering an indigenous culture and deciding there's no need to take the time to study its language or learn from its ways. There's so much more for the medical world to uncover about B_{12}.

Your liver is aware of what your ileum is doing, and your ileum is aware of what your liver is doing. They talk to each other; they communicate; they transfer information back and forth. When all is well, they work in perfect harmony to make sure that you don't lose your ability to methylate properly or receive and use critical methylated nutrients, all with the goal of making sure you don't end up with a nutritional deficiency. The harmony goes right until it goes wrong. When you lose your ability to methylate properly, it's common to receive a diagnosis of an MTHFR gene mutation. You may find a great practitioner who offers you recommendations such as good supplements to take, and that can be helpful. It doesn't tell you what went south to give you this diagnosis, though, and it certainly doesn't make you feel like you have the power to change your fate—not when it seems to be written in scientific stone that your faulty genes are to blame and there's no way to change them.

The methylation process goes awry when your liver becomes overfilled with sludge along the way. A percentage of that sludge could have been passed down from your parents, and then as time went by, your liver collected more gunk. It's the same usual suspects that you've seen throughout this book, including herbicides, pesticides such as old DDT still in the environment from years past, toxic heavy metals, antibiotics, other prescription drugs, and problematic

foods, that make your liver struggle in this case. These troublemakers alone are not enough to land you with one of the MTHFR gene mutation misdiagnoses, though; you need one more critical component: a virus.

That's right—it takes a virus in the mix to cause a true methylation disorder. Not just any virus; a virus in the herpetic family. This includes shingles, HHV-6, and even cytomegalovirus, though the main culprit is EBV. The virus, which for some is passed down from parents, can quietly live its life inside the liver, slowly building its numbers there and excreting poisonous viral waste. The viral waste buildup in the liver, together with the other liver troublemakers there, can cause the organ to become sluggish, which hinders its ability to communicate with the ileum properly and efficiently, store enough B_{12}, and prepare and deliver B_{12} throughout the body. As the liver becomes burdened over time, it needs more help from the ileum, which in turn overworks itself. If our diet isn't good and we don't choose foods wisely, the ileum will lose its capacity to create its own variety and coenzyme of methylated B_{12} for the survival of us and our liver.

It's this troublesome combination of the liver not having enough B_{12} already on hand, no B_{12} coming from the ileum's production line, and the liver being too compromised to produce B_{12} for itself that brings on a methylation condition at its worst. When the liver sends the other stored nutrients into the bloodstream for other organs to use, there won't be that glue, that pastry chef's flour—that bioavailable, perfectly prepared, methylated B_{12}—to come with them for maximum absorption that helps prevent deficiencies. Even if you get a blood test that shows high levels of B_{12} in your bloodstream, this doesn't mean enough B_{12} is present in your organs, central nervous system, and other important areas of your body. Medical research and science are unaware that the central nervous system and rest of the body can be deficient in B$_{12}$ even when it's high in the bloodstream. That high reading is also no reflection of the viability of that B$_{12}$—how methylated or usable it is. In fact, a large amount of B$_{12}$ in the bloodstream can indicate that the body isn't able to put it into use.

(By the way, while taking a supplement of methylated B$_{12}$ from a vitamin lab is good, and we need it when our body processes break down, nothing can compare to the methylation that your body performs when the ileum and liver are given the right tools to work as they should.)

Even when you have all of this going on with the ileum and liver, it doesn't automatically trigger a positive on an MTHFR gene mutation test or result in elevated homocysteine levels. That happens when someone has been viral for long enough that the liver can't hold on to all of the viral waste anymore. At this point, the small cloud of the virus's poisonous byproduct, viral casings, neurotoxins, and even dermatoxins leach into the bloodstream, elevating homocysteine levels and dirtying the blood.

Ultimately, it's dirty blood that's the true trigger for a positive on today's faulty MTHFR gene mutation tests. What those tests really detect are elevated inflammation markers due to the blood being filled with poisonous viral waste as well as other toxins such as heavy metals escaping the liver. They're just glorified versions of inflammation tests like the antinuclear antibody (ANA) and C-reactive protein (CRP) tests used to diagnose (and sometimes misdiagnose) chronic conditions such as lupus. (If an MTHFR test isn't triggered and homocysteine levels show up as high, that indicates a lower viral load inside the liver with a higher liver toxin load as well as a worsening condition of the ileum.) Remember: it's the high level of toxic debris, much of it viral,

in the blood that sets off the MTHFR tests, and that spreads the misinformation that your genes are altered and mutated.

CORRELATION, NOT CAUSATION

Oftentimes, MTHFR gene mutations are connected to preeclampsia—so if a woman develops preeclampsia, it will be blamed on a gene mutation. This is a classic case of the medical industry taking two aspects of our health that are not yet fully understood and gluing them together because they happen to be present at the same time. Suddenly, you're being told one causes the other. Medical diagnoses are riddled with these correlation-must-be-causation mistakes for hundreds of conditions. One aspect of your health takes the blame for another when they really have nothing to do with each other—or the connection is not what anyone realizes.

The true cause of preeclampsia is a viral condition. It's EBV sitting inside the liver and parts of the reproductive system such as the uterus. EBV is also what's really responsible for ovarian cysts, fibroids, and many other reproductive conditions and diseases. When a test says that a gene mutation is present, it's an easy source of blame for a problem that no one has understood the cause of all these years. Calling preeclampsia a product of a gene mutation is like having a reaction to a chocolate chip cookie and blaming the distinctive shape of the chocolate chips. The shape of the chips can indicate a certain brand, and that can help us track down its ingredients. It's not the shape itself that's the problem, though; it's only a sign. Positives on gene mutation tests and elevated homocysteine levels are both signs, and we can learn something from them. With today's medical information, we're still far from understanding the truth of what everything means.

Thrombosis is another condition wrongfully connected to gene mutations. The true cause of thrombosis is a stagnant, dysfunctional, sluggish, or even pre-fatty liver that's filled with toxins, viruses, and other pathogens. It's not caused by a gene mutation. This is another huge mistake developing in the medical industry, another example of chronic illness as a free-for-all. With thrombosis, we still need to remember that a weakened liver triggers off a mutation test. Since the liver is also what's responsible for thrombosis, that's why you see the two occur together. They're both products of the same underlying liver issue.

Various conditions are going to be connected more and more with gene mutation tests. Soon, someone could have a sniffle, get a positive on a gene mutation test, and be told that the sniffle is caused by a gene mutation. What no one will hear is that a gene mutation test is just a fancier version of the older inflammation tests. If only blood labs listed MTHFR reductase tests under inflammation, just like homocysteine tests, both doctors and patients would be able to see that they're not directly measuring gene mutations. That change may never happen, because the focus of medical research and science in this day and age is genetics, and that ignores the true causes of hundreds of chronic illnesses. Research and science are so close to making the real connections and finding the real answers—yet getting further and further away.

ALWAYS ON YOUR SIDE

It's true that when the liver and blood have been dirtied to the point of setting off an MTHFR gene mutation test, you likely have a methylation issue, because positives on these tests and dirty blood are both indicators that your liver is too strung out to methylate nutrients properly. What's not true is that there's something wrong with the fiber of your being. I'll keep saying it: Methylation issues are not gene problems. It was always outside troublemaking sources like viruses that were to blame, never your own body. For as long as it could, your liver stayed strong against them to protect you from methylation dysfunction. At a certain point, it became overwhelmed and had to switch over to its life-or-death functions in order to keep you in one piece. Your body was always on your side.

When your liver cleanses, revives, rejuvenates, heals, and strengthens, nutrients will absorb and process properly. They'll function like nutrients are supposed to function in your body. The ileum will strengthen. B_{12} will be more bioavailable. Since methylation problems really come down to how sluggish, clogged, and dysfunctional your liver is—how many pathogens and toxins are stored inside it—when that's addressed, your concerns about correlated diseases can dissipate. You no longer have to worry about what medical research theorizes is a connection between an MTHFR gene mutation and a higher risk of stroke, heart disease, or blood clotting, because you know the truth: that they're about the liver, and you're taking care of your liver. Viral loads that are responsible for preeclampsia, thrombosis, and positives on MTHFR gene mutation tests can decrease. Homocysteine elevations, if they were present, can disappear, and so can other markers of inflammation.

With a healthy liver, you can leave behind the limits of your diagnosis. With this knowledge, you're on your way to better health. Release the weight of thinking your very DNA is defective, and let yourself know peace again as you tend to your liver, clean up your blood, and reclaim your well-being.

CHAPTER 22

Eczema and Psoriasis

Modern medicine has given mysterious skin conditions different labels along the way: seborrheic dermatitis, other varieties of dermatitis, lupus rashes, hives, vitiligo, age spots, cellulitis, rosacea, actinic keratosis, scleroderma, lichen sclerosus, and, of course, eczema and psoriasis. Not everyone's skin condition looks the same, though that's not always taken into account. Take, for example, eczema. It's often approached as though there's one textbook variety. This leads to a flurry of misdiagnoses, including the label idiopathic (meaning cause unknown), when someone's skin condition falls outside eczema's narrow definition. The truth is that there are over 100 varieties of eczema and psoriasis.

Rosacea is actually one variety of eczema. When someone has a rosacea-style rash on the nose, cheeks, chin, or forehead, it's just a garden variety of eczema that happens to appear on the face, not yet another separate, mysterious skin condition. Lupus is a popular label, too. Instead of getting to the bottom of what causes this style of mystery rash, medical communities often tag it as autoimmune, explaining that your body's attacking itself, which is not correct. One misdiagnosis leads to another; one confusion to

the next. You don't know what the rash is, you don't know why someone has fatigue, so you put it in the category of lupus. And what's lupus? Medical research and science don't know, which makes it impossible to diagnose properly. It's an arbitrary word for a confusion of symptoms.

Hives are another mystery, understood on a basic level as a flurry of histamines causing a rash to develop. If you break out with an acute rash and head to the emergency room, the first thing the doctor's going to say is, "What did you eat?" If you say you had a turkey sandwich, the doctor will likely dismiss food as the cause, because turkey seems so normal. If, on the other hand, you tell the doctor you ate strawberries, the doctor will likely say it seems you're allergic to strawberries. If you ate a ham sandwich, the doctor will say it's not the cause of your hives; if you ate an apple, the doctor will blame the apple. If you ate a slice of pizza, the doctor will say that wasn't the problem; if you ate granola, the doctor will say the oats, nuts, or seeds are to blame. If you ate chocolate ice cream, the doctor will say that's not it; if it was raspberry sorbet, the doctor will say that's the source. That's the way doctors are taught to think, and their training will come across as certainty, even though those assumptions about which foods can cause a reaction aren't always right.

If there's no obvious, normal explanation and the hives are reoccurring with no discernible pattern and nothing to connect the dots, doctors will often throw them into the idiopathic, chronic allergy realm. Translation: "We don't know why you're having these reactions." If the skin condition persists, then these days, doctors are very likely to call it autoimmune—that is, to make that lupus diagnosis. If it's not enough to say that it's allergic or autoimmune, they'll blame it on genes. Telling someone you have a skin condition because your mother, father, or an earlier ancestor suffered with one makes surface-level sense that stops everyone from digging deeper. Even if your foremothers and forefathers didn't suffer from skin conditions, it will be called genetic. Doctors want to have answers for patients, which is honorable—and makes it all the more unfortunate that they're not always the right answers.

UNWANTED LIVER RESIDENTS

What do mystery rashes really stem from? Almost every single skin condition comes from the liver. The intestinal tract often becomes involved by default in a forced collaboration; however, conditions labeled eczema, psoriasis, rosacea, lupus, cellulitis, vitiligo, age spots, other discolorations, and more start and end with the liver. Even acne and cellulite derive from the liver. (More on acne in the next chapter.)

These conditions begin because something gets inside the liver that shouldn't be there. Is there anything inside your home that shouldn't be there? Dirt, clutter, garbage, spiders, dust mites, a gas leak? These problems seem to have a way of finding their way in, even when we don't

want them, and when they get there they can cause problems. That's how skin issues start—as unwanted guests in the liver. What type of skin condition develops depends on what type of poison or pathogen is there and how much has built up. Medical research and science don't realize this, because current scanning doesn't allow them to see when a liver is filled up with viral cells and various toxins. What they can't see, they can't understand. Meanwhile, the autoimmune theory that medical communities use blames skin conditions on your immune system treating your skin like an enemy, betraying you out of nowhere and starting to eat away at your epidermis, causing inflammation. This mistaken theory is impossible. While your body can get overloaded and its functions strained, it never betrays you.

One of the most antagonistic toxins when it comes to skin conditions is copper. Copper pipes are a common source of this heavy metal. Pesticides such as DDT and its modern-day pesticide cousins are also high in copper. You could have accumulated it from direct exposure throughout your lifetime and also have inherited it through your bloodline (mind you, not genetically) from ancestors who were saturated in it. Mercury in the liver is the next big instigator of skin conditions, along with pesticides, herbicides, solvents, petroleum products (even pumping gas at the gas station can expose you), antibiotics, and other pharmaceuticals.

As these troublemakers build up over time in your liver, the organ grows sluggish—and, as we just saw in the previous chapter, when the liver becomes overloaded, it can't detox as well as it should. Its functions slow down. Sometimes, these poisons in the liver can be enough to trigger a skin condition that confuses multiple doctors, though it may be nothing more than a random rash or itchy, dry skin that keeps you up at night once in a while.

THE DERMATOXIN EFFECT

When a pathogen such as EBV is also residing in your liver, that's when the more disruptive skin conditions appear. Different pathogens—and even different strains of the same pathogen—have different appetites for different toxins. Depending on which combination is present in your liver, you'll get a different rash. One strain of EBV can prefer copper's flavor, for example, resulting in a difficult case of eczema. Another EBV strain can prefer mercury, leaving you with fatigue and a hive-like, butterfly-shaped rash that sticks you with a lupus diagnosis. The skin reactions form because as EBV feeds off its desired food, it also eliminates it, releasing a much more toxic, destructive form of the original copper or mercury—that is, a dermatoxin.

A vaporized methyl toxin, this dermatoxin can travel through connective tissue and organs with ease. If your liver is in good working order, the methyl toxin will find its way into your small intestinal tract and colon and flush out relatively easily if you're also eating well enough, exercising, and eliminating properly. If you're like most people, though, then you have a sluggish liver, so this remanufactured poison can back up into the lymphatic system and reverse course back into the bloodstream. This doesn't automatically mean you'll have a problem. At first, most people's bodies are resilient. Even if the liver's stagnant, with toxins backing up and the intestinal tract not working well (perhaps constipation is occurring), the body will try its other escape routes for the methyl toxins—for example, through the bloodstream, into the kidneys, and out through your urine.

The backup plan can eventually run its course, and sensitivities can start to occur. Food allergies can be a sign that something is going wrong. Even basic histamine reactions like true hives can be indications that the liver is not functioning as it should be and poisons are accumulating. A small rosacea rash can appear. Or a larger, lupus-style rash can take shape, either accompanied by other lupus symptoms or on its own without other symptoms. For some people, a touch of eczema on the arms, elbows, chest, or back of one ear can develop. That's the beginning.

If the remanufactured methyl toxin form of copper and/or mercury—the dermatoxin—continues to proliferate due to the pathogen feeding continually, the body can become overrun. The toxins will really start to make themselves known, finding their way up to the skin more and more, leaving deposits in the subcutaneous fatty tissue and getting trapped there. It's unknown to medicine that the subcutaneous fatty tissue under your skin is actually your second liver. Here, you have a natural defense mechanism meant to work any toxins up through the layers of your dermis and epidermis so that they can finally make their way to your skin's surface and out of your body. Helping you rid yourself of toxins is one of your skin's true purposes.

Now, this natural process is meant for normal, everyday bodily toxins, not engineered, manufactured, man-made, or manipulated ones like viruses and the chemical industry's finest pesticides, fungicides, herbicides, solvents, and toxic heavy metals. We were never supposed to be up against the harsh chemical inventions that we are today—the liver's not supposed to contain them. Viruses like EBV were never supposed to take the destructive forms that they've taken as a result of feeding on those chemical inventions. By extension, the skin was never meant to deal with the dermatoxins created from virus cells fueling themselves on industrial brews. No one on the entire planet is supposed to have eczema. While it can feel like your skin is working against you, the truth is that it's still on your side, working in your favor, doing the right thing. Without those man-produced troublemakers, eczema couldn't develop.

What doctors ought to be telling you is, "We've taken a scratch sample of your skin cells and determined that you have a dermatoxin present. It's a remanufactured poison, in this case specifically a mix of mercury with copper that's 80 years old. Combined with the viral waste and its protein, which come from a virus called EBV that's actually feeding on copper deposits in your liver, this indicates that a virus-toxin reaction in your liver is the source of the mercury and copper taking on this more-toxic form that's causing your skin irritation. Your body isn't responsible for the problem. Your body's not attacking itself. Your genes aren't the issue, either. The treatment plan is to go after the virus and kill it off while starving it of its favorite foods in your diet. This will bring back your liver so that your skin can heal."

That's the explanation that doctors need to be able to say they learned from the finest, most elite medical schools. And yet that's not what's being taught. Unless a miracle occurs and modern medicine gets up to speed with this information in record time, that's not the talk you're going to get at the doctor's office anytime soon. It could take decades and decades for medical research and science to hand dermatologists what they need to correctly and fully inform patients about their chronic mystery rashes. Remember: at its most advanced, medicine is stuck back at the mistaken autoimmune theory that your immune system is attacking your skin.

That's the best reasoning out there right now. Think about how far there still is to go to catch up with the truth.

So releasing dermatoxins (formed by viruses feeding off heavy metals and other toxins in your liver) to the surface of your skin is your body's masterful way of protecting you. The skin knows your liver is getting overwhelmed, and in a panic, it pushes poisons up to the surface in a rush. The dermatoxins, which are at least far away from your internal organs now, do make life uncomfortable; they're highly inflammatory to skin tissue, causing blemishes, fissures, cracks, scabs, flaking, scarring, bleeding, and rashes of all kinds. The associated irritation occurs because of tiny nerve endings all through the epidermis. When inflammation occurs, the nerves get squeezed and pulled apart, causing the itchiness, discomfort, and outright pain of the rash. The level to which these symptoms disrupt your life can depend on the strain of EBV or other virus present, the levels of heavy metals or other toxins present inside the liver, how sluggish the liver is, and your current diet, which could contain unhelpful foods that are feeding the underlying cause, the viral strain.

WHAT'S BEHIND YOUR SKIN CONDITION

As I mentioned, different types of skin conditions come from different troublemakers in the liver providing different types of pathogenic fuel:

Eczema is a combination of half copper and half mercury with a virus, most commonly EBV.

Psoriasis is a combination of approximately three-quarters copper with one-quarter mercury with a virus, most commonly EBV.

Rosacea is usually mercury-based, with that mercury present in both the liver and the small intestinal tract, plus a virus, most commonly EBV.

Lupus-style rashes are also mercury-based, this time with more EBV involved.

Age spots are caused by dermatoxins made of one-half methylated aluminum and the other half a mix of methylated cadmium, nickel, lead, and mercury; different types of age spots depend on the composition of that second half.

Lichen sclerosus results from a virus in the liver consuming copper, mercury, and traces of inherited DDT. The resulting dermatoxins can go anywhere, though they tend to stay lower in the body, most of the time from the waist down. That's because the traces of DDT in the dermatoxins tend to pull them downward when they enter the bloodstream and settle in the lymphatic system, so when the dermatoxins surface at the skin level, that tends to be in lower areas of the body. Often confused with eczema, this condition is different; in lichen sclerosus, the skin becomes more fragile. It's also often confused with common dermatitis at first and then later considered to be an autoimmune condition when it doesn't improve. Make no mistake; this is a viral condition of the liver. It's not genetic, either, though believing so is a classic medical blunder. Any occurrence through the family line is because of DDT passed from generation to generation.

Scleroderma is a version of psoriatic arthritis, which is basically an eczema or psoriasis accompanied by deeper tissue pain, joint pain, and often sensitivity to cold and heat. Once again, the body's not attacking itself, and it's not genetic. In scleroderma, a different EBV strain than the common eczema ones is at work, and it's feeding on more mercury than copper. Common sources of mercury here include pesticides, insecticides, and fungicides. Symptoms come from dermatoxins and neurotoxins combined, with dermatoxins affecting the skin and neurotoxins affecting deep connective tissue and joints.

Vitiligo is another viral condition—not genetic or the body attacking itself. This one is different from rashing conditions; here, dermatoxins injure the cells that produce skin pigment, which are hypersensitive to these poisons. These dermatoxins come from a virus, HHV-6 or occasionally an EBV variety, sitting inside the liver feeding on formaldehyde as well as aluminum and some copper. Mainly it's larger deposits of aluminum interacting with traces of formaldehyde that makes the dermatoxic solution destructive to pigment-producing cells.

Seborrheic dermatitis comes from a toxic liver. In this case, there is no viral relation; it's not a pathogen causing the issue. It's a liver that is high in a little bit of everything that's also on the verge of becoming pre-fatty. The sluggish liver is resulting in dirty blood, and the toxins it contains coming to the surface is what causes the symptoms here.

Classic dermatitis is a garden variety of psoriasis caused by a virus inside the liver feeding off copper, a little bit of aluminum and pesticides, and traces of DDT. The virus is one of the more common mutations of EBV.

Actinic keratosis, in which patches of skin become tough, rough like sandpaper, or slightly bumpy and can come and go, is one of the many forms of eczema. Here, a specific EBV strain, one of the 60 varieties of the virus, is feeding on higher levels of mercury with some copper.

Cellulitis comes from a combination of strep plus dermatoxins. The strep has escaped to subcutaneous lymphatic vessels, and it's the bacteria's interaction with dermatoxins coming out of the liver from a virus there that creates this particular skin condition.

SYMPTOM CYCLES

The internal dermatoxins we're talking about in this chapter are different from the external ones usually associated with the word *dermatoxin*. These aren't detergents or other irritants inflaming the skin from the outside. Again, they stem from unwanted visitors inside the liver, and the internally produced nature of these types of dermatoxins explains why someone can go through cycles with a skin condition. As our skin, the largest organ, desperately purges dermatoxins to the surface, there's normally another round of dermatoxins being produced inside the liver. That means that one rush of dermatoxins can reach the surface, cause a breakout, and then subside, and meanwhile there's another batch brewing. If the liver isn't being cleansed or cared for, and the virus or other pathogen isn't being eliminated, then typically, just when it seems the skin has improved—this often happens on a six-week cycle—here comes another round of dermatoxins up through the subcutaneous tissue, preparing itself to surface at the epidermis and cause another flare-up.

Many people with severe skin conditions that require steroids find themselves with an even bigger reaction when they come off the medication, because the underlying liver problem was never addressed. Instead, more and more dermatoxins were building up in the liver and subcutaneous fatty tissue. The steroids didn't rid the body of these toxins; they got rid of the *reaction* to the toxins. When the steroids (or other immunosuppressive drugs) aren't there anymore, the dermatoxins still are, and so the body responds in kind.

It's completely understandable when someone goes on steroids for their skin. Some skin conditions can reach torture levels when they're at their peak, so it makes complete sense that someone would go on steroids to get through the hard times. What's important to understand is how they're really working. The medical world believes a steroid is stopping the body's immune system from attacking the skin. In reality, the medication is stopping the body from reacting to dermatoxins produced by a virus. The real reason steroids work for skin conditions is similar to why someone gets put on steroids immediately following cosmetic surgery: to stop the body from becoming inflamed as a reaction to the nose job or multiple incisions. Surgical wounds aren't a result of the body attacking itself, and neither are skin conditions.

A skin condition such as eczema or psoriasis normally isn't a quick reaction to a food just eaten. Like chemical sensitivities, it's more of a slow build, which means that it can make itself known at any time. We'll usually put the blame on whatever we were doing in the moment. Maybe it was an apple eaten yesterday or today. Maybe it was a certain salad ordered at lunch. Maybe it was a phone call from a friend. Maybe it was watching too much TV. We find all sorts of possible reasons for why our skin seems to give us trouble. Mostly, we go back to foods, which do play a role. And yes, the foods we eat matter when healing skin conditions, too. Dairy, eggs, and wheat can feed EBV and other pathogens—causing, for example, EBV to produce more viral cells that can feed even more on copper, mercury, and other toxic heavy metals found in sources such as pesticides, herbicides, and pharmaceuticals such as antibiotics.

As a result, the virus produces more dermatoxins that make the skin condition worse, sometimes in combination with virus-produced neurotoxins, which can create additional symptoms such as aches and pains, dizziness, tingles, ringing in the ears, numbness, or, as in the case of psoriatic arthritis, joint pain.

Like the doctor in the hypothetical ER scenario earlier, though, you'll likely guess that it was another food giving you a skin reaction—usually a fruit or a vegetable. Here's a common scenario: One day, you eat an egg-and-cheese sandwich and then take an antibiotic for your cough. This feeds the EBV in your liver, though you don't get a skin reaction in that moment. Two days later, the virus is actively using the antibiotic and the egg, cheese, and wheat to produce dermatoxins inside your liver. It's only then that your rash starts to get worse—except because you ate an apple your grandmother offered you that afternoon, you think it's the apple. Truth is, the dermatoxins causing your skin flare-up took time to be produced and released up through the skin. The apple was doing your health a favor, only it got the blame instead. This is just one example of the confusion that can occur with foods.

CLEANING HOUSE

It's imperative to look after, care for, address, coddle, and mind the liver to rid yourself of any skin condition. You'll likely need to pace the process of healing—because as the liver is cleansed, dermatoxins flush fast and furious to the skin's surface, causing the same symptoms you're trying to heal. If you flush them all at once, you'll be overcome with discomfort. Not only that, the skin has also grown accustomed to reacting to dermatoxins, so it needs to be given time to calm down. Someone with the worst case of eczema or psoriasis has a little extra copper and mercury and viral waste matter stored deep in the liver, so it takes longer for the skin condition to heal. If that's you, have patience as best you can.

Diet means everything. Above all, no matter the severity of your skin condition, keep out the unproductive foods in Chapter 36, "Liver Troublemakers." As time goes on, you will see results. For some, they'll happen immediately. For others, they'll be delayed. Eventually, as the liver cleans house, toxic heavy metals will be released and pathogenic loads will reduce to the point of minimizing the skin condition, or freeing yourself from it altogether.

CHAPTER 23

Acne

When acne is present, it means that the liver is harboring a chronic, low-grade level of *Streptococcus*. Strep lives in the organ when the liver holds an abundance of food for it. Antibiotics are one of strep's fuels of choice—and one of the liver's greatest enemies. As it happens, they're frequently handed out to those who suffer from acne, along with other medications that can be hard for the liver to bear. It can become an endless cycle, with antibiotics feeding the very strep that causes acne and acne causing the dermatologist to write a prescription for more antibiotics.

So what comes first, the chicken or the egg—the acne or the antibiotics? The answer is clear: the antibiotics. Our livers' storage bins of this and other pharmaceuticals can go back to childhood and even babyhood. Like so many other liver troublemakers, they can also be inherited through your family line from foremothers and forefathers, so you can actually enter life with antibiotics stored in your liver. Then your early years often bring with them antibiotic prescriptions. Ear infections, for example, are caused by strep, though normally diagnosed as general bacterial infections that call for antibiotics.

(When ear infections go too far, doctors often prescribe liquid steroid drops and sometimes insert ear tubes to prevent the canals from closing up and stopping the administration of those steroids in times of inflammation. This can be helpful if the infection has become severe. With a baby's first ear infection, though, it normally isn't that bad yet. At that early point in time, the infections can usually be handled easily with natural antibacterials and antivirals such as elderberry syrup, lomatium root, zinc, goldenseal, vitamin C, and mullein-garlic ear oil. These can head off the need to use antibiotics down the road, because they take care of the underlying strep.)

Here's the thing: conventional, prescription antibiotics don't kill strep as they should, because strep has an unbelievably adaptable nature. It becomes resistant to many varieties of antibiotics. So as we move through the various infections that can occur in life, from those first ear infections to respiratory infections to sinus infections and beyond, with antibiotics prescribed continually for their treatment, the strep in our bodies becomes immune—and can even strengthen over time. Urinary tract infections (UTIs) and bacterial vaginosis (BV), which are both caused by strep, are frequently mis-diagnosed as yeast infections; that is, *Candida* proliferation, because that's what's apparent to doctors. Antifungals are often recommended. (*Candida* itself is never the problem; it's only the messenger. For more on the truth about *Candida*, see *Medical Medium*.) When UTIs or BV are accurately diagnosed, antibiotics are recommended. This is a great mistake in modern medicine today that's strengthening strep bacteria and causing continual, chronic UTIs and yeast infections in so many people, mostly women, as well as BV. The more prescription antibiotics and even antifungals build up in the liver and the fatty subcutaneous tissue beneath the skin, the more strep can use them to build up its immunity and the more someone can suffer in the long run.

ANTIBIOTICS ALWAYS COME FIRST

What does all of this have to do with acne? Everything. Acne is a result of early wars that go undocumented in people's lives. Everyone who deals with a true acne condition has a history of taking antibiotics before any antibiotics they took for acne. This is the chicken-and-egg part: antibiotics always come first. For the very few who struggle with acne and yet never had antibiotics prescribed in early life—not even pre-memory, for example, for a cough at age two—then the antibiotics were passed down through the bloodline or came into the body through animal protein.

It isn't just that strep becomes resistant to antibiotics; it also learns to use them as fuel. (When someone afflicted by cystic acne doesn't take antibiotics for it, the strep can still find other sources of fuel. More on what those are soon.) Refined petroleum, basically a form of engine oil, is in all antibiotics—not because it needs to be; it's because industrial deals were made and business contracts were signed, probably long before you were born. Plastics, as well, are in antibiotics, and of course, let's not forget GMO (for "genetically modified organism") corn grown for medical use. This type of corn is much different from the GMO corn grown for food. Strep learns to consume these antibiotic ingredients, feeding itself off the very treatment meant to kill bacteria.

Antibiotics don't just disappear from your system once you've finished a round of them. They stick around, becoming part of the space junk stored inside your liver. That's "space junk" not just in the sense that your liver is like space polluted by man-made debris; it's also space junk in the sense that it's junk taking up space. What happens, in life, when your home gets too full and cluttered? You step on or trip over something that shouldn't be there—you get hurt. Leftover antibiotics and so many other toxins and poisons are there in the liver, keeping strep nice and happy in its very comfortable environment. Meanwhile, they edge out space for the good.

Strep throat is one form that strep in the system can cause. It's not only common in children and teenagers; there are also cases of adults dying from strep throat infections that in truth go back to brand-new strains of highly antibiotic-resistant strep they happened to ingest at a restaurant or contract in a bathroom. Tonsillitis happens when people have EBV (which takes the form of mononucleosis, or mono, in one of its early stages) and the virus's cofactor, strep. Chronic allergies happen because of elevated strep deposits in the body. Sties in the eye are, for the most part, caused by strep. Sinus infections are caused by strep. In children, strep can take the form of PANDAS (pediatric autoimmune neuropsychiatric disorders associated with streptococcal infections). Again, what does this have to do with acne? Everything. They're conditions that very often affect young people, prompting prescriptions for antibiotics and giving strep a chance to take hold in the system so it can eventually blossom into acne.

Your immune system is constantly monitoring and trying to control your body's environment, so low levels of strep bacteria find places to lie low and hide out of sight. The liver is its ideal hiding place. Most strep gets policed and destroyed by the liver's immune system as it enters the liver. Some of the bacteria, however, escape, slipping by the armed guards and taking refuge in the garbage department of the liver. This is the refuse heap, where tons of junk are placed in hopes that the person belonging to that liver is given the information to do the right thing and cleanse it out.

Your liver always wants you to do the right thing, like drinking a glass of lemon water every day; eating more fruits, leafy greens, and other vegetables; and sipping celery juice when you can. That's not what we learn to do, though. Instead, we're told to increase our fats by experts who have no idea what causes chronic illness to begin with. You couldn't get away with that lack of knowledge as a pilot flying a plane; you can with chronic illness. The standards are vastly different. And so we get more and more of these garbage piles, and they get bigger and bigger, and strep finds it easy to locate a little nook or cranny where it can make itself at home: inside a section of the liver's connective tissue or the middle of a lobule alongside toxic copper from pipes, aluminum from cans, mercury from tuna and pharmaceuticals, poisons from the batteries inside our devices, plastics, pesticides, herbicides, fire-retardant chemicals from clothing, carpet chemicals, nano–particulate agents

from nanotechnology sprays, or strep's favorite, antibiotics.

If you think you've never consumed an antibiotic and neither has anyone in your family line, think again. Have both you and your ancestors never, not once in your lives, consumed a piece of regular chicken? A hamburger at a chain restaurant? A conventional turkey at someone's house on Thanksgiving? These are all sources that are regularly pumped through with antibiotics. If you try to outwit the reasoning of how these pharmaceuticals enter your system, you'll only outwit yourself of your health. Because it's when these space-junk antibiotics in our system meet strep—and we're exposed to strep all the time—that they give the bacteria a chance to reproduce and multiply in the liver's garbage heaps.

HORMONE BLAME

Acne is often blamed on hormones. It's one of the most common, accepted, bread-and-butter concepts out there and one of the greatest mistakes in modern medicine today: hormones cause acne. (Many doctors are now suggesting that some cystic acne is autoimmune; this is also wrong.) The timing of acne hitting at adolescence is indisputable, so it's understandable that the medical world makes the hormonal mistake. In truth, it's strep taking advantage of puberty. With puberty, the immune system lowers. This allows strep, an extremely adaptable type of bacteria, to leave the liver unnoticed, escaping into the lymphatic system to do battle with the lymphocytes. Strep detects what's happening because it can actually taste the hormones flooding the teenager's system; it knows that the body's hormonal shift means the lymphocytes are at their weakest point. While the lymphocytes can destroy some of the strep, many strep cells escape and make a run for the subcutaneous tissue. Like a gold rush that spurs people on past bears, wolves, wildcats, deadly snakes, and brutal weather conditions in search of their destination, teenage hormones spur strep to do whatever it takes to get past the lymphatic system's white blood cells to their ultimate destination, the skin.

Acne breakouts that occur with the menstrual cycle are another reason that the medical world mistakenly tags acne as hormonal. The truth is that a woman's immune system lowers around her menstrual period, which is why acne cysts can show up before, during, or even after menstruation. It's not over then. Next, ovulation comes—the middle of the cycle—and once again, the immune system lowers, strep makes a break for it, and acne occurs. If women are not on healing foods, herbs, and supplements and avoiding triggers, they become more susceptible. Many women in menopause or postmenopause wake up one day and realize they don't have acne anymore. It's not because of hormones; it's because their immune systems aren't lowering on a steady twice-a-month schedule anymore to let strep escape to their lymphatic systems and, in turn, their skin.

HOW ACNE FORMS

Let's talk more about how strep causes those acne cysts on common spots like the face, neck, hairline, chest, back, shoulders, armpits, and upper arms. Do you have a favorite route to travel when you're taking care of business on your way to a celebratory destination? A main thoroughfare that takes you past the doctor's office, the grocery store, the nail salon, and the post office until you finally get to the movie theater and a great restaurant? The lymphatic system is that favorite path for strep—a string of highways it can use to enter the subcutaneous tissue beneath the skin's surface and feast there.

Like what you see when you cut into a piece of raw chicken and find that yellow layer of fat beneath the bumpy outer skin, our skin has a fatty layer under the surface—it's part of the subcutaneous tissue. It's meant to be there, only it happens to be a refuge for poisons and excess fat cells—just as they accumulate in the liver, they accumulate here. Dairy products tend to find their way to our subcutaneous tissue, giving strep plenty of delicious food. So do eggs from breakfast omelets, fats from chicken dinners, antibiotics in these foods that were fed to the animals to fight off strep infections at the farms where they were raised, and antibiotics from the public water system. This is the promised treasure of the gold rush, the lure that has strep calling, "There's gold in them hills!" as it fends off your lymphatic system's immune system to get to your skin. Strep tends to take the path of least resistance, so it takes the lymphatic highways that are weakened and haven't been replenished by lymphocytes and are therefore less policed. Its route of choice determines where acne will eventually surface. This is why Jimmy gets acne on his chest and back while Sarah gets it on her forehead and chin while Jessica gets it on her upper arms and armpits.

Before acne even develops, strep stays in its happy place for a while, feasting on tasty treats, slowly working its way through the subcutaneous fat and re-strengthening itself for the new fight ahead. Finally, it enters the bottom level of the dermis. The skin's personalized immune system starts to gather sebum oil as a quicksand-like agent to deter the strep from getting any higher. Because the strep has been well fueled and is extremely vital at this point, the sebum oil isn't enough to stop it. Now the skin's immune system kicks into higher gear, prompting the production of sebum oil at even larger volumes as a last attempt to trap the bacteria and safeguard your skin—because your immune system doesn't want your skin to become scarred. When strep is strong and mighty, it fights through even the extra sebum oil and survives the lymphocytes and killer cells just below the epidermis. It climbs up into this outer layer of your skin. *Voilà*, cystic acne shows itself.

In many cases, these outbreaks are mild and temporary. In extreme cases, they're devastating. So much goes into what determines a mild versus aggravating versus extreme case of acne, including how many strains of strep you have, how many toxins such as heavy metals are present in the liver and subcutaneous tissue for strep to feed on, how many antibiotics you have used or otherwise ingested over a lifetime, what happened before your lifetime that you inherited, what kind of adrenaline surges you experience in daily life, pesticide exposure, and of course, what your diet's like.

Today's alternative medical communities believe that dairy products such as milk, cheese, and butter, as well as grains such as wheat, are problematic because they're allergenic. (Although cheese is making a comeback. The high-fat trend is now promoting cheese as a healthy longevity food.) They observe that the more acne patients eat wheat and dairy, the more they break out. This correlation isn't really because of an allergy. These acne breakouts happen because strep loves wheat and dairy. When they're in the diet, strep goes into a frenzied feast, launching new, low-grade attacks on the skin that eventually display themselves as cystic acne. While dairy products are notorious for creating a sluggish lymphatic system, that doesn't make it harder for strep to travel along its preferred route. In fact, it becomes even easier, because when the lymphatic system is sluggish, your defense mechanisms, lymphocytes, are trapped and minimized. The lymphatic highways with the least amount of lymphocytes due to higher amounts of strep-friendly foods like milk, cheese, and butter become strep's paths of least resistance.

When acne is treated with antibiotics, the liver must then soak them up, which can weaken the liver's personalized immune system and allow for more gangs of strep bacteria to hide in the garbage heaps among old, stored antibiotics. Further, the strep can feed on the antibiotics. The process will repeat itself. Fortunately, our bodies are resilient and have a fighting spirit.

Even medical research and science know by now that there's more than *Streptococcus* Group A and Group B. While medically recognized groups stop partway through the alphabet, the truth is that there are enough strep groups to go beyond Z. These different groups contribute to the different varieties of acne someone can exhibit. The very aggressive types of strep, for example, cause scars and large clusters of cysts. Throughout life, it's very easy to pick up multiple varieties of strep bacteria through intimate contact, restaurant food, bathrooms, and more. Along the way, you can pick up a variety that became very resistant to a strong antibiotic someone took in her or his lifetime. And some women who experience a new sexual partner later in life will develop their first UTI, or a tougher-than-average UTI, due to picking up a hard-to-beat strep variety that requires strong antibiotics to get under control.

RELIEF WITHIN REACH

This is why building up strong immune systems throughout your body is a critical step in addressing and preventing acne and other strep-related ailments such as SIBO, which you'll read about in the next chapter. The most important place to start is your liver. Being proactive and making this internal organ a strep-unfriendly environment will go a much longer way toward protecting your skin than treating yourself with the best facial, the best face wash, the best lotion, the best pill, and the most sought-after blemish potion combined. Bolstering your lymphatic immune system will also make a huge difference. The lymphocytes you rely on to stop strep in the lymphatic highways feed off vitamins and minerals from fruits, vegetables, herbs, and spices. That makes food a big part of healing acne. In Part IV, you'll find just the immune-enhancing, liver-strengthening, strep-killing guidance you need to finally find relief.

CHAPTER 24

SIBO

SIBO, which stands for small intestinal bacterial overgrowth, is one of the hippest new diagnoses out there today. Though you'll hear the term everywhere, the questions of which bacteria are actually involved, why this condition plagues patients, and what to do about it remain a mystery to medical communities. To really understand it, we need to look past the label and consider the truth of how the body works.

GASTRIC JUICES

When your stomach acid is out of balance, various gut health issues can occur. One in particular is your hydrochloric acid becoming sparse, weakened, and ultimately ineffective. Hydrochloric acid is the glue, the balancer, the leader, the parent, the uniting agent of our gastric juices, so when it's low or diminishing, the strength of our gastric juices can weaken substantially. Where does hydrochloric acid come from? Not from the liver. It comes from the stomach, produced by glands and stomach tissue there. So why bother mentioning it in a liver book? Because low hydrochloric acid is an indicator of a liver problem. Medical research and

science are not there yet with understanding this truth.

Medical communities do know about the greenish, yellow brown liquid called bile (composed of elements such as bile salts, bilirubin, and cholesterol) that's produced by the liver, stored in the gallbladder, and delivered to your digestive tract as needed to help digestion. There's more to it than they've yet discovered. For one, there are more components than they realize, such as cluster minerals; that is, trace minerals that stay huddled together in a sticky, filmy solution secreted by the liver in one of its over 2,000 chemical functions. Cluster minerals strengthen the bile so it has the ability to stay active even in the deepest parts of the small intestine.

One of bile's roles, breaking down and dissolving fats, is critical: it keeps fats from saturating the intestinal lining and going rancid. When fat does go rancid in the digestive tract—it can happen with any radical fat source, whether pork, lard, butter, French fries, nut butter, avocado, or the purest oil—it can feed pathogens. Not only can SIBO result, so can other gastrointestinal conditions such as irritable bowel syndrome (IBS), Crohn's disease, colitis, ulcers, and *H. pylori* proliferation.

When the liver is weakened, sluggish, becoming pre-fatty or fatty, or filled with poisons from before birth through the present, it can't create sufficient or strong enough bile. It calls out for help, using yet another of its miraculous chemical functions to protect you, in this case sending chemical compounds through the bile duct to the duodenum, from which they travel up to the stomach like messengers. They sound the alarm to the stomach that too many fats are intruding and bile is diminishing and losing its function. This puts pressure on the stomach glands to overproduce hydrochloric acid and the other components of gastric juices, and then to disperse them outside of their normal reach, as far as the entrance to the small intestine. It's all for the purpose of lowering the bloodstream's fat ratio to prevent the liver from becoming too toxic and the blood from becoming too thick, which would translate to less oxygen for the heart and even less critically needed glucose for the brain.

Eventually, the hydrochloric acid supply starts to wane. We can't blame the liver for asking for help when it was in dire need. Instead, we need to look to diet. A standard modern diet is not enough to support the stomach's extra production of hydrochloric acid and other components of gastric juices. In truth, someone's diet might have been a big part of how the liver and bile weakened and created the need for extra gastric juices in the first place. Not even the trendy, "healthy" diets popping up every week are enough, because the makers of these eating plans aren't aware of how bile production and stomach acids really work, so they can't gear the food plans to support these critical tasks of your body. When someone doesn't know which foods to eat to support the stomach's

hydrochloric acid production and rejuvenate the liver, that protocol is going to be less effective. Diets can only be supportive when the people designing them are truly familiar with the liver, not just pretending to be.

Even celebrated high-protein diets aren't as effective as we would want them to be; they can even make matters worse, because the more protein in a diet, the more fats are in it. Protein almost always equals fat, and snacks and meals full of fat are going to be trouble when someone is dealing with low hydrochloric acid. Medical research and science have not yet discovered that hydrochloric acid does more than just break down protein. The liver also gives permission to the stomach via chemical compounds transferring information to partake in breaking down fats. This is different from breaking down protein; this is license from the liver for hydrochloric acid to prepare fats in the stomach to be more easily and properly broken down and dispersed by bile salts and fluid, so that there's less chance of rancid fats sticking to the lining of the small intestinal tract and rotting, and so that blood doesn't become thick from fat. (As you've read, once blood becomes thick, it becomes hard on your heart. That's critical to remember: if you're not taking care of your liver, not only are you not taking care of your gut, you're also not taking care of your heart.)

Hydrochloric acid's readying of fats for bile's next phase with them is part of an undiscovered process of separating fats from proteins inside the stomach. By the time proteins and fats reach the small intestine, they're meant to be separated, though that doesn't always happen—because of what we eat. The food combinations, eating habits, and outright gastric bombs we choose, get stuck with, or are persuaded into can be too much for even robust hydrochloric acid production and a strong liver to counter.

Imagine, then, if your liver is sluggish and/or you have low hydrochloric acid, how much fat and protein descend into the small intestine without being separated first.

Why is this separation important? Because while breaking down fats and making them as valuable and safe for the body as possible is certainly within the liver's domain, the liver is not responsible for breaking down dense proteins such as those that come from animal products. The liver's bile can't as effectively break down, digest, and disperse the fat when it's still bound to protein. And when too much fat, whether healthy or unhealthy, mixed with too much protein, whether healthy or unhealthy, enter the small intestine together, calamity occurs. For one, a feeding frenzy can begin. *Candida* and other microorganisms will begin to fight for food.

If you're strong as an ox, don't think calamity is out of reach for you—not if you're eating abominable concoctions of food. A surf-and-turf special with some fritters washed down with a bottle of beer is enough to throw off the stomach's process of fat and protein separation for the best of us. Remember: your liver gets drunk before you ever feel a buzz. And when the organ gets tipsy, its bile production drops dramatically while hydrochloric acid gets diluted fast, faded like an old Polaroid picture from the '70s. Though you may still feel perfectly clear-headed and fine at the helm, if your liver were driving and got pulled over, it would fail the test of walking a straight line. It's important to know that the liver gets intoxicated from even one glass of wine so we can also know that when we're eating fat and protein with alcohol, the separation of that fat and protein isn't going to happen in the stomach. They're going to enter the small intestine largely undigested, and that's how problems such as SIBO begin.

SIBO IS THE NEW *CANDIDA*

For the last 30 years, *Candida* has been a health craze. Bloating and other stomach discomfort, digestive issues, yeast infections, constipation, diarrhea, loose stools, IBS, nail fungus, UTIs and other infections, fatigue, brain fog, rashes, and more have all been blamed on it. *Candida* very often still gets the blame today.

As I've always said, *Candida* isn't the source problem. Yes, *Candida* is often present in the body, though it's with good reason. This beneficial fungus works only in your favor; without *Candida*, we can't thrive or be truly healthy. One critical role it plays is breaking down nutrients to allow for their proper absorption into the organs and throughout the rest of the body via the bloodstream. Another of its jobs is to devour nonuseful foods and debris in our system, cleaning up hazardous waste that would otherwise harm us. *Candida* is directed to do this by a force that medical research and science will never in human history be able to explain, an undeniable force from above that guides it to work in our favor.

Yes, *Candida* can proliferate too much if we're eating unproductive foods and not taking care of ourselves. It can become cumbersome and even seem like it's getting in the way. And so, out of misunderstanding, it's chosen as a bad guy, picked out of the crowd by health professionals and deemed a culprit of symptoms and disease. If only they knew that it's a crucial, even heroic, fungus.

Candida is part of the sanitation department of your body. Have you heard of the historic garbage strike in New York City, when hundreds upon thousands of garbage bags littered the streets? Rats descended by the millions to feast on the trash, scavenging and breeding disease. It was madness. That is, until the sanitation department reached an agreement and garbage collectors sprang back to action, carting away the trash and getting the streets cleaned up again. *Candida* is the garbage man on his normal rotation, removing the trash before the rats can overtake the city. It means that *Candida* takes food away from the rats. In your body, that translates to *Candida* feeding on trash that if left around will feed bad bacteria, viruses, and evil forms of mold and fungus. It's when these and other unproductive microorganisms get around the reach of *Candida*—when they spawn like rats from the garbage in our guts of poor food, rancid fats, drugs, and antibiotics—that we have to worry. That's when they create the condition SIBO.

It was never *Candida* behind people's bloating, digestive discomfort, constipation, yeast infections, and the like. And yet turning over a new leaf as medical communities have done lately, calling the problem bacterial overgrowth and throwing the label "SIBO" on it, while progress, still isn't enough of an answer.

SIBO should be renamed "small intestinal streptococcal overgrowth," because the truth is that *Streptococcus* is the leading type of bacterium that causes SIBO and in many cases the only type of bacterium involved. Better yet, overall diagnoses of strep should replace diagnoses of SIBO—the focus shouldn't be limited to the small intestine. Strep overgrowth is not stationary. If strep is in the small intestinal tract, chances are it's in the colon and rectal area, too, and also in the stomach. You may hear that within the gut, bacteria can only thrive in the intestinal tract, not the stomach. This isn't true. Bacteria can thrive in the stomach for years or even decades when hydrochloric acid levels are low enough; they can even create ulcers in the stomach and scar tissue at the bottom of the esophagus. Strep can even travel farther up,

which means that someone with SIBO could in fact have strep proliferation from the mouth all the way to the rectum. It can make its way to the pancreas, too. And let's not forget that there's likely to be a whole pocket or more of strep hiding out in the liver, sustaining itself on the garbage storage bins there. In particular, old antibiotics sitting in the liver contain petroleum byproducts that give strep plenty of food so it can thrive there.

Here's what your doctor would be telling you if she or he only knew: "SIBO goes all the way back to an unsupported liver." As we just examined, when the liver gets overburdened, bile production weakens in turn, which means that the liver needs to call on hydrochloric acid for help digesting fats. If the liver isn't given the chance to improve over time with strengthening foods and instead its condition continues to worsen, and the right foods to strengthen hydrochloric acid aren't consumed, either, the stomach glands' production of hydrochloric acid eventually diminishes, too. Undigested fats and proteins end up heading into the small intestine together, and there, the fat grows rancid, making it a delicious food for pathogens.

Candida is the next line of defense, fighting the battle for your body, acting as a helpful scavenger and even a messenger and feeding on any bugs that are thriving in the intestine. Strep is one such bug, and it's an old adversary that could have been in your system for years, if not your entire life—plus we're exposed to new strains of strep in our everyday lives. *Candida* sees strep as an enemy. It won't always attack strep, though, unless that strep is weakened. If *Candida* is getting stronger and growing in number from scavenging toxic foods and substances in the intestinal tract while strep is losing fuel and starving, that's when *Candida* will strike and try to trap and suffocate strep in corners of the intestinal tract. Once the strep dies, *Candida* will devour the dead bacterial cells. It's a natural, symbiotic war working many times in your favor, and it goes unseen. All that's seen is *Candida* growing in number—neither doctor nor patient knows why it's growing or what the symptoms of this war mean.

Hydrochloric acid is meant to knock out any bugs like strep before they get to the intestinal tract. When this element of gastric juices is not being produced at the strength and level it should be, though, it can't kill off the strep and other bugs in the stomach, so the bacteria slip into the small intestine and join the party. It's also possible for strep to detour to the gut when it's making its way from the liver to the skin to cause acne. (That's why acne and SIBO commonly occur together; strep causes them both.) Eventually, when the state of bile and hydrochloric acid production drops beneath a certain low point, not even *Candida* can save us. Strep takes over, and SIBO blooms.

It's only right that you understand this reality of how SIBO develops. Not knowing what's really wrong, we get cheated out of extra immune system fighting abilities. With the general labels and makeshift diagnoses out there like "bacterial overgrowth," we do get some relief. Still, there's a higher wisdom inside of us that knows that's not the whole truth—and also knows that discovering the truth is half the battle in healing a problem. The vague tag of "SIBO" is not enough. We get better from having answers.

It's critical to understand that strep is the type of bacterium behind SIBO and that it's not just bacteria in general going haywire in the small intestine. Think of it this way: You take your child to a country fair for what's meant to

be a fun Saturday afternoon. There's a stable of ponies and the opportunity for your child to choose one for a short ride. You hear that one of the ponies is untamed, rowdy and reckless to the point of being dangerously unpredictable. It still lives in its wild state of mind and needs more attention, love, training, and discipline before it's a reliable ride. As a parent, would you want to know which pony in the stable that is? Or would you be comfortable with the risk of putting your child on any of those ponies, taking the chance that it could be the wild one? Knowing exactly which is the feral animal—so you can keep your child away from it—could change your life and your child's forever. It could spare your child from injury and spare you both from emotional trauma and lifelong fear. That's the importance of knowing that strep is behind SIBO. It activates your immune system to go find strep and tame the rogue bacteria, and it tells you where you need to keep your eye to stay safe in the meantime. Strep has more of a history of causing problems than anyone knows.

Another issue with the SIBO label is that it's becoming one of those catchall diagnoses like *Candida*, with symptoms such as fatigue, aches and pains, and brain fog being classified as SIBO when they really aren't—nor were they *Candida*. These health complaints are frequently viral issues, which I've written about in detail in my previous books. Strep is a very common viral cofactor; that is, a tagalong to viruses, which is why people so often experience SIBO alongside these viral symptoms. It's important to distinguish bacteria from viruses so they can both be dealt with, just as it's important to zero in on strep as the cause of SIBO, rather than letting it go as merely "bacterial."

THE ANTIBIOTIC DILEMMA

Antibiotics are the leading treatment for SIBO and the leading SIBO mistake. The story of strep here is the same as the story of strep and acne from the previous chapter. Much of the time, when strep is hanging around in the system, it's due to past antibiotic use or antibiotics inherited through the family line. Most people's strep starts in childhood, maybe even passed down from a parent at conception; a newborn can enter the world with strep already in her or his system. A child can also get strep from day care or school, as it's easily passed from child to child—as well as adult to adult. Because strep is a type of bacterium, antibiotics do seem like the obvious choice to treat it. Here's the crucial point to know about strep, though: long ago, before the antibiotic revolution, strep used to be one strain of bacterium. Strep is not and never was a superbug. It's much more forgiving, because in its original state back in the old days, it wasn't working against us. It even had the potential to work for us—unlike superbugs like MRSA, which have worked against us from the start.

Strep is no longer one strain. Over decades and decades of being a victim of antibiotics, it found a way to survive: to adapt. Adaptation didn't just mean getting stronger. It meant mutating and spawning different strains and varieties, each one able to defend itself against the stronger and stronger medications that research and science have developed. Along the way, strep got classified as having a Group A and a Group B. The medical world now identifies strep all the way through Group H, though as you read about in the acne chapter, the truth is that they would need to invent new letters in the alphabet to cover all the groups of strep that the population carries. There are also strains within the known groups that are as yet unidentified and undocumented.

Even if a gifted and talented lab technician discovered that there were more strains and groups of strep than are currently known, the breakthrough would go unrecognized. The scientist would not be able to find funding for this area of critical medical importance—because right now, funding is too tied up in misled areas like how genes relate to disease.

What you need to know is that strep is responsible for so many conditions you've read about—SIBO, cystic acne, ear infections, and UTIs and BV that are often cast off as yeast infections, as well as actual yeast infections and *Candida* proliferation. These conditions keep coming back for people after they're treated because they're really caused by strep that's not being eliminated through any of the medical treatment plans. Then there are sinus infections and other sinus-related issues like chronic allergies—even if there's something additional like pollen irritating the sinus cavity and causing histamines to rise, it doesn't mean bacteria's not already present, creating the inflammation and sensitivity to begin with. Pelvic inflammatory disease and sties in the eye, as different as they may seem, are both strep-related. Even chronic appendicitis is strep; hundreds of thousands of appendectomies are precipitated by strep causing the appendix to deteriorate and become inflamed. For constipation and inflammation of the colon or the rest of the intestinal tract, strep can also be responsible. (See the next chapter for more.) Tonsillitis is a combination of strep plus EBV.

As with acne, you'll almost always find that someone suffering from SIBO was treated with antibiotics at some point in her or his younger years. Often before that person can even remember, whether for bronchitis, an ear infection, or even a basic cold or flu, chances are there was an antibiotic prescription. Since it was never a true healing protocol, there was likely a recurrence at some point, so even more antibiotics were used. If you've been treated with antibiotics for any reason, even a basic cold or flu, strep inside your body has had the chance to grow even stronger and more antibiotic-resistant and to linger in your system into adulthood.

Don't get me wrong; there's a place for antibiotics in today's world of medicine. There are emergency situations that call for them, like an infected injury from stepping on a nail in the woods, or a bleeding UTI with severe kidney infection. The goal is to strengthen the immune system and avoid emergency situations as best we can so antibiotics aren't needed in the first place. I know what a dilemma it can be. When the immune system is low and we're not taking care of ourselves the way we could be, whether because of resources or education, we can fall victim to medical communities' lack of knowledge about strep, getting chronic UTIs or sinus infections that can only be tamed with continual use of different varieties of antibiotics. Eventually, we can end up in the ER or urgent care with an emergency flare-up that calls for even more antibiotics. It's not your fault if this is happening to you because along the way, no one understood that what was causing your underlying issues was antibiotic-resistant strep.

It's not your fault if you have SIBO, either. It, too, can become a vicious cycle that we want to avoid if at all possible. If medical communities knew that strep is the rowdy, unpredictable pony in the stable causing so many different health problems, they would think about other options for treating SIBO that didn't perpetuate the condition. It's not a foreign concept in medicine that strep can become antibiotic-resistant;

researchers and doctors know this. If they knew that strep is the problem behind SIBO, they wouldn't want to add gasoline to the fire by prescribing so many antibiotics.

So strep is not a superbug, because unlike MRSA and *C. difficile*, which had evil beginnings, strep had a docile background and only through antibiotics did it get turned into something more sinister. Antibiotics suppress many emergency conditions; it's no wonder we use them in our times of need. Learning the answers so you can move forward and truly heal and prevent many of those emergency conditions is critical. Knowing that we can go after the strep in our system and work on healing SIBO, or any other strep-related condition, is key. Whenever there is a key, there is a door to open—a door of opportunity to heal.

MYSTERIES OF DIGESTION

Nowadays, doctors check for strep as a safety measure when a woman is pregnant or planning to become pregnant. While vaginal strep tests are not guaranteed to be sensitive and accurate enough to give us answers, it is progress that doctors are trained to look for and identify this hard-to-understand bacterium in certain situations. With strep throat, it's harder to detect than you'd think. You can have a later stage of strep throat, where the strep has burrowed too deep into the lining of the throat and/or tonsils to be detectable in a throat swab and culture. And with SIBO, it's virtually impossible to identify strep as the individual bacterium responsible. The small intestine is too far outside the reach of a simple swab for diagnosis to be straightforward—at this point, it's impossible for doctors to diagnose definitively. It will remain that way until medical researchers can someday land funding to develop new ways of testing for bacterial overgrowth in the small intestine.

As I often say, medical research and science do not understand the full picture of what happens to food when it enters the stomach. It's a mystery. They know theoretically about enzymes. They know that digestion and assimilation of nutrients occur. They know about hydrochloric acid breaking down proteins. These discoveries remain crude, like oil drilled from the earth that needs to be refined before it can be put to work. So much more still remains beneath the surface, waiting to be extracted in the first place. One of the great reasons why the medical world doesn't know more about the true miracles of digestion is because God plays a role in the digestive process. Medical research and science don't like the meddling hand of God as an answer. If they stay with that mind-set, they may never discover all that happens with digestion.

To say "see you later" to SIBO, it's important to know a little more about our gastric juices. Medical research and science are unaware that hydrochloric acid is not one single entity; it's actually a complex blend of seven different acids. That means that even if you get a test for hydrochloric acid and your health professional tells you it's strong, you may have other blends of hydrochloric acid that are compromised and hindering the digestive fluid's ability to do its job. If parts of your seven-acid blend are weakened and you ingest any type of foreign microorganism like bacteria or a parasite that enters your stomach, your stomach acid may not be strong enough to kill it off. The one type of hydrochloric acid they test for registering as high doesn't mean the entire composition of the stomach acid is what it needs to be. Three out of the seven could be low, weak, or partially diminishing, and yet that test could still show high hydrochloric acid. There are many people

with stomach ulcers caused by bacteria that are having a grand old time in the stomach because much of the seven-acid blend is dwindling, which actually translates to low hydrochloric acid, and meanwhile their tests will say they've got adequate hydrochloric acid. While this may sound complex, it doesn't even scratch the surface of the infinite amount of undiscovered information about what really happens when food enters the stomach. What you need to remember is that you can't rely on hydrochloric acid tests to give you an accurate snapshot of your gut. Because medical research and science don't realize that the seven-acid blend exists, there's no test to weigh or measure the six blends of hydrochloric acid they don't know about and no test to determine if someone's gastric juices are truly adequate.

BACK TO BALANCE

One reason that I brought celery juice to the world's attention years ago is because it is so beneficial and restorative to the gut. Its undiscovered cofactor micro trace mineral salts actually restore the missing acids in the seven-acid blend and, at the same time, are themselves toxic to unproductive bacteria. That gives celery juice double power: (1) as a stomach acid replenisher so that gastric juices can once again kill invaders and (2) as practically an antibiotic (and antiviral)—one to which detrimental bacteria such as strep cannot become resistant or immune. After the stomach, the mineral salts in celery juice drop down to the small intestinal tract, knocking out bacterial overgrowth such as strep that's present there, too, which is why celery juice will be your new best friend if you have SIBO. In fact, celery is specifically a weapon against strep. The power of celery's mineral salts doesn't stop at fighting bacteria in the small intestine. They continue traveling onward into the colon, where they can continue to fight overgrowth. Plus they're absorbed into the walls of the intestinal tract and from there travel through the bloodstream, acting as an antiseptic to strep along the way to the hepatic portal vein and inside the liver.

Rather than uncovering and pursuing the remarkable healing power hidden within celery, medical research and science instead focus on theories like your genes being responsible for why you're sick. Remember: scientific research's focus is all about where vested interests lie, so celery remains uncharted territory. Health professionals regard celery juice as simply a source of salt and have no idea of the complicated structures of beneficial sodium that it really contains.

Celery juice enhances your entire body's immune system. Your liver's individual immune system also relies on the undiscovered types of mineral salts inside of celery; it uses them specifically to strengthen its lymphocytes (a type of white blood cell), allowing the liver to fight more battles for us and have a better chance of ridding us of strep and other SIBO bacteria that can tag along with it. The white blood cells absorb the mineral salts through their cell structure as nectar and then use them as an offense mechanism, not just a defense mechanism. You know how in the old days, salt was put in a wound to disinfect it? There was something to be said for this topical treatment. Internally, table salt isn't the right type for disinfecting; the mineral salts in celery

are. Your liver's lymphocytes use celery's mineral salts to create a chemical weapon to harm unproductive bacteria such as strep. You'll often hear me say that certain truths will take decades for medical research and science to discover. This one will take hundreds of years.

I always say that finding out what's really behind your suffering is a huge part of healing. That's because your immune system receives information from your thoughts and your soul. I realize some people may prefer to slap a Band-Aid over a wound without looking too closely, to get a general name and a pill for what's going wrong and leave it at that. Yet when you know what's really behind your health struggles, your immune system thrives. There's a confidence that happens internally when you figure out that the bacteria you're going after are strep. Which is to say, if you're suffering from any of the conditions we've looked at in this chapter or the previous one, you're already well on your way to feeling better simply because you've now zeroed in on this pathogen.

The immune system can arm itself better from your knowledge alone, and then your white blood cells strengthen even more when you provide them with the resources you need, such as celery juice. When you become aware of your needs, your awareness can even enhance the chemical compounds that the immune system forms from celery's precious mineral salts—while it enhances all the other healing tools you'll find in Part IV.

CHAPTER 25

Bloating, Constipation, and IBS

As you just read about, gut health starts with one of the liver's top roles: producing bile. It's bile's responsibility, along with hydrochloric acid made up of a blend of seven different acids in your stomach's gastric juices, to engulf food to help you digest it. Given the ideal support, the fluids work together at full strength and in perfect harmony.

When the liver weakens or becomes sluggish in any way, such as when pathogens like EBV and poisons like toxic heavy metals come to visit or when fatty liver develops, it produces lower-quality bile at a lower quantity, too. This is not a proud moment for your liver. For the liver lobules, quality control is number one. So if the liver is releasing bile that's less-than, it truly is a sign that it's burdened. Even when compromised, it's using every reserve it has to produce the strongest bile it can. Still, it's got over 2,000 chemical functions to perform, and some of them, like immune system support, are more important than bile. Lower levels of less powerful bile mean that breaking down food becomes a problem.

There's also the adrenaline factor you've seen come up in other chapters. If someone's under a tremendous amount of stress, it can

cause the liver's bile production itself to weaken. With adrenaline production always in high gear, the stress hormone can saturate the liver at a rate it can't neutralize, straining its bile function as the organ works on sopping up and storing away the adrenaline to protect the other parts of your body. When this happens repeatedly, the liver can become oversaturated with adrenaline, like someone who prunes up after swimming in the ocean for too long.

As we examined in the previous chapter, hydrochloric acid can weaken when the liver calls out for preemptive help as its bile production flags. Excess adrenaline also lowers hydrochloric acid production. Emotional attacks, mental abuse, continual arguments with a spouse or partner, dissatisfaction at work, and high-pressure deadlines can cause ongoing adrenaline rushes that interfere with your stomach's gastric juices. Adrenaline is like a monkey wrench thrown into a delicate, intricate Swiss grandfather clock. It's like a neighbor dumping a bottle of beer into your pot of soup simmering on the stove that you made using your grandmother's perfected recipe.

With lower bile production, lower bile salt content in that bile, lower hydrochloric acid production, and lower levels of precious mineral salts in those seven blends of stomach acid, food going down the pike of your digestive tract doesn't get massaged enough, altered enough, and prepared enough for full digestion. It's like a soufflé falling flat because it came out of the oven too early. The small intestine isn't able to absorb the nutrients it's meant to: while there are enzymes that help with digestion in the small intestine, they're not meant to do the whole job; their function is hindered when food isn't broken down enough. Ultimately, overall digestion in the gut weakens.

WHAT'S BEHIND BLOATING

When this occurs, bloating starts to happen. Part of bloating is the gut coping with poorly digested food. Another part is that when the liver is unhappy and stagnant to the point of lower bile production, it means that it's also overburdened with toxic materials that are leaching out into the bile, so they end up back in the intestinal tract, or they're being excreted from the bottom of the liver, floating down, saturating lymphatic vessels around the colon, and absorbing into the colon through its intestinal walls. Bacteria and viruses' waste matter, such as old viral casings and the sticky jelly-like sludge produced by toxins combined with pathogens, are among the materials that can bleed into the intestine. So is heavy metal oxidative runoff. These all coat the lining of the small intestine and colon, causing more bloating as it hampers any good bacteria that are present and feeds bad bacteria and other unproductive microorganisms. Ultimately, it can get to the point where overgrowth of strep causes SIBO to develop, with strep flourishing in pockets

of the intestinal tract, creating gas that pushes the intestinal linings outward and contributes to bloating. Someone can live with this for a long time before SIBO actually gets diagnosed, if it ever does, and in any case, strep won't be identified as the cause.

Due to low bile and hydrochloric acid production, undigested food debris composed particularly of fat and protein enters the scene and ultimately feeds the pathogens as well, coating the intestinal tract and creating total calamity. A condition I call *ammonia permeability*—which medical communities confuse with leaky gut—develops, with food decomposing in your intestinal tract and producing ammonia gas that both causes even more expansion of the intestinal tract (creating bloating, cramping, discomfort, and distension) and also rises up the gut into your stomach, contributing to further diminishment of hydrochloric acid and even the reserves in the stomach glands and tissue of the components that make hydrochloric acid.

Bacteria such as *H. pylori* can proliferate in this environment, causing ulcers and even lesions to form. Other bacteria, such as *C. difficile*, *E. coli*, and *Staphylococcus*, can prosper, too. *Candida* may also rise—though as you already know, it's only trying to help you by feeding off undigested protein, fat, and other food particles to break them down faster so they don't rot and feed more pathogens. It goes into high gear not because it's out to get you; it's to prevent invaders like strep, *E. coli*, staph, and dangerous funguses from getting strong. While all this is happening, chronic gastritis can occur, whether diagnosed or not, and gas can also sit stationary in the small intestine or colon, not necessarily feeling like gas because it barely moves, yet causing more bloating.

CAUSES OF CONSTIPATION

A common cause of constipation is the intestinal tract narrowing and expanding in different areas due to inflammation brought on by pathogens getting to feast on their favorite fuel. Many people, when they feel mildly constipated, will rub the abdomen and be able to feel where they're blocked as a mass or lump. When it's severe, they may not be able to feel the blockage because it could be filling up the entire colon.

Pathogenic fuel includes items such as wheat gluten, eggs, and dairy products, as well as other foods we've ingested that weren't broken down well enough before reaching the intestines. Those first foods—gluten, eggs, and dairy—are sometimes considered inherently allergenic, when the truth is that they create inflammation and other reactions because they feed pathogens, and it's the pathogenic activity and waste that give people symptoms.

When inflammation of the intestinal tract occurs, peristaltic action weakens and constipation can begin. Sometimes it's only temporary, and sometimes it's chronic, depending on how weakened peristalsis has become and to what degree pathogens are prospering in and inflaming the intestines. A sluggish liver that's producing less bile and becoming fatty and overburdened can also release viral casings, jelly-like film, neurotoxins, dermatoxins, other viral and bacterial sludge, toxic heavy metal runoff, and old, rancid fat deposits, mostly through the hepatic veins and also through the bile, and from there they find their way to the intestinal tract, contributing to a sluggish colon and constipation.

The part of the lymphatic system that surrounds the gut can also get overburdened, causing lymphatic fluid buildup that creates pressure against the intestines that's enough to slow down peristaltic action and create narrower areas that make it more difficult for food to pass through. This alone can create mild bloating, causing the belly to become hard and pushed out.

Pathogens, along with their toxic debris and sludge as well as heavy metals, can find their way into the ileum along with food that hasn't been digested and broken down properly, causing this final section of the small intestine to become inflamed and contribute to constipation. In truth, it's the most common area of the intestine to be inflamed; scar tissue can also form here.

For a man, constipation can lead to what feels like a prostate condition, with frequent urination and pressure on the bladder, or he can experience no additional symptoms besides bloating and constipation. For a woman, it can be much more challenging. For one, constipation can get more intense and uncomfortable around ovulation and menstruation. Women with PCOS, cysts, or fibroids can also experience great difficulty from constipation that results when an inflamed or cystic uterus or ovary presses up against the intestinal tract, narrowing the passageway. It can also be an inflamed colon pressing up against the uterus and ovaries, causing discomfort, pain, cramping, and constipation. An inflamed colon can press up against the bladder, too, causing the feeling of urgency for women, due to the construction of nerves that makes women's bladders more sensitive than men's. When someone has endometriosis, whether diagnosed or undiagnosed, the intestinal, stomach, and bladder symptoms can be even more uncomfortable.

If someone has had her or his appendix out, a scar or adhesion can form on the bottom right of the colon, making it more difficult for food to get through the ileocecal valve and causing a particular variety of constipation.

And when the colon is inflamed for any reason, it can kink slightly around its different bends. The top of the descending colon, on the left side of the abdomen, is a very common spot for a kink. So is the bottom of the descending colon on that left side. A kink can also occur at the top of the ascending colon when there's inflammation. While these spots can contribute to constipation, pain, and discomfort, they're not true obstructions or blockages.

THE TRUTH ABOUT IRRITABLE BOWEL SYNDROME

When someone is eating a lot of trouble-making foods such as dense proteins, dairy, eggs, gluten—and for people who are more sensitive, any type of grains—the problems you've just read about can intensify and lead to irritable bowel syndrome, known as IBS. In medical research and science, it's a label for bowels that aren't functioning as they should, with cause unknown.

(Celiac is another instance of mystery intestinal inflammation, with some functional medicine sources calling it autoimmune; that is, the body attacking itself. That's not an accurate explanation. In truth, celiac is inflammation caused by the same sources as much of what we've discussed in this chapter: pathogens. Gluten in particular is a problem for those with celiac because it feeds bacteria and viruses so they can prosper and cause more symptoms.)

IBS results when the colon is lined with pathogenic waste product, elevated levels of strep, *E. coli*, other pathogenic varieties, rotting food that wasn't digested properly due to low bile and hydrochloric acid, and ammonia gas. Contributing to it all are unproductive foods that feed the condition—for example, dense fats and proteins that bile and hydrochloric acid can't break down anymore entering the intestines and feeding pathogens rapidly, then reaching the colon, the final dumping ground for the mess. Inflammation that prompts pain, constipation, and/or diarrhea results, and even hemorrhoids, polyps, and fissures can form from the strain, as well as an itchy rectum from the irritation.

GUT HEALING

Not only are the symptoms and conditions in this chapter uncomfortable; the gut also can't absorb, alter, and deliver nutrients at its full capacity when it's in distress. That means the liver doesn't get all the sustenance it needs, which contributes to someone's overall suffering. At the same time, if someone has any kind of gut disorder, it takes longer to heal when the liver has lost its own ability to absorb, alter, and deliver nutrients throughout the body. The gut and liver, meant to rely on each other, end up each paying the price for the other's vulnerability.

Figuring out how to heal is no vicious cycle or chicken-and-egg conundrum. The answer is clear: helping the gut starts with helping the liver. The liver is essential to healing any kind of intestinal issue, and lending it a helping hand with the tools you'll find in this book will finally give you digestive relief.

CHAPTER 26

Brain Fog

When you hear that someone has brain fog, it doesn't sound all that serious if you haven't experienced it yourself. It's easy to say, "Snap out of it," or, "You're tired? Get some coffee and get through it."

Those who have brain fog know it's not as simple or easy to beat as it sounds. True brain fog—not just grogginess from a late night out that has you reaching for an extra serving of caffeine to get you through the next day—can be very disruptive in someone's life. It can be detrimental to the point of diminishing people's vitality and keeping them from accomplishing what they want to accomplish. I've seen brain fog stop students from getting their degrees—not just in higher learning; I've seen it cause high school students to drop out. I've seen brain fog stop moms from being able to take their babies for walks in the park. I've seen people lose their jobs and careers over brain fog—resigning or being handed a pink slip and let go. So when we talk about brain fog, it is serious. It has affected a lot of people's lives.

THE GUTS OF THE MATTER

When brain fog isn't being blamed on the thyroid, it's often thrown in the category of gut health these days, with articles and professionals saying that it's all about *Candida*, yeast, mold, and other fungus in the intestinal tract. A fuzzy mind, confusion, and lack of focus that take away a person's vitality and ability to function like she or he used to: it's considered digestive.

The truth is that people can have the dirtiest, nastiest small intestines and colons, filled with bacteria, yeast, loads of *Candida*, mold, and other fungus—and yet not experience brain fog. That's right; these people could be using the public restroom, with mucus from bacterial byproduct discharging from their bowels, leaving behind two kinds of strep on the toilet for the next person to come and get and still experience no brain fog. If they did have any brain fog, it would be a version so mild they wouldn't even think to call it that. Then you could have someone who does have a track record of yeast, mold, and other fungus in the intestinal tract and who does experience brain fog. Or you could have someone whose intestinal tract is clean as a whistle, with no serious gut problems, and still has a problem with brain fog. This is all because brain fog is not a product of the gut. It's just a trendy misbelief and a mistaken hypothesis that brain fog is gut-related, and it's sent thousands of people on a wild goose chase for answers.

We still want to keep our guts clean—it's not as if bacterial and fungal overgrowth in the intestines *helps* our health. A proliferation of strep in the intestinal tract does contribute to constipation, gastritis, other inflammation, intestinal scar tissue, diverticulitis, diverticulosis, colitis, IBS, diarrhea, intestinal narrowing and expanding, upper intestinal distension, a sense of burning in the stomach, sharp pains and stitches in the abdomen, cramping, and bloating. What about the people with these digestive discomforts who don't have brain fog, though? We can't package this topic up in a tidy bow, leave the liver out of it, say, "Oh yeah, brain fog is all about gut problems," and call it a day. The few who say, "I don't leave the liver out of it. I consider the liver part of the gut," still don't know the real reason for brain fog—which is why it's time *you* knew.

REAL REASONS FOR BRAIN FOG

Brain fog mostly stems from the liver and partly from the brain. As you know by now, the liver harbors certain troublemakers—for example, the pathogen EBV. Many, many people carry an EBV viral load in the liver without realizing it. If your liver is also filled with other troublemakers, they'll provide food to the virus. One such food is adrenaline, which you know the liver soaks up like a sponge in order to protect you from this stress hormone scorching your central nervous system when you're in fight-or-flight (even the

milder forms of it, like driving in heavy traffic). That fear-based adrenaline is one food source for EBV. Toxic heavy metals and pesticides are other favorite viral foods. The very reason that viruses such as EBV camp out in the liver is because the food sources there are so plentiful. When EBV consumes them, it releases different forms of waste matter, one of which is a neurotoxin. As the liver fills up with these neurotoxins, it reaches capacity, at which point they escape into the bloodstream as blood is flowing from the liver. Neurotoxins have a unique travel ability, an infiltration quality, almost like a fumigant, that allows them to easily transport themselves to different places—it's what lets them cross the blood-brain barrier. In the brain, they can cloud up, interfere with, and short-circuit neurotransmitters. Neurotoxins in the blood and cerebrospinal fluid are a big factor in brain fog.

Medical communities are unaware that neurotransmitter chemicals are supposed to be clean and pure in order to work. Neurotoxins make them dirty. Harboring homeopathic, minute levels of mercury and other metals and toxins, neurotoxins are polluted; when they enter into neurotransmitter chemicals, they pollute them, too. As an electrical impulse runs down a neuron using an impure neurotransmitter chemical, it doesn't burn clean; the impulse is shorted out, diminished, or left to run on less power. That makes neurotransmitter chemicals dirtied by neurotoxins a recipe for brain fog. This will take at least 50 years to uncover.

EBV neurotoxins are not the only cause of brain fog, though. Someone could have adrenal issues from prolonged periods of excess stress, and that adrenal dysfunction could have resulted in erratic spurts of adrenaline that the liver then sponged up, causing it to become more stagnant, which in turn could have lowered energy, allowing for a mild brain fog. Adrenaline can also get into the brain, where it can be highly corrosive to neurotransmitter activity by quickly diminishing neurotransmitter chemicals and electrolytes as it courses through. Over time, our ability to create new neurotransmitter chemicals can also diminish due to poor diet and the condition of the liver.

The list goes on. You can also develop brain fog from toxic heavy metals such as mercury and aluminum in the brain that oxidize and create a metallic runoff that can saturate brain tissue, short-circuiting electrical impulses and hindering neurotransmitters. This type of brain fog is a little different from others. It comes and goes, with moments of clarity and then confusion—though it's not the everyday, mild type of confusion that we might call a brain cramp.

Brain fog can also develop when the liver has become toxic with other types of troublemakers, such as solvents, prescription drugs, and toxic chemicals. People with this form of nonviral brain fog experience less fatigue and tire less easily than when a virus is in play.

A viral liver, EBV neurotoxins, adrenaline surges, toxic heavy metals, and other liver troublemakers: these are the various reasons for brain fog. Everyone's brain fog is different and deserves to have its real causes recognized and identified individually. What brain fog is not about for anyone is the gut.

CLEARING UP THE CONFUSION

When someone with brain fog visits a practitioner, that health-care professional should not fall prey to the belief that it's gut-related. It's an easy mistake to make: Say a practitioner does tell a patient that her or his brain fog is really a gut problem. What's the next step? Clean up the diet. As a result, that patient could see improvements, so it's going to seem to everyone that the gut hypothesis was correct. This is where the confusion lies.

What really happens is that when we clean up the diet, removing junk food and fast food and processed foods, we're unknowingly boosting the liver, allowing it to detox more efficiently, and offering the adrenals a little more support than usual. Though it likely cleaned up the gut, too, that wasn't what cleared up the brain fog. Case in point: There are people with very high viral loads and sluggish livers congested with neurotoxins who improve their diets according to what health-care professionals believe is good for gut health and still suffer with brain fog. That's because these diets aren't specifically aimed at getting the viral issues out, strengthening the liver, extracting neurotoxins, fortifying the adrenals, and rebuilding neurotransmitter chemicals.

It ends up being hit or miss whether various popular diets do any of this, which means these diets are hit or miss for alleviating brain fog. What really helps brain fog is knowing what's really causing it, so you can directly address viral issues, liver saturation, toxic heavy metals and other troublemakers, and adrenal overload.

LIFTING THE FOG

Brain fog is a big part of our world. It affects a lot of lives, both of the people who experience it directly and the ones around them. It's time they all knew what's responsible for brain fog.

So many mistakes are made in this area; so many people are blamed for their brain fog and called lazy, irresponsible, uninspired, or unpassionate. People are called silly and even stupid because of brain fog. Children are misunderstood and misdiagnosed because of brain fog. When young adults can't find the right words to express themselves, and the words that come out of their mouths don't come out the way they want—that can be brain fog. Adults often feel inadequate or useless—that can be brain fog. When anyone has difficulty making decisions and feels like the process sucks the life out of them—that can be brain fog. It was never supposed to come to this.

Understanding brain fog for what it really is, we can identify the issues people are struggling with and stop misunderstanding and mislabeling them. We can stop misunderstanding and mislabeling ourselves. You're not guilty of bringing brain fog upon yourself. There are reasons you've experienced it, and with the tools in Part IV, you can free yourself from it. It's time we lifted this fog so we can all see the truth.

CHAPTER 27

Emotional Liver: Mood Struggles and SAD

When we call people "emotional," we usually mean that we think they're being too sensitive or even acting ridiculous. In those moments, we decide whether we're going to hear these people out and listen to their emotional concerns because we care or need to work with them, or we're going to keep our distance and not poke into their emotions. Either way, there's usually an element of judgment that we attach to that word *emotional.*

If you're the one experiencing an emotional issue, you may doubt yourself. While you may be able to point to a trigger for a mood swing, like a package that didn't come on time or a significant other acting out of sorts, you may also know that's not the real problem and say to yourself, *I've never been that sensitive before.* You may decide it's hormonal, given the hormonal blame that's been thrown upon women for decades. If you stay in a funk too long, a friend or loved one may tell you that you need to seek help and talk out what's really making you emotional. What no one ever considers in all of this is that the real instigator could be the liver.

THE STORY OF SEASONAL AFFECTIVE DISORDER

A good example of liver-related emotional struggle is the condition seasonal affective disorder (SAD). The symptoms of SAD range from feeling kind of sad, gloomy, devalued, lonely, or lost to feeling hopeless, severely depressed, discarded, or even devastated for no apparent reason. It can reach the point of mental torture and suicidal feelings. A range of physical symptoms can develop, too, from low energy that makes you a little tired and sluggish to a feeling of fatigue that makes your arms and legs heavy to the point that you can't even walk easily—almost an arthritic feeling—as well as aches and pains, focus and concentration issues, and possibly a little weight gain.

When the cause of someone's suffering isn't obvious, the way it is when an MRI reveals an aneurysm or a tumor, the medical industry struggles to figure out what's wrong with patients. In the absence of answers, it's human nature for medical communities to look for outside possibilities and excuses. SAD falls into that category. Enough people went to their doctors complaining of the onset or worsening of the symptoms above that the SAD label developed relatively recently as an easy explanation that blamed the change of weather that comes with autumn and winter.

That's how it started out. When researchers present a hypothesis, it doesn't always mean that the medical establishment is going to recognize it; SAD had no guarantee of making it to the mainstream. The medical industry recognized and adopted the SAD label because it was a reason to stop looking deeper for answers behind chronic illness and save funding for other causes. Though recent history, it was an early enough time that it wasn't all about genes yet—this was just before the raging everything-is-genes theory started to dominate—and chronic illness was even less respected than it is today, with "It's all in your head" even more common. With SAD, medical communities acknowledged people's symptoms, yet the tag became a decoy that negated what people were really experiencing.

The way it's conceived of now is that as winter comes, our melatonin and serotonin levels drop, bringing on SAD symptoms. Many also believe that it's a lack of vitamin D in winter. How to explain, then, all the people it affects at other times of year? And all the people taking high doses of vitamin D and still experiencing SAD? Over time, doctors realized that these symptoms weren't just affecting people in the colder, darker months; they were also coming on in spring and summer, and so the definition of SAD was expanded to avoid funding the search for deeper issues. Any time of year now, the SAD label can apply—pick a month, pick any part of any season—which should tell you that there's something amiss with the way research and science conceive of this condition.

The truth is that there are hundreds upon hundreds of different variations of it. If medical communities started categorizing them, they'd realize something else is going on.

What is SAD, really? Many people experience 10 years of SAD symptoms, whether in winter, summer, or any other time of year, and each year it slowly worsens. Someone can progress from that arthritic feeling I mentioned to severe aches and joint pain, leading to another confusing diagnosis: rheumatoid arthritis. For that person, it was never SAD to begin with; it was a very, very mild form of RA, which, if you read *Medical Medium* or *Thyroid Healing*, you know is an EBV-related illness. Were the seasons playing a role in agitating the RA? It's possible. Winter is hard on the body. Most any condition you have will tend to feel worse in this season.

Another example of a condition misdiagnosed as SAD is sinus cavity sensitivity. When the weather turns cool, the dry, hot air inside of buildings can aggravate the sinuses and cause them to ache only in late fall and winter. What someone could really be experiencing is chronic dehydration that causes the sinus membranes to be dry and sensitive or an old deposit of strep in the sinuses from a sinus infection injury decades ago—one that could have scarred the sinuses. Low-grade strep infections are common in the sinuses, and they create sinus sensitivities such as seasonal allergies, headaches, and nosebleeds that are not diagnosed properly as strep. These bacteria are very elusive and can hide inside the sinus cavities for a lifetime.

The SAD label is one of the saddest misdiagnoses out there. It takes advantage of the fact that we do all feel a boost on beautiful, sunny days with moderate temperatures and low humidity, and it ignores everything else wrong with people. That deprives them of the opportunity to get better. Yes, a seasonal change can affect our health. When winter comes in a cold climate, we don't take as many walks in nature; we don't eat the freshest food—we don't get in our farmers' market trips and feast on a pint of strawberries here or there. That is, we don't do what we normally would to support the immune system. So if we're not upping our game in other ways as the weather gets colder, any problem under the surface will peek out its ugly head a little more. Almost all people with SAD end up getting worse, with new labels and diagnoses along the way over the course of a lifetime, because the underlying problems aren't being addressed. It's not just RA or sinus issues that get ignored. Someone who's had low energy for the last five winters may develop deeper fatigue in the sixth year and finally receive a diagnosis of Lyme disease. While it may be a misdiagnosis, nevertheless it's a diagnosis brought on by the fact that symptoms are worsening. SAD is a way of not taking seriously the early symptoms of what could turn into an aggressive and progressive health condition.

Let's talk more about the symptoms attributed to SAD. When you're dealing with depression, anxiousness, anxiety, sadness, nervousness, fatigue (whether mild or severe), or aches and pains, know that these are often neurological. In truth, almost every symptom associated with SAD, except for weight gain, can be neurological. Whether it's feeling suicidal or feeling sad and lost or experiencing physical discomfort, the brain or another part of the nervous system is being affected by some deeper cause to create these symptoms, and it's not a change in season—while the season could be a trigger, it's not the cause.

Aches and pains in the feet occur when the tibial and sciatic nerves are inflamed. Headaches, migraines, and tingles and numbness that cold air or heat and humidity can trigger to worsen are caused by the trigeminal, phrenic, and vagus nerves. Focus and concentration issues are related to weakened neurotransmitters. Anxiety and depression can come on when the liver gets viral and starts releasing neurotoxins, or when the liver gets overloaded with prescription drugs such as antibiotics and starts releasing oxidized heavy metals, which go to the brain and short-circuit neurotransmitter activity. The emotions that go with SAD, whether they have you feeling angry, frustrated, abandoned, crushed, forgotten, or the like, have to do with your brain being affected by the true story of what's occurring inside of your liver.

The liver's unhappiness is the foundation of our emotional instability—all of those neurological symptoms that are blamed on the seasons actually originate with the liver. For one, when the bloodstream is filled with neurotoxins, which are created when pathogens feed on toxic heavy metals such as mercury in the liver, focus and concentration can go awry as these toxins soak into the brain and wreak havoc, causing electrical impulses there to short-circuit. For another, emotions such as frustration and anger can arise from a sluggish, pre-fatty, or fatty liver—a liver that's burdened with fat, struggling, losing its strength, and fighting for its life. That's right; the liver has emotions, and we can feel them. The liver experiencing a down time is almost enough to give us a bodily sensation of sadness, concern, disconnect, or crankiness on its own. Then add in the poisons that enter our brain at any given moment as well as what life throws at us every day, and you can have an instant condition that a doctor may diagnose as SAD or give another label.

OUR EMOTIONAL LIVERS

Now, you could say, "How is it possible that the liver has emotions?" The answer is that with the sophistication of being able to perform over 2,000 chemical functions comes the ability to think for itself. The liver decides when to access the power of these chemical functions—it can make its own decisions. It also stores the information of our lives. Given that level of ability and responsibility, how could it not have emotions? We're not robots. Our livers aren't made out of metal, wires, and plastic. They're flesh and blood, with intelligence. When someone receives a liver transplant, she takes on the patterns that the donor exhibited. The liver recipient becomes emotional in ways she never did before. She experiences new desires, new thoughts, new beliefs, new habits, new expressions, new food cravings, new hobbies, new dreams at night— she could have the same dreams the donor had when she was alive—and new dreams in the sense of goals and aspirations. That's the power the liver holds—because it's a living, emotional, thinking, breathing, functioning part of our bodies. In fact, whether it was a liver you received via transplant or one you were born with, your liver has to make more decisions than you do in any given day. With so much to do, again, how can it not get emotional?

The liver plays a huge role in our emotional state of being. A prime example is when the liver goes into spasm; it's similar to when a person throws a tantrum. Liver spasms are the organ's attempts to free itself and ignite new energy when it feels confined or held back. Sometimes the spasm will even set off your own emotional reaction, causing you to feel caged or trapped, to feel the need to get out and go for a run, or to have the sensation of wanting to crawl out of your own skin.

When the liver gets toxic and it's holding on to a tremendous amount of poisons such as radiation, pesticides, herbicides, nanotechnology materials, toxic heavy metals, bacteria, viruses, and pathogenic waste matter (like dermatoxins), some of the poisons can leach into the bloodstream and intestinal tract, as you've read before. They can cause some of the issues we've examined like eczema, psoriasis, and dry, cracking skin that are also mistakenly blamed on SAD because they get worse in winter. These poisons can travel through the bloodstream to the brain, causing problems there such as an "up one minute, down the next" feeling that can result in a diagnosis of bipolar disorder.

Adrenaline has come up in previous chapters, and this is another instance where its interplay with the liver is important. Breakups, betrayals, being stabbed in the back—your liver wants to prevent you from becoming intoxicated by adrenaline when this steroid races through your bloodstream during these and other traumatic moments. Your liver becomes so nervous and even scared for your life that it releases a hormone undiscovered by science that draws excess adrenaline into the liver so the organ can sop it up to protect you from stroking out, from neurotransmitters in the brain burning out, and from hemorrhage. When the liver soaks up excess adrenaline from the bloodstream during bouts of intense stress and other adrenal triggers, though, it's only a temporary solution. Over time, it must release the adrenaline stores bit by bit to be eliminated through the kidneys and intestinal tract so it can be prepared to receive a new batch the next time you have an adrenal surge. As the adrenaline leaves, you'll experience the information stored within it in a nostalgic or almost surreal way. Even if the adrenaline was from a month ago, six months ago, or a year ago or more, you'll feel a little loss, frustration, or anger to accompany it.

The liver tends to release its storage bins of adrenaline with the change of seasons. It will send out a little spurt to prepare for fall, and a little extra spurt as a detox to prepare for winter. The liver will often let go of a heavy amount of adrenaline for spring, and that release can last throughout late spring and early summer, so you may find yourself processing emotions from up to nine years ago, making you feel lost as adrenaline holding on to that information slowly circulates out of your body. When your liver took on this adrenaline originally released during your emotional trials and tribulations, it also took on and held on to your emotional experiences. Its release can trigger the same painful feelings you had when the adrenaline was first released at a time of struggle, because it holds this emotional essence. As the liver lets go, you let go, too.

(Touching back on liver transplants, a transplanted liver is usually filled with adrenaline. When a new person receives that liver, she'll experience the sadness, loss, emptiness, or other emotions stored inside when the liver is ready to release the hormone. As adrenaline flows out of the liver, the donor's experiences of emotional hardship will ring through the recipient's body, and the recipient could experience the feelings associated with the ups and downs of the donor's life. If the liver was hungry for a certain food that it never got from the donor, when it's transplanted it will keep asking for that food, which may even change the appetite and palate of the person who received the liver. More on cravings in a moment.)

I'm not trying to undermine SAD itself. The symptoms are very, very real. When you're tricked and fooled with a cover-up label, though, you get cheated from stopping the condition, whichever condition it may be for

you, from getting worse. Another sad part about SAD is the amount of antidepressants people are offered when they suffer with these symptoms—antidepressants that saturate the liver more, giving it a heavier burden that makes SAD symptoms worse. For many people, these medications can take a case of SAD that once came only during the liver's annual winter release of adrenaline and extend it all year. That's not to take lightly the importance of antidepressants for some situations. Medication is indeed critical in those severe cases where someone is feeling suicidal, until natural solutions carefully brought in alleviate the situation. We need to know where this is all stemming from if we want to give someone long-term relief. We can't stamp the SAD label on real symptoms and conditions that are developing in people for real reasons and act like that's a solution. Experiences of SAD are experiences of liver issues.

AN UNEXPECTED FACTOR

Here's the most common reason that SAD sufferers experience symptoms in the late fall and early winter: dietary changes. The light and temperature changes alone have us going into hibernation mode and eating differently from normal. Then Halloween comes, and with it, candy everywhere. Soon after, we get the time change that puts us off-kilter and drinking a little more coffee to stay alert later. This loads the liver up with caffeine, one more item it must store to protect you. Less than a month later, it's Thanksgiving, and instead of the strawberries, walks, and salads of summertime, we're eating heavier food. Already on Black Friday, the rush of the holiday season begins, with cookies set out at the office; parties that encourage a few too many glasses of wine, champagne, or eggnog;

and other treats around every corner. While it may seem like only an indulgence here and an indulgence there, it adds up. People don't realize how much extra work they give their livers to do at this time of year. As you've read throughout this book, they also don't realize how burdened their livers become from years of toxin exposure and not eating well. The holidays can push the liver over the edge. The influx of liver troublemakers can force the organ to take on the extra fat of fall and wintertime treats (that extra fat is why people tend to gain weight at the holidays) or to overspill and release.

This second factor, release, is one reason why you'll feel extra emotional as you get toward the end of the calendar year. Just as adrenaline that's released on the liver's schedule is attached to emotions, the adrenaline that's attached to toxins that the liver is forced to let go of can bring out emotions. It could be that at a funeral eight years ago, you ate a ham sandwich to wash down your sorrows. All this time, your brain has stored away the memory within its database, even if you can't consciously remember it, and your liver has stored that emotional information along with the cheap ham's ammonia, nitrates, other preservatives, and fat that it neutralized and took on to protect you. Now overburdened from all the present-day holiday treats, the liver needs to release some of what it took on from that sandwich long ago, giving you a mild feeling of sorrow again as the old troublemakers that you consumed in a time of grief travel through your bloodstream. That's just one of hundreds of examples.

As organized as the liver tries to stay, with different compartments for different types of stored toxins, it does keep a miscellaneous storage bin. Back in Chapter 5, "Your Protective Liver," I mentioned that the liver can end up like a trash dump. Have you ever seen the junk area

at a dump? There will be toilets and sinks in one pile, bikes and scooters in another, cans and bottles lumped together, and then, inevitably, the miscellaneous pile, where people have tossed beds, mattresses, cardboard boxes, windows, roof shingles, motorcycles, baby carriages, car tires, and more, all of it meant to be sorted eventually. If there's just one person tending the dump, though, and more refuse keeps rolling in, that miscellaneous pile will keep getting bigger until it overflows.

That's how it works for your liver and its miscellaneous storage area, which it uses for those moments when it's truly bombarded by toxins and fats, trying to take in and process them as fast as it can. It will throw in items like the troublemakers from a funeral-reception ham sandwich, hairspray from a prom that went bad, air freshener from a waiting room where you were awaiting bad news, chemically treated fire-pit wood and excess alcohol from a cookout where your relationship broke up, and even little bits of adrenaline. The liver is not being sloppy in throwing them all together; it's being as efficient as it can in the moment, with the goal of using chemical functions to sort out the miscellaneous pile and categorize its contents properly later. The liver can only get to that organizing stage when we treat it well. Most people aren't on track to give the liver the break it needs to do this—we leave it to be the lone worker at the dump instead of teaming up with it because we don't know otherwise. And since organizing the miscellaneous pile is last on the liver's to-do list, it often doesn't get to it. When it comes time to purge to make room for more, it's this pile that gets emptied. Out come the ham sandwich's troublemaking ingredients and any of the other miscellaneous junk the liver sees fit to toss out—and with them, out come cravings. Along with the sorrow, which you probably won't be aware traces back to the funeral, you'll likely get a hankering for ham.

Any time you detox, whether in a healthy way endorsed by the liver or when it's forced to empty some of its miscellaneous storage bin to make room for more in the moment, emotions can come up as the toxins leave. It happens both during the liver's stress bomb time that is the never-ending indulgence buffet of fall and winter and also, as we saw, in those seasonal shifts when the liver releases previously stored excess adrenaline. Cravings are a subject you'll recall if you read *Life-Changing Foods*. A craving for a honey-baked ham, a double bacon cheeseburger, or other burdensome food for that matter is not your body telling you that you need iron or protein. The best way to handle these cravings is *not* to give in to them and instead to opt for nourishing comfort foods like the recipes you'll find throughout the Medical Medium series.

ALWAYS FORGIVEN

Your liver also possesses the memory bank we examined earlier in this book, a catalogue of what you've experienced as well as the ebb and flow of your lifestyle. This means that on top of everything else we've looked at in this chapter to explain why symptoms often come with the seasonal shifts, your liver also anticipates when it's your pattern to get sad at the holidays. It knows whether the end of the year was tough for you growing up because of certain family experiences, and so when that time starts to roll around again, your liver can start to become emotional, too, which you'll pick up on without knowing it. This means that the holiday season, rather than a time to trash our livers, is actually the time when we should be taking care of them the most.

Luckily, the liver is very forgiving. It has great patience. At the same time, it has a challenge: your mind, if it doesn't have forgiveness and patience built into it yet. Your liver, extremely intelligent and emotional, has the smarts and reason to know that your mind may not be looking out for it. When the mind behaves irrationally, without logic, it makes decisions that burden the liver, whether poor food choice, drug use, or adrenaline-rush activities. In these cases, the liver must become even more forgiving, sensitive, and heart-ful—because yes, your liver has heart, since the liver's number-one job is to protect the heart. In order to protect your ticker, the liver must relate to it, just as a mother or other primary caregiver for a baby must be attuned to the baby's every need. When the mind is reckless, immature, unreasonable, irrational, or egomaniacal, the liver balances it out with supreme fortitude.

The emotional liver lives inside of us: in you and in me. It has heart. It has smarts. It has feelings. Know this for certain: we *can* live with it, and we can't live without it.

CHAPTER 28

PANDAS, Jaundice, and Baby Liver

We come into this world with compromised livers. While we think of infants as beginning life with a clean slate, the truth is that a developing baby's liver takes on the past. In utero, and even at the moment we were conceived, we inherited liver troublemakers from our parents, their parents before them, and so on down the family line. Any poison or pathogen that an ancestor has carried can end up in our livers before we're born. Plus, early standard medical treatments for babies can fill newborns' livers with troublemakers. So instead of being born with our livers functioning at 100 percent like they were in indigenous cultures centuries ago, or even 90 or 95 percent as they were in more recent history, the average healthy person today is born with a liver running at 70 percent at best. Since we don't learn how to care for our livers, that percentage gradually drops over the course of someone's lifetime, for some more quickly than others, depending on exposures. It can already start to slowly reduce early in life—and early liver trouble translates to many of the mystery health conditions that arise in babies and children.

SIGNS AND SYMPTOMS OF BABY LIVER

One is gastric distress. It's not uncommon for newborns to display an inability to take in liquids, whether breast milk or formula, without chronic acid reflux. When a baby's intestinal tract is freshly developed and that baby starts to receive its food supply orally after birth, it's a shock to the system. Though taking on nutrients like this to survive and thrive is a natural progression of life, it comes as a digestive disruption early on that can cause the baby to regurgitate the liquid (that is, spit up). Sometimes, a baby spits up so frequently that it becomes alarming and sends the mom to the doctor's office with baby in tow. The doctor will often diagnose the problem as acid reflux and in many cases offer an acid reflux medication.

What's really causing the problem, though? Most every pediatrician dreads this visit, because to medical research and science, infant acid reflux is a complete mystery and there's not a lot to offer besides a good bedside manner and antacids. They have theories: Theories that the baby's intestinal tract or stomach hasn't developed properly, isn't kinked right, or is still developing. Theories that the baby's intestinal tract is so soft and pliable that sitting at certain angles puts pressure on the duodenum (the top of the small intestine), creating a very slight impediment that causes reflux. In almost all cases, the pediatrician will say that your baby will grow out of it, and most of the time it does pass. Within a week, a month, or a year, the GERD (gastroesophageal reflux disease)-like symptoms will seem to dissipate. What never goes away is the conundrum of why it happened in the first place. In some cases—if the baby was nursing when the problem developed—the mom's breast milk gets the blame. This disheartening theory could cause her to switch over to one formula, then to another, only to find that the acid reflux still won't go away and there was never anything wrong with her breast milk. After that guessing game, confusion, and fear, she likely has to build back her confidence in her ability to mother.

What's really behind a baby's acid reflux are the liver and gallbladder. It's a sign and symptom of what I call *baby liver*, when the liver struggles from the beginning of life because of all it's inherited. In particular, a baby's acid reflux is a baby's liver that's struggling to produce its first rounds of bile. Baby livers do not naturally produce a lot of bile at the beginning. They only need small amounts, because breast milk is more sugar than fat. The small amount of fat that is in human breast milk is the only fat in existence that needs very, very little bile, so it's easy to break down, digest, and disperse. It is also structured in such a way that it can coexist with the breast milk's sugar and not cause insulin resistance or clash the way fats combined with sugars normally do in our diets. (This is similar to how the sugar and fat in avocados coexist, and it's one of the reasons that avocado is the closest food to breast milk.)

Babies' stomachs only produce small amounts of hydrochloric acid at the beginning, too, because breast milk is very low in protein, and the protein it does contain is more assimilable than any other protein on the planet. Since breast milk is basically nourishing sugar water, and that sugar has a predigested factor, a baby doesn't need to use much digestion to break it down, so not much hydrochloric acid is needed.

That said, what little bile and hydrochloric acid a baby does need to produce is still important. When a baby's liver is weak from the start, it can create a digestive issue, because baby liver translates to bile underproduction and low hydrochloric acid. When a baby's liver is sluggish or stagnant right from the start, born with poisons and toxins and hampered by the effects of standard medical treatments from birth and continuing through early life, bile and hydrochloric acid will diminish even more. What little fat and protein there are in breast milk, the baby will have a harder time digesting on a micro scale, resulting in those GERD-like symptoms that are a mystery to doctors.

WHAT REALLY CAUSES JAUNDICE

Now, if a baby also has jaundice (another symptom of baby liver), with yellow in the skin, eyes, or tongue, doctors will instantly know they're dealing with a liver problem. Still, they won't connect the dots that the acid reflux is also liver-related, because it's not in their training.

The theory with jaundice in newborns—that's right; it's only a theory—is that a baby's liver is so brand new that it hasn't developed enough to fully handle the normal liver responsibility of processing, dispersing, and detoxing red blood cells. That's not what jaundice is about. Jaundice is actually a baby's liver trying to overcome a highly toxic load, to rev its engine and function in the face of obstacles that are not understood by medical research and science—because early medical treatments the baby first receives are some of the obstacles. The others are inherited troublemakers from the family line.

Meanwhile, jaundice is a baby's liver that's in shock, trying to start up its over 2,000 chemical functions and short-circuiting in the process. Imagine a farmer goes out to a field and tries to start up an old tractor she hasn't used in years. As she turns the ignition, the engine pops and fizzes, maybe blows some smoke, and certainly misses a beat as it tries to cough out buildup. That's exactly what's happening with baby liver. Troublemakers inherited and exposed to at the beginning of life are like old engine oil in a baby's liver—yes, it's possible for a newborn's liver to be dirty, since it inherits toxins at conception and in the womb. It could have been the parents' diet 20 years ago, poisons that have been passed from generation to generation, or any number of other factors that led a baby's liver to take on troublemakers.

The medical establishment doesn't have a reason to look past its theory that jaundice is a newborn's liver that hasn't caught up to speed yet, since jaundice eventually dissipates, red blood cells detox, and the overabundance of bilirubin reduces. What's really happening is that most babies' livers, after the initial struggle starting up, are able to overcome the obstacles and find an acceptable balance pretty quickly. Jaundice disappearing doesn't mean complications of baby liver have gone away; it doesn't mean a baby's liver is functioning perfectly and that there aren't *other* signs of liver trouble that no doctor is going to connect to the liver. Baby belly, that bloating and distension in little ones, is a sign of baby liver. Stomachaches and intestinal issues that ultimately get diagnosed as

parasites, *Candida*, celiac—really, the liver's a big part of why they're happening.

A HORNET'S NEST OF ANSWERS

Most of the time, a baby's gastric condition occurs without jaundice. Another liver condition may occur, such as eczema or psoriasis, only doctors won't know this is liver-related, either. Usually, the baby's liver will eventually recover, strengthen, and heal as she or he grows older, the acid reflux will disappear, and no one will ever realize a liver problem was afoot. If liver problems resurface later, no one will connect it to that person's struggles in babyhood. This is how the true story of somebody's health gets lost along the way, with the connections we're supposed to be able to make so we can understand our lives instead buried, lost, or undiscovered.

There's a reason that it's completely off the radar of medical research and science that babies are born with compromised livers all the time. If the inherited poisons we receive from our forebears were identified, catalogued, and documented properly, all the way down to which chemical factories how far back in history created each toxic chemical in each toxic solution that's ended up in our everyday environment—from pesticides sprayed on our grandparents' lawns to nanotechnology materials sprayed on manufactured items to plastics and even to viruses that have fed on all of this—every mom on this planet would have a new cause to fight for. Moms would truly make change happen. Knowing that her baby had been hindered in part by what had collected in her liver and her parents' livers and her grandparents' livers and her great-grandparents' livers without their consent, knowing that these industrial mistakes were the reality behind her baby's emergency room visits and nights with no sleep, each mom would demand that the rightful sources be held accountable. There would be hell to pay. Medical research and science want no part of unleashing that. It would be their greatest nightmare, because without the gene theory or the body-attacking-itself theory to lean on, the medical industry would be held accountable to moms and babies for the first time in history.

SIGNS AND SYMPTOMS OF CHILD LIVER

Poking that hornet's nest of answers would also reveal that it's not just babies these liver inheritances affect; it's children, too. Unexplained constipation, stomach pain, intestinal spasms, and gastritis—these are liver-based symptoms that you've read about in previous chapters. When they happen to a young child, they mean she or he started life with a sluggish, stagnant liver from the get-go. If the child's also eating troublemaker foods like gluten or dairy or taking antibiotics regularly, the digestive situation can worsen. The food itself will get the blame, when the truth is that it's the gluten and dairy and antibiotics worsening the liver condition that's already there or feeding early pathogens inside the liver, preventing it from performing as it should, and leading to constipation or other intestinal issues.

Other problems that can develop as a result of what I call *child liver*—a compromised liver in childhood that occurs as the result of inherited poisons and pathogens—include Crohn's disease and colitis. In the case of colitis, it's one of the 31 varieties of the shingles virus getting

its start in the liver and then launching a new, successful life in the colon. Many other pathogens, including strep, reside in children's livers, because the liver collects them to try to keep them from spreading to other parts of the child's body. The liver's goal is to destroy the unproductive viruses, bacteria, and more that live within it; however, if there's enough food there in the form of toxins, including heavy metals such as mercury and aluminum, the pathogens survive and sometimes become unruly. After sitting in wait, the viruses and bacteria can go rogue and escape from the liver, causing IBS, other inflammatory issues in the digestive tract, or problems elsewhere—such as early mono, strep throat, ear infections, acne, bronchitis, random rashes with pustules, mysterious boils, hives, random swollen glands, fever, and blisters.

Child liver determines more of children's health and well-being than we know. In addition to the above and many of the symptoms and conditions you'll find throughout Parts II and III, child liver can generate a lot of liver heat, especially when the organ is filled with toxic heavy metals. That can translate to unexplained irritability, anger, frustration, and even tantrums in young ones that leave many parents and caregivers feeling powerless. When it's struggling, the liver can lack glucose storage at a young age, creating a hungry liver that creates the mystery hunger we looked at in Chapter 13. That liver starving for glucose can also get little ones very cranky, with low blood sugar episodes, fatigue, and seemingly random tiredness due to the adrenal output required when the liver's glucose storage is low and blood sugar drops. Around age three, four, or five, it's common for the liver to come out of stagnation and for symptoms and conditions to go away, at least temporarily.

PANDAS

PANDAS is another confusion in medicine today, which is unfortunate, because when it comes down to our children especially, we want things done right—we don't want a mystery aspect. At this point, PANDAS (pediatric autoimmune neuropsychiatric disorders associated with streptococcal infections) is openly theoretical. The associated symptoms include tics, spasms, twitches, and acute attacks of OCD, with the reasoning that strep triggers autoimmune responses in the body that create these neurological issues.

Medical research and science have found that prior to the onset of PANDAS, children often experience a strep infection, sometimes in the form of a fever with rash—so then it's automatically assumed that strep is the trigger. The only real connection between strep and these symptoms is that both can be found in some children. Strep can also be found in children without these symptoms. When it *is* present, it's a coinfection, and two other very important factors that go ignored are really behind children's struggles in this area.

PANDAS is, in truth, a viral infection, because only viruses can create a factor that can be responsible for OCD, tics, spasms, and twitching: neurotoxins. When strep is present at the same time, it's merely a coinfection to a virus. It's not the strep causing the neurological symptoms, nor is the strep triggering an autoimmune response that creates the symptoms. Neurotoxins are the cause, and strep cannot produce a neurotoxin. Even if strep created any kind of brain inflammation, that could not cause tics, spasms, twitches, and OCD. Only viral neurotoxins can.

When PANDAS develops in little ones, it's because they were exposed to a large amount of mercury at roughly the same time they were developing a viral infection. One of the main viruses responsible for PANDAS is HHV-6 and its many mutations. HHV-7 causes a smaller percentage of cases, shingles an even smaller percentage, and lastly, EBV, though it's not as commonly the cause. Mostly, HHV-6 is the cause, and it's having a feeding frenzy on a child's mercury exposure, wherever that mercury came from. Early medical treatments could be harboring mercury, and a child could also be born with mercury deposits in the liver inherited through the family line.

With the combination of the virus plus mercury, a near explosion occurs. As the virus feeds on mercury, it releases an extremely elevated degree of neurotoxins. When these neurotoxins rush up to the brain, they immediately saturate neurotransmitter chemicals, short-circuiting electrical impulses, and that's what can cause obsessive-compulsive symptoms, tics, spasms, switches, and even difficulty communicating.

Strep infections happen to be nearby because strep takes advantage of a lowered immune system. Strep is not only the cofactor to EBV, as you've read earlier in the book; it's also cofactor to HHV-6, the very cause of most PANDAS cases. It's classic for the medical industry to blame it all on strep and the body attacking itself, though. It would be a little more fitting if the industry blamed PANDAS on strep *and* mercury, which is instead avoided. It would be completely accurate if the industry blamed PANDAS on HHV-6 feeding on mercury, creating a neurotoxin.

The rashes associated with PANDAS come from dermatoxins also exploding from the virus as HHV-6 has a feeding frenzy on mercury. They're viral toxins that surface to the skin—so the rashing that medical communities associate with strep is not really strep-related.

By the way, scarlet fever is not bacterial, either; it's also viral. That scarlet fever is caused by strep is another mistake of the medical industry. In truth, it's another version of HHV-6 or even early-onset EBV feeding off a child's large deposits of mercury in the liver or elsewhere in the body and releasing neurotoxins and dermatoxins that cause the scarlet rash.

The medical establishment does know that roseola is viral. HHV-6 and sometimes HHV-7 are the true causes. Unlike with scarlet fever and PANDAS, medicine is not focused on strep infection with roseola, though it is actually there as a coinfection, too, just much milder and not enough to come through in testing. Children can still experience tics, jerks, spasms, and OCD along with a heavy roseola rash—because it's a virus behind all of them, creating neurotoxins and dermatoxins.

It just so happens that with PANDAS, medical research and science are focused on strep, which is merely a coinfection and not the cause or trigger of neurological symptoms. For PANDAS to develop, a child must have high mercury in the body from some source or another. If mercury weren't there, chances are the viral explosion would not have erupted so early in the child's life. It would have been saved for down the road, taking the form of another viral illness that's covered in the Medical Medium series.

THE TRUTH IS IN THE LIVER

Inherited liver problems can follow us into adulthood—for many of us, the liver problems we experience in adult life started out as baby or child liver. Let's be clear that this inheritance is not genetic. It's a passing down of poisons and pathogens, both from the father at conception and from the mother throughout the baby's development. A baby's liver has a lot to do with a mom's liver. When a mom's liver and reproductive system are high in heavy metals such as nickel, cadmium, aluminum, and lead, a developing baby's liver can take them on. Also, when a mom's liver is stagnant, it creates that dirty blood from Chapter 10 that's not gauged with any scientific model because medical research and science have not yet caught on to this type of blood toxicity. When the mom has dirty blood and the baby gets nutrients for development through the umbilical cord, they'll be coupled with higher levels of toxins. Since the mom's liver isn't filtering blood properly in this case, the baby's liver will become a filter for it. In the process, the baby's liver will take on some of those toxins.

None of this is the mother's fault. It's not her fault that industries created toxic chemicals and fueled viruses and bacteria that we find ourselves exposed to in everyday life. It's not her fault that she didn't learn in school how or why to care for her liver. It's not her fault that doctors don't know how to test for sluggish liver and dirty blood and how to clean them up. It's not her fault that pediatricians aren't given the training to get to the root of babies' and children's mystery digestive, skin, and other conditions. It's not the father's fault, either, or the doctor's. Say it with me: it's not your fault!

What's important is that finally you know where the truth lies, and that truth is in the liver. Your liver, your baby's liver, your child's liver: these are precious jewels to guard with your life—and now you have the tools to protect them.

CHAPTER 29

Autoimmune Liver and Hepatitis

When illness affects the liver and doesn't ring any of the normal alarm bells that help doctors identify what's wrong, or when the liver doesn't respond to treatment, it leaves behind the classifications of hepatitis A, B, C, D, or E, and doctors often diagnose it as a mysterious autoimmune situation. It's a prime example of how chronic illness gets misunderstood and the mistaken autoimmune theory gets employed. Some doctors who think outside the box sometimes label this mystery situation as *autoimmune hepatitis*, believing that even though it isn't an easily identifiable form, it hasn't completely left the realm of hepatitis. They're onto something. Any liver inflammation that gets called autoimmune still has everything to do with hepatitis.

LIVER INFLAMMATION

With any inflammation of the liver, diagnosis is a gray area. There's no magic button you can press to determine which letter of the hepatitis alphabet you should get. Blood work doesn't separate them out, because what blood work really tests are liver enzyme and bilirubin levels to see whether there's liver

dysfunction, possible antibodies present and white blood cell count to see whether there's a blood disorder, and, overall, whether any inflammation is present. If elevated counts of the killer cells and other lymphocytes, as well as basophils, neutrophils, monocytes, or tests for immunoglobulin (IgG) indicate a new infection or post-infection of some kind, that's not enough to distinguish among the different types of hepatitis, so you move on to the next test: When the doctor presses on the liver, does it feel like it hurts? Is the liver area tender? If the answer is no, then as the doctor stands there palpating the area, she or he will be perplexed and maybe start to rule out the possibility of hepatitis A, B, C, D, or E. The third test is what the liver looks like when imaged through an MRI, CT scan, PET scan, or ultrasound. Does it show scar tissue? Cell damage? Is there a mass? An obstruction? These questions all factor in to a hepatitis diagnosis—or nondiagnosis. With everything they factor together, you're still not going to get a diagnosis that's 100 percent transparent and correct.

If the liver inflammation someone is experiencing has been long term and is acute in that moment, plus a scan shows that there's not a lot of scar tissue, then it may be classified as hepatitis A. If the inflammation is short term and acute and accompanied by a slight fever, tenderness in the liver area, and an elevated white count, it could also get a hepatitis A diagnosis. If someone's condition seems more chronic, with longer-term inflammation that's not acute, a little more scar tissue damage showing up on an MRI, CT scan, PET scan, and either elevated or low, weakened white count accompanied once in a while by a very mild fever and some off-and-on pain in the abdomen, it could be classified as hepatitis B.

If someone's scan reveals more damage, injury, or scar tissue in the liver, like a fibrosis or a mild cirrhosis, and elevated liver enzymes in the blood work show what appears to be long-term inflammation while antibodies show evidence of a possible past infection or elevated white count, it could be diagnosed as hepatitis C.

And if the liver exhibits extensive, chronic damage, with fibrosis and cirrhosis in various parts of the liver and mild noncancerous lesions as well as chronic inflammation and swelling plus bilirubin issues and extremely elevated enzymes, then the diagnosis will most likely be hepatitis D, with a hepatitis B background. Again, these are just conditions of the liver being eyeballed, with theories behind the eyeballing. It's rare in chronic illness that you ever get a straight answer that's right.

Finally, chances are you'll get a hepatitis E diagnosis if you walk into the doctor's office experiencing a persistent fever, acute abdominal pain on the right side, weakness, and extreme fatigue as well as elevated liver enzyme and bilirubin tests, a CT scan, PET scan, MRI, or ultrasound that detects inflammation, and you've been traveling extensively. If you haven't been traveling, those factors could initially lead to a hepatitis A diagnosis, though if you become sicker and it can't be tamed, then the diagnosis could change to hepatitis E.

See how there's no "hepatitis A virus," "hepatitis B virus," "hepatitis C virus," "hepatitis D virus," or "hepatitis E virus" that determines each classification? Diagnosis is all based on the guesswork of interpreting symptoms, external examination, imaging, and indirect blood test results. Some of the other usual indicators a doctor looks for are flu-like symptoms, fever, and jaundice (yellow in the eyes and skin tone). If nothing adds up to make textbook sense, then the patient's condition is usually thrown in the idiopathic (meaning unknown) pile of autoimmune liver disease with no hepatitis. Hepatitis A, B, C, D, and E are actually mysteries, too; they're just labeled, which makes them seem better understood than they are.

The miracle is that the medical system actually realizes hepatitis is viral. That's a massive, positive breakthrough. While there's not one separate virus for each, which is how they conceive of it now, there is a virus involved. That it's only one virus is unknown to medical research and science as of today, even though with those "hepatitis virus" labels, they make it sound, even to doctors, as though they've singled out one virus for each letter. The truth is that they've identified variations in symptoms, not different viruses; medicine has no proof that there are five separate hepatitis viruses, and they don't even know which virus *is* involved.

DIAGNOSIS BIAS

The most common information you'll hear about hepatitis C is that you can have it for decades and not develop problems until later down the road; that if you're worried you have it, you can run to your doctor to get an easy hep C test; and that 1 in 30 adults will eventually be diagnosed with hepatitis C. This is a misleading and incomplete understanding about what's happening inside someone's liver.

Let's break it down a bit. First, that "easy test" is not so clear-cut. It's the same collection of diagnostics we've already examined: How does the liver look in an ultrasound, CT scan, PET scan, or MRI? How's the blood work? Are there elevated liver enzymes? And so on. None of this identifies a so-called hepatitis C virus. If they *were* looking for a specific virus, they'd be stuck, because they don't know what virus to look for yet. The viral concept is only a theory—a good theory in this case, yet not a fully developed, proven answer. Even when they show images of what they've pinned down under the microscope, they don't understand it. It's part of where they go wrong with understanding hepatitis C and the other hepatitis varieties.

Some more on diagnostics: After the blood test and the hands-on check for tenderness, there's the imaging. If there are visible cysts or tumors, or if the organ's enlarged, they'll often order a biopsy to collect some tissue and examine it for damaged, scarred liver cells or cancer cells. If cancer is ruled out, not a lot of inflammation is present, blood work seems relatively normal, and only benign cysts are present, there won't be a hepatitis C diagnosis. On the other hand, for some doctors, even one test coming back positive is a yes for hepatitis C, because the condition is trending. The slightest dysfunction of the liver, and you could land yourself a hepatitis C diagnosis with a snap of the finger, before your doctor has even had a second cup of coffee for the morning.

An exception is when there's degenerated liver tissue. If scarring or fibrosis is detected, patients will likely face the question of how much alcohol they imbibe. If they answer that they drink in quantity pretty regularly and that they've done so long term, they'll likely be ousted from the hepatitis C diagnosis and thrown into the category of cirrhosis. The gray area here is vast. If the person exhibiting liver symptoms drinks martinis and other cocktails on weekends only, she'll be told she has hepatitis C, while the person who drinks a few beers every night will hear he has cirrhosis. That's a subjective measure. If medical research and science had really identified the hepatitis viruses, they'd be able to test for them and make a real, accurate, definitive conclusion in each person's case instead of being stuck in the guessing game of gray-area theories. There would be no gray area. A diagnosis wouldn't be eyeballed based on lifestyle. That's not how diagnosis works, though. In the medical industry, hepatitis C is a grade, not an identification. It's a partisan disease.

The same keeping-you-in-a-box thinking happens when you've used drugs. If symptoms develop like a mild fever, an achy liver area, and elevated enzymes, plus you have a history of recreational drug use (rather than prescription drug use), you'll likely be given a hepatitis B or C diagnosis and told it's the unclean lifestyle that's to blame, rather than the non-hepatitis diagnosis that a non–drug user with the same symptoms would get. Even if that other person uses prescription drugs regularly, they may not get a hepatitis diagnosis. It's subjective.

And here's another older medical misstep: If you experience a bit of discomfort in your liver area, a little inflammation shows up in an MRI or ultrasound, and your blood work shows slightly elevated liver enzymes or an imbalanced white blood count and you're also gay, your symptoms will likely be diagnosed as hepatitis A, B, or C, while someone with the exact same symptoms who wasn't gay would possibly receive no hepatitis diagnosis—because once again, medical communities are not identifying a virus that allows them to definitely identify what's really happening. Doctors' training in the earlier days taught them to factor people's sexual orientations into their diagnoses. I've seen these biased diagnoses happen to many people over the years, and the bias is not talked about in the wider world. While it may not occur today as much as it did 15 or 30 years ago, it does still—unfairly—exist.

With drug use, the truth is that just as many people who live what's called a "clean lifestyle" get sick livers as those who struggle with drug addiction. Any kind of drugs, whether recreational or prescription, weaken the immune system. If you're a patient who has been prescribed 10 drugs for various conditions—painkillers, sleeping pills, antidepressants, antipsychotics, blood pressure medication, diabetes medication, and so on—the liver is going to face just as much of a challenge as the liver of someone shooting up street drugs. With lowered immune responses, you'll both be just as susceptible to viral infection. The difference is that the heroin addict is going to be told she has hepatitis B or C, even if she swears she uses brand-new needles with each use because she's OCD about germs. The doctor may not trust her. They call it a different virus based on what you're doing differently.

WHAT REALLY CAUSES HEPATITIS

So medical communities are taught that there are different viruses when it comes to the liver—the hepatitis A virus, the hepatitis B virus, the hepatitis C virus, the hepatitis D virus, and the hepatitis E virus—and they're almost right to believe it. There is a virus behind hepatitis, although it's only one virus with many different strains and mutations. That virus is none other than Epstein-Barr, the same virus that causes mononucleosis. The same virus that enlarges the spleen in many people who also have liver conditions. The same virus that I wrote a whole book about called *Thyroid Healing*, because it's at the root of thyroid conditions, too.

EBV purposefully likes to make a home inside the liver and can lie dormant there for years or even decades for many people. When practitioners say you could have had hepatitis C for ages and not known it, they're right. You can have EBV inside your liver for a lifetime before it rings the alarm bells in your body that alert your doctor to investigate.

Throughout a person's life, EBV develops a relationship with her or his liver—an ongoing relationship, both fruitful and nonfruitful. In its early days, EBV was a beneficial virus that kept the immune system in gear. When the liver isn't taken care of, though, and a person's immune system isn't looked after and replenished, then as you've seen throughout this book, troublemakers can get inside and cause problems. When just the right stage is set, with adrenaline from hardships, prescription drugs, and not having the resources or teaching to eat right, then over time EBV can create damage to the liver that can eventually be seen through medical testing and diagnosed, often, as hepatitis. On the other hand, if you're eating right, caring for your body and liver, EBV can become helpless and stop causing harm so you can heal.

So many people live throughout their whole lives with a low-grade viral condition of the liver that eventually leads to a diagnosis or a confusing nondiagnosis. Many people get diagnosed with hepatitis because of their viral livers. Hundreds of millions of people don't get any diagnosis, and they just walk around with a low-grade viral infection of the liver, never knowing what's causing their symptoms and other health problems.

Not everyone with EBV automatically develops hepatitis. It's only certain varieties of the virus that, if left untamed and not taken care of right, can cause extensive damage to the liver. With hepatitis E, for example, it's a severe viral infection of a very aggressive EBV mutation that for the most part someone picks up from an outside source rather than living with it since childhood. Even in that extreme case, you can gain back control.

THE FUTURE OF HEPATITIS

Until medical research and science zero in on EBV as the cause of hepatitis, which strain of EBV causes which variety of hepatitis, *and* how to detect EBV in the liver, not just the blood, they won't be able to improve their diagnostics. The differences among the different EBV strains and mutations that cause hepatitis A, B, C, D, and E, as well as autoimmune hepatitis, can be subtle. There are over 60 varieties of EBV, and some cause more liver damage than others if conditions are right, which still leaves a gray area. Add to that the condition of your immune system, how you take care of your body, what other pathogens and liver troublemakers you've inherited and been exposed to along the way, and the factors in your environment, and there's more subtlety that influences how one individual's case of hepatitis presents itself versus another's.

Medical research and science will become more and more attuned to the differences among cases of hepatitis and keep expanding the hepatitis alphabet continually as they see

there's more to the liver condition than anyone expected. They'll keep seeing more and more mutations of EBV—without realizing what they're seeing—and they'll keep adding on to the string of hepatitis letters, just as they've done with strep. As they keep adding letters to the hepatitis alphabet, it will only be evidence that medicine hasn't yet identified the real virus behind it all. If they did, they'd name it the proper herpetic virus it is: EBV. Remember that the letters assigned to hepatitis are just placeholder schematics for a condition that hasn't yet been discovered in full. Letters only identify different viral paths of disease inside the liver, not the virus itself, which to this day they have not identified. And they may never—because if different types of hepatitis are tagged as different mutations of EBV, it will attract too much attention to this virus that they want buried and forgotten. EBV has a forensic trail that can incriminate a tremendous number of industries.

AUTOIMMUNE LIVER

Let's put hepatitis aside for a moment. A viral liver doesn't only cause hepatitis. It can go in another direction instead: a viral liver plays a huge role in every autoimmune disorder there is. If you have celiac, RA, lupus, Lyme disease, PANDAS, sarcoidosis, rheumatic fever, mono, scleroderma, Sjögren's syndrome, type 1 diabetes, lichen sclerosus, vitiligo, ulcerative colitis, Graves' disease, Guillain-Barré syndrome, Hashimoto's thyroiditis, fibromyalgia, autoimmune hepatitis, Addison's disease, optic neuritis, stiff person syndrome, Ehlers-Danlos syndrome, endometriosis, Crohn's disease, Castleman's disease, Raynaud's syndrome, restless legs syndrome, interstitial cystitis, juvenile arthritis, MS, Ménière's disease, ME/CFS, polyglandular syndrome, or any other autoimmune condition or disease, the virus that's really responsible resides in your liver.

We're told instead that these are all instances of the body attacking itself. That's not the case at all. Your body is always on your side and would never turn against you. These symptoms and conditions are very real, though, and they're all signs of a viral activity. No matter what autoimmune issue you have, there's a virus behind it, and one of that virus's homes in your body is your liver. Different viruses and different viral strains and different viral fuels cause different autoimmune illnesses and symptoms, so a viral liver doesn't automatically translate to hepatitis. A viral liver could take a completely different form, one that doesn't even show much evidence in the liver. No matter what the virus or the problems it's causing, though, if you take care of your liver in light of the realization that it's harboring pathogens, you're on the road to doing something about your autoimmune issue, rather than living in fear of what your body could do to you next. Your body loves you unconditionally.

SPLEEN INFLAMMATION

People who develop enlarged spleens without a physical injury are dealing with a viral condition, too. Any kind of spleen sickness is viral, and there's only one virus family that causes spleen inflammation: the herpetic family. Every single type of herpes virus, ranging from simplex 1 to the undiscovered HHV-10, HHV-11, HHV-12, HHV-13, HHV-14, HHV-15, and HHV-16, and all their mutations, can inflame this organ. The most common virus behind spleen inflammation is EBV and its over 60 mutated strains.

Oftentimes, anyone who has any kind of liver condition has also experienced some kind of spleen inflammation at some time in their life, whether they knew it or not. It could range from mild, going completely undiagnosed and diminishing on its own, to extreme, forcing an emergency splenectomy. If your liver condition reached a detectable stage, identified as either hepatitis or an idiopathic autoimmune condition, your spleen was most likely affected in some way by the same chronic viral infection causing the liver issue.

REGAINING CONTROL

Now you have control, understanding what creates a liver condition or a hepatitis diagnosis or an autoimmune liver or even an inflamed spleen. You can either get blindsided at the doctor's office 10, 20, or 30 years from now, or you can clean up your liver right now in life and completely avoid a liver condition—or heal and reverse the hepatitis or other liver condition you already have. That's the force of knowledge. To move forward, it's all about taming viral activity. Knowing what's really going on now instead of falling prey later to not knowing how to protect yourself the way you need to can mean everything.

CHAPTER 30

Cirrhosis and Liver Scar Tissue

When we hear the term *cirrhosis of the liver*, we often get a stigmatic image of a person who's lived an "unclean" life related to alcohol or drug abuse. This isn't how we should view the condition. Yes, it's true that alcohol and drug addictions are often catapults to liver disease. As you read about in the previous chapter, when a virus is present in the liver, drug and alcohol abuse can lower the immune system so that the virus can take advantage. Their abuse can also do its fair share of slowly injuring the liver over time. The combination can create scar tissue that begins the process of liver damage. Keeping our focus on condemning certain folks for their struggles, though, not only prevents us from lending them compassion. It distracts us from a dirty secret.

PERICIRRHOSIS

Let's give the medical world the benefit of the doubt on this one and say that the reason this secret hasn't been unveiled is because medicine doesn't know, either, that millions of people—over a billion globally—walk around with what I call *pericirrhosis*, a condition that may take decades for medical science to discover. This is a transition period before cirrhosis that can occur subtly in various tiny spots in the liver and go unnoticed long term.

Drug and alcohol use is everywhere. A huge part of the population drinks, and a huge part of the population takes prescription drugs. Not to mention that most of us have viruses in the liver. Pericirrhosis can happen for that person who has a glass of wine every other night and eats too much steak or has been on prescription medication for 20 years. And in many cases, pericirrhosis and cirrhosis don't even happen as a result of drug or alcohol damage to the liver. Many more people are on the edge of pre-cirrhosis than anyone realizes. (Pre-cirrhosis is a condition starting to get some recognition in medicine; it's a mild, early form of cirrhosis that's visible in imaging. Pericirrhosis occurs at a much earlier stage and is not yet detectable by medical scans.) Should everyone just be condemned and live with the stigma?

The signs of pericirrhosis are not in plain view at your doctor's office, especially since it's not a documented condition yet, so physicians aren't given the tools to detect it. With any liver condition, because the organ is so good at persevering through struggles, the signs don't often show themselves early given the limits of today's technology for testing and examining the liver. Imagine you're driving down the road. You can't get lost, since your car's computer or your personal device can easily provide direction. The gauge on the dashboard will keep you updated on your fuel level. You can check your personal device if you want to know the forecast, and your car's thermometer tells you the temperature in the moment. If a tire starts to lose air, the sensor will alert you. Now, what if all these warnings were gone? You'd have no gas gauge to tell that you were running low on fuel, no idea of what the weather could bring, no sense of direction, not even a paper map in the glove compartment like in the old days, and no signal if air was starting to escape one of your tires. What if your oil stick even went missing so you couldn't tell how much oil was in the engine? You'd be driving blind, aimlessly wandering until finally something—a flat tire, a dead end, an overheated engine, a blizzard—stopped you. That's the state of the liver in today's medical research and science.

As you read in Chapter 9, the current state of liver testing is merely guess testing. There's no reliable means of detecting trouble until you wake up one morning with a problem. An acute attack of pain on the right side of your abdomen and some nausea, and you're off to the doctor, where an MRI, CT scan, PET scan, or ultrasound could reveal extensive damage that's been building up for years. With the limits of modern equipment and the limits of modern understanding of the liver, they couldn't have caught it back when it was still at an early stage—when it was still pericirrhosis and hadn't stopped you in your tracks. The liver's not an important part of the medical world's agenda right now. It's

sitting on the back burner, so looking for very early phases of disease in the liver is not considered important. That's why you have to take matters into your own hands when it comes to your health. This is your body and your life that you're protecting.

When you're living with hidden liver damage, it comes down to that one lightning bolt in a storm that can finally split the old oak tree down the middle, showing us the rot that had been spreading inside for decades. When liver damage is building, one more of anything can overload the organ and push it too far. That's life for someone with pericirrhosis. Is one more of this or that going to be the strike that finally causes it to break down? We use the expressions "Don't be so hard on your friend" and "Don't be so hard on yourself." We should be telling each other, "Don't be so hard on your liver."

Throughout our lives, we're given prescription drugs to help our problems. Meanwhile, they can create their own problems if we aren't careful. If you're taking medications that you were prescribed by a well-meaning doctor who understands the full scope of your health, that's rightfully so. You don't deserve to live with aches and pains and anxiety and the other symptoms that cause doctors to reach for their prescription pads. When you're on medication, you do have to be a little gentler with your liver in other ways to balance it out. If at the same time you're taking pharmaceuticals, you've also got an overload of toxins inside your liver and a low-grade viral liver infection, like almost everyone has, and then you have a few too many social drinks, that could tip the balance. The liver trouble may not be as quickly evident as for someone who's addicted to and abusing alcohol. What it will be is a slower progression headed to the same place in the end.

SCAR TISSUE IN THE LIVER

Cirrhosis is a process of liver cells becoming damaged faster than they can be rejuvenated. Plain and simple. Millions of Americans alone have scar tissue in the liver. People's lives, situations, and circumstances can vary in the whole process. When someone's liver is stagnant from holding on to too many toxins, that's one way for scar tissue to form.

In many cases, an elevated inflammatory reaction happens due to one or more viruses inside the liver. If an aggressive virus or bacterium that's not easy to neutralize escapes past the white blood cells assigned to the liver's portal vein and hepatic artery, the pathogen can avoid becoming incarcerated, using its freedom to cause trouble. The Epstein-Barr virus, for example, can roam the halls of "school" without a hall pass, slowly making mischief and causing its own variety of scar tissue, which is off the radar of medical communities.

Liver scar tissue builds up chronically when liver cells aren't rejuvenating in enough time before the next round of instigators appears, whether they're from toxic food, toxic substances in the bloodstream, pesticide or other chemical exposure, prescribed medication, or the like. For many people, it won't be until the liver is fully loaded with troublemakers—that is, poisons and pathogens—before scar tissue can be diagnosed at the doctor's office. In all cases that aren't alcohol or drug abuse related, they'll never know what's really causing the scarring.

The microadhesions I mentioned in Chapter 6, "Your Purifying Liver," can contribute to the liver scarring I'm talking about here, though only when the liver's state of overload gets out of hand. While those natural microadhesions are created as a protective measure to wall off a controllable level of poisons, when the liver is pushed to a certain point, viruses and highly toxic troublemakers can also create their own microadhesions or even lesions. When the liver is dealing with this kind of rapid cell death, it goes into survival mode. Healthy liver cells cannot exist in danger zones, so the liver must protect you and itself by walling off whole areas that have become too filled with too many toxins, as when an entire radiation zone is walled off, or when a submarine springs a leak and a compartment must be sealed off even with people trapped inside. The life of the liver must back off from these areas that have lost their vitality—it must go beyond its natural process that it needs to function and operate instead at an out-of-control level, because what's coming at it is out of control. It groups together whole areas of microadhesions, and more scar tissue forms. Luckily, the liver also has a built-in safety mechanism.

MORE PROTECTIVE MEASURES

Protective membranes run through and across our livers. These thin, fine, delicate strips act as barriers so that the entire liver does not become injured at once. It's unknown to medical research and science that the liver tries to keep, for example, pesticide damage to one area of the liver so one exposure won't flood the entire organ in a wave. The membranes are living walls that adapt, learning how to close themselves off at the right moments so troublemakers don't get to cross the liver on the easy route. Think of one of those classic stories from elders about trips to school in the old days, walking seven miles in the cold and snow, with holes in their shoes, books in their arms, no gloves, walking hours out of their way because of a farmer's high fence that they had to walk around. That's the goal of these microscopically thin membranes: to make troublemakers take the long way so they don't all hit at once. Or think of them as levees that hold back the poisons as long as they can.

This is why cirrhosis occurs quietly and slowly and only in some areas of the liver at a time. The liver's built-in safety mechanism of these membranes allows the rejuvenation of cells to continue in certain areas while other areas are being damaged. Otherwise, the whole liver would become pickled at once. This is also why blood alcohol takes a bit of time to rise when someone is drinking. The membranes keep the alcohol partitioned at first so that the liver doesn't become saturated in one go. As the alcohol takes the long way around, and if someone drinks more and more of it throughout the night, more areas of the liver become more saturated.

A DOSE OF COMPASSION

When people have scars on the outside, they're always looking for that magic ointment that will heal them faster. No one even wants a blemish or a wrinkle. They'll go to incredible ends to figure out what to put on the skin. In truth, it's dirty blood on the inside that keeps scars from healing. When it's toxic and filled with poisons, like from drinking too much alcohol, oxygen doesn't get to the deep level of the derma where scar tissue lies, which limits the body's ability to mend scars from beneath. Everybody's trying to heal the skin's scar tissue

from above, when it's the liver they should be tapping into to mend the skin.

In the liver, it's all inside and out of reach, and so the healing must all be done from within. Dirty blood can similarly prevent the healing of internal scar tissue, and since dirty blood comes from an overburdened liver, if you don't take care of your liver, it's hard to heal the scar tissue.

This is when good, natural, cleansing, antiviral food really does matter. Pushing pathogenic invaders out to an area of the liver where the armed guards (white blood cells) of the liver's immune system can tag the virus for destruction or capture, or even push virus cells out through a flush-like technique to be caught by adjacent white blood cells that roam the borders of the liver—that's a big step toward healing. The powerful antivirals that you'll read about in Chapter 37 can give you just the boost you need. You also need antioxidants for healing scar tissue, because they essentially stop your liver from dying. There are antioxidants in fruits and vegetables that haven't even been discovered by research and science yet that are critical for softening scar tissue and bringing back the liver. If you keep your fats low and bring in the most important foods to heal your liver, you can stop the progression of pericirrhosis or even cirrhosis.

The saying "knowledge is power" couldn't be more true, especially when it comes to living with a condition that isn't shown enough compassion. Come back to this chapter when you need to remember what's really going on inside your body, so that you can truly move forward.

CHAPTER 31

Liver Cancer

You're going about your life when out of nowhere, you develop a symptom that sends you to the doctor's office, or you're at a routine checkup and your doctor recommends a CT scan, PET scan, or MRI. A mass is spotted in your liver. The first thing you're going to ask is, "How did this happen?" In other words: Where did it come from? Is it lifestyle? Hereditary? Chance? Why me? Why cancer? Why now?

If your physician is a liver expert, you'll likely get an answer that's close to reality and slightly productive. While so many medical truths remain undiscovered, in this area, there's a truth rumor among doctors, and that's that viruses play a role in liver cancer. Doctors aren't certain. They don't have a guarantee. It's not an etched-in-stone theory. Still, to them it's a possibility because they're aware that problems such as hepatitis B and C are viral and can lead to cell damage and cancers such as hepatocellular carcinoma (HCC). (There's an offshoot of HCC called fibrolamellar hepatocellular carcinoma [FHCC] that occurs more often in women.) Viruses do indeed have a great deal to do with liver cancer—so there's a lot of hope that medical discovery around this will keep advancing in the right direction.

The fuller truth is that liver cancer forms as a result of a virus fueling itself on toxins in the liver. Here's the equation: Virus + Toxins = Cancer.

Not that every time you have a virus and toxins present in your body, cancer will form. It takes particular mutated strains of certain viruses to create cancer, and they won't go cancerous unless they have strong enough toxic fuel. The most common and dominant virus that creates liver cancer is Epstein-Barr virus (EBV), which you can read about in detail in *Thyroid Healing*. Again, only some mutated strains—of its over 60 varieties—can form cancer cells, and only when they consume a particularly strong brew of toxins, so having EBV does not automatically translate to developing cancer. Other viruses such as HHV-6; HHV-7; the undiscovered HHV-10, HHV-11, HHV-12, HHV-13, HHV-14, HHV-15, and HHV-16; shingles varieties; cytomegalovirus; and all their mutations and undiscovered strains can create a stir inside the liver that contributes to cancer.

A VIRUS'S PARADISE

You'll hear that becoming ill has everything to do with lifestyle. Oftentimes in alternative medicine especially, everything is simplified to belief systems, where if you don't eat this version of "healthy" or that version of "healthy," or if you eat foods labeled "bad," then something unfortunate is bound to happen. If they don't understand how cancer really works, though, how can they say what's healthy or unhealthy? If they don't know which foods viruses feed on, how can they say what will safeguard or doom you? They can't. Not with their current state of understanding, anyway.

One of the biggest problems we have in medical research and science that has been passed down to health-care professionals is a law written in stone: a virus cannot eat anything. This great mistake—a theory that's never been definitively weighed, measured, tested, and proven—has nonetheless been grandfathered in as a commandment. Believing this incorrect information holds us back from knowing how to stop certain liver diseases such as cancer and even benign liver tumors and cysts. When medical research and science someday break this law that was paid for and invested in back in the old days and finally allow new, brilliant scientists to open doors and study viruses properly, they'll discover that a virus does need food to stay alive and thrive. They'll find that all liver growths, no matter how large or small, cancerous or benign, need those two elements in order to form: a virus (very often EBV) and food for that virus.

For a virus, the liver is like a Garden of Eden. Tons and tons of delicious food are all around, and as long as it doesn't taste the one type of food that can kill it, that virus can flourish. Its fueling foods include compounds and agents from dairy products; lactose from dairy; proteins and fats from eggs; toxic heavy metals such as mercury, aluminum, lead, cadmium, nickel, steel, arsenic, and alloys inherited through the family line; solvents; insecticides and other pesticides; herbicides; old medicines such as antibiotics stored up for years; plastics; petroleum fuel; industrial, chemical-laden oils; conventional household cleaners; and many more. They form an abundant smorgasbord of options.

Then there are the forbidden foods: fruits, vegetables, leafy greens, certain herbs, tubers like potatoes, and roots. If the virus feeds on any of those, there's a good chance it won't gain energy. With many of them, such as with any fruits, if the virus consumes some, it will even self-destruct. I know what you're thinking: it's not like a whole apple just ends up in the liver. Very true. It's digested and broken down in the digestive tract, its phytochemical compounds extracted and assimilated in a godly way, and it's these that find their way through the bloodstream of the hepatic portal system to the liver.

Forbidden foods' phytochemical compounds are tempting to a virus. Some viruses, depending on the variety or strain—the ones that aren't so smart—will even take a crack at sampling them. That's right; different types and mutated forms of viruses have different intelligence systems. There are a lot of EBV varieties that will have a go at an apple's forbidden compounds, which have glucose and what I call *hyperantioxidants* attached. Hyperantioxidants are an undiscovered variety of supercharged antioxidants, amplified to kill bugs such as viruses inside the body. When these curious strains of EBV and other viruses such as HHV-6 as well as bacteria sample that apple by absorbing the food through their cell structure, they choke and die. Smarter viruses, like others in the EBV family and the herpetic family in general, ignore the apple and other fruit compounds and move on to the foods they know will fuel them. Some very intelligent virus varieties won't even hang around the liver when it's clear someone is consuming enough fruit—they'll run from those hyperantioxidants and try to find fuel in other parts of the body. When the virus cells travel, they expose themselves to eager white blood cells in the liver that identify and destroy them. In this way, hyperantioxidants indirectly stop viruses as well.

If it's only one apple a month that someone's eating, Mr. Intelligent Cancer-Causing Virus will happily stay and just avoid that single apple. Here in paradise, Mr. Virus and his family are finding abundant resources with which to build a home for themselves. Those building materials are the liver tissue cells, which Mr. Virus fabricates and manipulates by poisoning some with toxic byproduct and turning others cancerous, using them to construct his perfect habitat. In order to do all this—both to have the energy to build his dream house and to excrete enough toxic waste to keep the pipeline running—Mr. Virus needs food. Luckily for him, he's in the Garden of Eden that is the liver, with delectable, tasty delights at his fingertips to keep him and his viral family of cousins strong. He has all the food he needs.

HOW LIVER CANCER FORMS

Cancer doesn't just appear. There's a complicated underworld constantly evolving inside the liver. Invaders like that virus speed down its streets and your liver's immune system chases after them. When the virus comes upon a hyperantioxidant from an apple or another liver ally such as red pitaya, it's a red light that sends the virus in the opposite direction. It's a busy city, your liver.

Or think of an ant farm—did you ever have one as a child or look at one in science class? It gave you a window into an otherwise hidden world, and you could see that the ants were always on the move, their world continually changing. Never again could you look at an anthill the same way, because it was like you had X-ray vision now and could see underground. It's that same perspective that we need to bring to the liver so we can understand what's happening inside of it. Does a liver tumor just appear? No. It takes poisons and a virus for them to spark the process of liver cancer's formation. Here's what I mean:

When a mutated virus strain that has the potential to cause cancer enters the liver, it continues to mutate if it has the right toxins to feed on. It takes in toxins and processes them, remanufacturing them to become even more poisonous before excreting them as byproduct into the liver tissue that surrounds it. These more-poisonous toxins can then serve as fuel again to any virus cells that come upon them, making their byproduct even more toxic. This creates a continual cycle in which only the strongest virus cells survive and multiply.

As this increasingly venomous byproduct saturates an area of liver tissue, it damages it and can even kill it. Benign tumors and cysts can start to form at this point from the dead tissue alone. The virus will also start to feed on dead liver tissue, and since the tissue is saturated with high-octane, remanufactured poison, it will be deadly to a certain number of virus cells. Fifty to 70 percent of the liver's viral load could actually reduce at this point.

For these tough-as-nails surviving virus cells, another feeding frenzy will begin. They'll feed on old and new toxins and byproduct in the liver and saturate liver tissue with the even more potent byproduct they excrete, and that will kill off more liver cells, which virus cells will then consume. Because the dead liver cells are more toxic than ever, the surviving virus cells will be that much stronger.

This can all occur in slow cycles, on and off, for years, depending on multiple factors that include emotional adrenaline releases and other triggers occurring in someone's life.

In the third round of virus cells feeding on dead liver cells that they've poisoned with even stronger viral byproduct, the result changes a little. This time, virus cells that consume the saturated tissue reach their mutation capacity when faced with its toxicity. Struggling for life, the virus cells produce an enzymatic chemical compound that transforms them into active cancer cells, giving them an afterlife. Newly structured, these viral cancer cells go back to eating the saturated liver tissue, and they reproduce and multiply as cancer. As they do, they'll release a new enzymatic biochemical into surrounding healthy liver tissue, slowly morphing the human cells into cancerous ones, too.

The cancer cells, both those that used to be viral and those that used to be human, are living, and they group together to survive. In their quest for food, these cancer clusters form tiny blood vessels to draw up nutrients past the microscopic membrane holding them together. (The formation of blood vessels is a process called angiogenesis, and as a broad concept, medical science and research have discovered it, though they don't yet understand these specifics.) At the same time, there are still active virus cells in the liver that haven't yet gone through as many cycles and reached their mutation capacity yet. They're devouring and eliminating toxins, then devouring and eliminating that poisonous byproduct, and that's continuing to kill off living liver tissue. Through their tiny blood vessels, the cancerous cell masses nearby are sucking up both the byproduct and the dead liver tissue, using them as fuel—and that's how a malignant liver tumor or cyst forms, grows, and expands.

PRIMARY, NOT SECONDARY

Liver cancer is always primary, no matter what else you hear. While medical research and science believe that liver cancer is often secondary, meaning that it metastasizes to the liver after first developing somewhere else in the body, that isn't the truth about how it works. Liver cancer develops directly in the liver through the process we just examined, not from cancer cells spreading from the prostate, lungs, reproductive system, or elsewhere.

Viruses love to make their early home in the liver. Before they end up venturing out and causing problems anywhere else in the body, their original base camp is the liver. If a growth develops in the lungs—forming from the exact same process that liver cancer forms—it means the virus was and still is inside the liver, its primary location, too. It just so happens that the virus could have been held back from creating a noticeable cancerous growth in the liver because of a strong liver's immune system, when meanwhile, the virus also traveled in the body and found a weaker link elsewhere, such as the lungs, where it could form cancer. It was the virus cells traveling, not cancer cells.

Eventually, if the liver weakens over time, the virus can also form cancerous growths there, because the virus has been in the liver all along. Certain cancer therapy treatments are one factor that can weaken the liver's immune system, allowing viruses that have been living there long term to take advantage and turn cancerous. Since the growths are developing after cancer formed in another spot in the body, it will seem to doctors as though the cancer itself spread to the liver, and they'll call it secondary cancer.

Remember, though: no matter how long it takes to develop, liver cancer is always primary. The liver is where the viruses such as EBV that create cancer like to nest first in your body. Knowing this means knowing that the liver is the place to focus in order to protect yourself from other cancers. Killing off pathogens in the liver before they have a chance to advance within your body, as well as minimizing the toxic viral fuel that builds up in your liver, is your first line of defense against cancer, period.

THE POWER OF YOUR NEW WISDOM

Everybody's liver is different, with different levels of poisons that can serve as viral fuel to different viruses, if they have any at all. Some people have more DDT for a cancer virus to feed off and proliferate. Some have more mercury. Some have more petroleum. Some have more antibiotics. Some have more fats and less oxygen. Some have more derivatives from eggs because of a very egg-heavy dietary routine. Many people have viruses that can create trouble, just not cancerous trouble; the strains they carry don't create tumors and cysts. No two people have the same liver underworld.

Eating poorly doesn't guarantee that cancer will develop, because even though someone may eat junk—or what she or he believes is healthy and is still junk—that person doesn't necessarily have a virus in the liver. Now, that liver could be dirty and nasty. It could be like the worst smelling pair of shoes you can imagine, with the kind of odor that people buy toxic sprays to cover. (Toxic sprays that get absorbed back into the liver as troublemakers, by the way.) That liver could be completely stagnant and develop the problems you've read about in the previous chapters. Yet it won't develop cancer if there isn't that cancer-causing virus to feed. For cancer to form, the perfect scenario with one of those relatively rare particular viral strains also has to be there. It's like a mite or a fungus that found its way into those dirty shoes, feeding itself from the grime in the moist toe box, creating a real infestation.

Or someone can have a clean-as-a-whistle liver, having properly cleansed all their toxins using the Liver Rescue 3:6:9 in Chapter 38 and maintained the organ by continuing to eat lots of fruits and vegetables and avoid high quantities of both plant and animal fats and proteins, and they could still have a virus sitting in there. Because the liver's so healthy, the virus won't have a lot to go on. It can't create a tumor or cyst because it's surrounded by forbidden fruits, with no real foods around to fuel it and allow it to create toxic byproduct. The old poisons from pharmaceuticals and pesticides and toxic heavy metals and other troublemakers have mostly been weeded out. This is no Garden of Eden anymore, even if the virus is still causing other problems such as ME/CFS, fibromyalgia, RA, or MS.

Which is why it takes more than just saying, "Maintain a healthy lifestyle to prevent cancer." You need to know exactly what "healthy" for your liver is, and the keys to unlock that are in Part IV, "Liver Salvation," in chapters like "Liver Troublemakers," so you can discover the timetable for cleansing various toxins, and "Powerful Foods, Herbs, and Supplements for Your Liver," so you can figure out what other foods will serve as big, old stoplights for virus cells.

Learning about viruses and cancer itself is not something to strike fear into your heart. The truth is that this information gives you the ultimate control. You don't have to be the person who says, "I don't want to know about that bus until it hits me," then gets blindsided. You don't have to live your life with that looming possibility of cancer getting you as you get older. The truth about cancer that you've read in this chapter puts you in touch with the power of your free will. You can be the person who knows exactly how to avoid the bus. You can be the person who knows how to protect your liver so you can prevent both liver cancer and other cancers throughout your body—and so you can work on protecting your friends and your family with your wisdom.

CHAPTER 32

Gallbladder Sickness

Your gallbladder, that little organ tucked beneath the right side of your liver that kindly stores its bile, contains a puzzle to solve. It has a story to tell. It has a dirty past. It has a long history of battle wounds and tales of war to share and teach. It has a treasure trove of knowledge and information inside of it.

To the medical world, it's Pandora's box. They don't want to open it, because its truths may be more than it wants anybody to know. We're not talking here about well-meaning doctors, who seek only to give patients relief; it's the medical *industry*, operating above doctors, that's wary of what secrets the gallbladder would divulge.

The medical establishment points to the stones that can form inside the gallbladder as decoys to keep us busy. Now, gallstones are entirely real. It's just that we're supposed to stay focused on those and those alone so we don't look further for answers. If we did look further, we'd find the gallbladder's battle wounds and the truths they hold.

Think of scientists assessing a pond. One way they measure its health is to analyze the mud at its bottom. Chemists, biologists, and naturalists alike know that the mud is teeming with information about the life of that pond. Inside our gallbladders, there's a secret pile of debris, muck, and sewage that's often viewed by medicine as simply "sand." When it shows up on an ultrasound, CT scan, or other imaging, a surgeon will likely call it just piles of tiny stones and then focus only on any visible gallstones. This muck, while acknowledged by medical research and science and sometimes called *gallbladder sludge*, is not sifted through or scrutinized enough. If they took a deeper look, it would tell a profound, hidden story, similar to the story that dirty blood has to tell us.

It would be shocking to see what's inside our gallbladders. In this sludge is a trail of our everyday exposures, including hundreds of preservatives and thousands of toxic chemicals at the most minute level that we get from contaminated air, water, and food. It would tell the true story of what we've faced over our entire lives, from the smog and pollution we already know about to the much deeper and wider pool of contaminants that are kept hush-hush. If we knew what it really takes to make a piece of plastic wrap from start to finish or to refine petroleum into gasoline or what certain pharmaceuticals contain or what sorts of pathogens cross our paths—if we knew what lies inside our livers and gallbladders—we would be in an uproar. We would never look at our world in the same way.

Instead, the gallbladder sits on a shelf like a dusty old library book, long forgotten. Opened properly, with the right funding and intentions, that book would tell us of the toxic warfare we encounter in our daily lives, its evidence buried in sludge at the bottom of this organ. It would lead us to chemical companies that have been around since the birth of the Industrial Revolution. And it would lead us to see that the gallbladder, though small, deserves plenty of attention.

GALLBLADDER INFECTIONS

Food poisoning is a global theme. Anywhere that food-borne pathogens exist, people can get food poisoning from these bacteria and other highly toxic microorganisms—and often food poisoning comes along with an unknown strike against the gallbladder. Whether it was a case from 20 years ago that gave you diarrhea, vomiting, fever, and extreme abdominal pain and put you in the hospital, or a mild case where you vomited for a day or two and then slowly recovered, the gallbladder likely sustained an injury. That's because the pathogens behind food poisoning don't remain solely in the stomach and intestinal tract. They also find their way into the gallbladder.

Often, people survive a food poisoning attack that affects the gallbladder because the liver kicks in with stronger bile production. The bile produced by the liver has an unknown strength factor that enables it to destroy unproductive microorganisms such as bacteria in the gut while protecting the good bacteria and other beneficial microorganisms. Bile is actually

the greatest probiotic. The healthier the liver, the stronger the bile will be, with the right acid balance and the right pH. As we get older, the bile may weaken. Add in that our gallbladders also weaken from an accumulation of stones, sediment, or sludge (more on this soon), and our bile won't be able to enter the gallbladder with the right timing and strength—which means that with the next case of food poisoning, we may not be so lucky. We could end up with an inflamed gallbladder or chronic gallbladder spasms from the food-borne pathogen finding its way into the organ. In cases of severe food poisoning that require hospitalization, patients will often extend their stay a little longer in order to undergo gallbladder surgery. (Pathogens look for weak spots, so if someone has a sensitive appendix and bacteria are raging through the intestinal tract looking for places to interfere, they could create appendicitis, too, adding to the pain and prompting a surgeon to call for an appendectomy.)

So food poisoning is one source of gallbladder damage and infection (which goes undetected, seems only like inflammation to doctors, and gets a label of cholecystitis) and damage. We can carry bacteria in the gallbladder from old cases of food poisoning long term, because they like to nestle themselves in there. We also carry the wounds, like scar tissue, that can come along with even mild cases of food poisoning in which we didn't exhibit any symptoms of an infected or inflamed gallbladder.

And we can have strains of *Streptococcus* bacteria inside us that have been passed down from our parents, that we've had since a childhood case of strep throat, and/or that we've picked up along the way (more in Chapters 23, "Acne," and 24, "SIBO"). This strep can enter the gallbladder and, over time, weaken its lining, creating scar tissue that allows for crevices and pits to form.

An important side note is that strep and *E. coli* are what create diverticulosis and diverticulitis, through a similar process to how the gallbladder becomes scarred. These bacteria are the divot makers inside the colon, making crevices and pits called *diverticula* in the intestinal lining that they can then infect. It's sort of like the way a woodpecker's holes in a tree create cozy burrows for spiders, ants, nematodes, and other creepy-crawlies to inhabit. In the colon's diverticula, bacteria can bury themselves and hide away from the immune system. When unproductive foods cruise by, the bacteria will reach out and grab some to fuel themselves. When healthy foods sweep past, the bacteria will do their best to sink down so they don't get ousted. A powerfully medicinal fruit, vegetable, or herb acts a bit like a woodpecker, getting in there to extract the bugs.

Back to the gallbladder. Strep loves to nestle into any openings before the organ has a chance to heal. In this case, the woodpecker that can dislodge the burrowed bugs is bile. Remarkably enough, healthy, strong bile also holds the building blocks for tissue repair inside the gallbladder. This is unknown to medical research and science. Good bile is, in truth, filled with a treasure trove of vitamins, minerals, and undiscovered chemical compounds that work continually over time to heal the inner lining of the gallbladder.

Here's the thing: oftentimes in our world today, people don't have good bile. Say a farmer looking to buy some land with hard-earned money from seeds she's sown and reaped walks into the middle of a field she's thinking about purchasing. She sticks her hand in the earth, grabs some, and has enough experience to know that she doesn't need to run that dirt

through a lab test. She can smell it, feel it, and even taste it, and know in that moment that this land hasn't been respected; it's bad dirt. That's what we've ended up with, the way we treat our livers: bad bile. If it were that sample of dirt that the farmer inspected, she'd turn down the deal.

While the harmful microorganisms of food poisoning can cause immediate problems in the gallbladder, day-to-day strep that ends up there doesn't wreak havoc instantly. It nestles itself in there over years and even decades, taking advantage of the rocky road the gallbladder has faced and our high-fat diets that have burned out the liver's bile production. In time, the strep finds its opportunity for a gallbladder infection, causing it to become mysteriously inflamed and prompting a doctor to order an MRI, ultrasound, CT scan, PET scan, or X-ray. And actually many times, the chronic, low-grade gallbladder infection will be missed.

If it is caught, there's often not enough evidence to call for its removal, which isn't a bad thing. Still, it creates a very confusing situation for both doctor and patient. It especially confuses doctors when the patient has either no or few gallstones, because they expect someone exhibiting gallbladder issues to have a whole pile of stones in there, like the pouches of gold and silver carried around inside the suit jackets of old-timers. Coincidentally, it was the practice to hang these pouches on the right side, same as where the gallbladder is situated, so that if they got into a fight, they could protect themselves with the stronger right arm (if they were right-handed) while guarding their treasure with the left. Like a coin pouch, when the gallbladder fills up with stones, it gets heavy, which can create pressure on the right side; doctors know this. What throws them is when they find sludge, muck, or sediment in the gallbladder instead— if they find it. While they can come across it in ultrasounds, this material isn't as identifiable as gallstones, so it seems like a worthless discovery to doctors. Meanwhile, the sludge is finding its way into any crevices in the gallbladder's lining, and since weakened bile doesn't have enough woodpecker power to extract bugs from their burrows, chronic infection is occurring that's creating mysterious spasms that bring on periodic pain.

Sometimes, as I said, no one will detect the infection and inflammation at all, so the gallbladder won't be removed. Sometimes surgeries are ordered for gallbladders that didn't really need to come out; they just needed a better diet—one that didn't follow the trend of high fat—and a chance for healing. Even if someone isn't aware of exactly what's ailing her or him, chronically inflamed gallbladders can still heal. Not that gallbladder removals (known as cholecystectomies) are always unnecessary. If not caught early, a dysfunctional liver with weak bile production, an injured gallbladder, and the amount of bacteria we come across in our lives, including brand-new varieties of strep as well as *E. coli*–tainted food, can add up to an infected gallbladder, to the point of becoming obviously gangrenous in an imaging scan.

GALLSTONES

What about if you're not dealing with a gallbladder infection, and instead you're only dealing with gallstones? Let's talk about those stones. Medical research and science know about two types: *cholesterol stones* and *pigment stones* (also called bilirubin stones). First, let's consider those pigment stones, which are made from the bilirubin of discarded red blood cells. They're created when the liver is coping with constant toxicity. With troublemakers such as solvents,

pesticides, heavy metals, medications, alcohol, and plastics in the liver plus a high-fat diet, the liver must constantly detox, which can accelerate the death of red blood cells, and it struggles as it detoxes. Dead red blood cells that would normally be tossed out begin to collect instead, forming a soft, jelly-like substance. Like a ball of clay, the cells stick together.

Now, if your liver is highly toxic, its internal temperature is higher than it should be. Liver heat is a concept recognized in Eastern medicine, though not yet fully known or understood. There's actually a good type of liver heat, a warming of the liver that happens when it's being supported in a gentle detox. When it's overwhelmed with material for detox, though, and pushed continually with no breaks whatsoever, then it starts to overheat. Imagine a friend borrowing your car. Before he even leaves your driveway, he sits there with his foot on the gas, revving up the engine when it doesn't need to be revved. Once he finally leaves your driveway, you notice him revving it again at the stop sign. You decide that when your friend returns, you'll tell him you'll never lend him the car again—then 10 minutes later, you get a call from him saying he's on the side of the highway waiting for a tow truck. When you meet him at the mechanic's shop, you see that the engine overheated to such a degree that the metal became malleable and two pieces of the engine forged themselves together. The amount of coolant in reserve had not been enough to sustain misuse.

When the liver overheats from trying to detox so much at once, a colliding of liver responsibilities can occur. Chemical compounds from poisons it's been storing to protect you can smash into dead red blood cells, and the intense heat can forge them together. The liver pushes out this forged material to the gallbladder, because bilirubin is disposed of in bile. Since the gallbladder's temperature is lower than the liver's, an undiscovered cooling process occurs in transit—that's what transforms a jelly ball into a pigment stone. If medical research and science analyzed pigment stones thoroughly, they would reveal secrets of what's happening inside the liver.

Cholesterol stones are forged in the same way. Bad cholesterol (there's more than just one) coupled with toxic matter in the liver bind together when the liver overheats, and then these masses cool in the gallbladder, creating stones. Actually, even good, healthy cholesterols can contribute to a cholesterol stone if the liver is struggling and bile production is low. A high-fat diet (keep in mind that any high-protein diet is high-fat) helps contribute to cholesterol stones.

It's important to understand this, because it means that the more toxic the liver, the more heating and then radical cooling occurs: the hotter the liver is, the colder the gallbladder has to be. The gallbladder sits in an area underneath the right side of the liver, where in good circumstances, it has enough blood and fluid between it and the liver to try to keep its cool. This is a fluid that hasn't yet been identified and is instead mistaken by medical communities for normal blood. In reality, it's not just blood between the liver and the gallbladder; there's also a very thin layer of protective coolant that has a mucus-like, gel-like consistency, like a paste or a jelly, that acts as a lubricant cooling shield between the two organs. It's actually one of the liver's chemical functions to produce this chemical agent for its underside. You can't see it with the naked eye; if medical research and science were aware of it, though, they could swab it and study it under the microscope. So between this blood and fluid, the gallbladder has a coolant shield from the liver—and the body fights to keep that gallbladder as cool as possible, whether stones have formed or not. If you're in an earlier part of life and you don't have gallstones, you could still have massive liver heat developing and a gallbladder that wants to go stone cold to cope.

Oftentimes, the liver becomes so burned out that it can't produce as much of the jelly shield. The gallbladder's not supposed to overheat, and so the body must fight to keep the gallbladder's temperature down, which can forge more stones. Plus, the more toxic the liver is, the more radical cooling must occur in the body. It creates a constant tug between hot and cold that can bring about the classic symptom of hot flashes, which are too often mistaken for a hormonal issue caused by menopause. The real reason these hot flashes happen to occur around the time a woman ceases menstruation is that it takes a good number of years before someone's liver gets that toxic. When it does, which is often by pure timing also when a women happens to be entering menopause or perimenopause, the constant hot and cold of the liver getting revved up and then trying to expel that heat can cause for many—in addition to hot flashes—random sweating, loss of digestive strength, emotional ups and downs, intense mood swings, irritability, depression, sadness, anxiousness, and sleeping issues. The same symptoms can occur for men, too—because they're not really menopause symptoms. (For the explanation behind why so many symptoms are misattributed to menopause, see *Medical Medium*.) Women are often prescribed hormones in answer, which gives the liver an even harder time. Whether standard hormone therapy (HRT) or bioidentical hormone replacement therapy (BHRT), the steroids bombard the liver without anyone realizing it. Instead of giving the liver a hand, hormone replacement burdens it more.

Over time, the liver can lose the ability to create that excessive detox heat, and that's not good, either. If your liver's staying cool because it's so healthy it doesn't need to rev up, that's one thing. If it's been overheating for decades and becomes so sick and burned out that it can't get hot anymore, that's not what you want. It means it can't detox with the same strength anymore.

When the liver is working well, the body has a built-in feature to prevent stones, and that's bile. One of bile's jobs when it's strong is to disperse bilirubin, watering it down like turpentine thins paint. As the liver sends bile into the gallbladder, it disperses red blood cell pigments so they won't clot problematically. It does the same with cholesterol, thinning it in the gallbladder to prevent cholesterol stones. Strong bile also means less heating of the liver, which translates to less need for the gallbladder to cool, which creates fewer gallstones. A liver that gets overloaded, however, leads to weakened bile production, and we lose this fluid's protective measures. The undiscovered chemical compound that the liver produces for the bile to help thin out and disperse red blood cells and cholesterol also diminishes.

Thousands of people deal with this mysterious, chronic pain in the abdomen or rib cage. If a doctor can't find gallstones or gallbladder inflammation, only a gallbladder filled with sediment and sludge, there's often no diagnosis. The truth is that when the gallbladder is filled with stones and sludge, its placement can actually shift from the heavy weight. It rests in an area of hypersensitive nerves around the liver and colon, so when it moves, it can not only put pressure on the gallbladder's neck; it can also put pressure on, irritate, or agitate surrounding nerves, any of which can trigger gallbladder spasms or random pains. When people with this discomfort lie on their side or sit up in bed in a certain way, it can help alleviate a spasming or painful gallbladder. The gallbladder's weight shifting around is the unknown explanation for how people find moments of peace and relief in the midst of this mysterious pain. Castor oil packs around the rib cage are another way of calming spasms and pain. Everyone's a little different, so the placement of those packs will depend on what's comfortable for you; the right side of the abdomen or around the ribcage to the back are helpful spots for them.

GALLBLADDER FLUSHES

Flushing the liver and gallbladder in order to purge stones is a popular trend. One technique, which I do not endorse, is to drink a large quantity of olive oil at once. What happens when we drink 4, 6, or even 12 ounces of oil, depending on the recommendation we find? What if we drink more than is called for, guzzling from the bottle without measuring? Why is this all a bad idea?

When people drink oil, they often think they see flushing results, because they pass jelly-like balls and "stones" in their feces. These masses are really made of the oil they just drank coagulated with debris from the gut—your digestive system uses mucus to package the oil into those little balls, which can end up different colors due to the food that was near the oil in the intestinal tract when it was encapsulated. They're not gallstones or liver stones miraculously expelled from the body. They're a sign of the body pushing the oil out. (More on liver stones in Chapter 34, "Liver Myths Debunked.")

Why doesn't your body look kindly on all that oil when you're trying to do it a favor? Because when you drop an excessive amount of radical fat into the stomach, it forces the liver to produce an extremely large amount of bile.

There are several reasons why this isn't a good idea. One is that if your liver's already weakened, it puts it under enormous stress to use all of its reserves to produce an emergency supply to send to the gallbladder for delivery to the digestive tract. (And if your liver is weakened already, who would know? It's not a developed science yet; we're not yet at a place where you're going to find out at the doctor's office. Don't think you're free of liver problems because you haven't received worrying liver enzyme test results.) Still, the liver must uphold its responsibility to protect the pancreas at all costs, so it will go to this exhausting, dangerous level where it was never meant to be pushed.

As you know well by now, most people have low bile production because their livers are sluggish, weakened, slightly disabled, or struggling in some other way. While in this state, the liver still has the ability to create bile as needed and balance its reserves, though it will also need to make less (and less-strong) bile. The liver curbs bile production because it has so many other chemical functions to perform—so it gives the body enough bile to take care of at least 50 percent of its normal breaking-down-fat needs. Anything lower, and the liver knows the pancreas will start getting hurt. The degree to which the liver must lower bile will be different for every person. So if it's a healthier liver, it can produce stronger bile in more quantity, allowing less sacrifice to occur in other areas of the body and ensuring that the pancreas will not be threatened by fat. If someone had a sluggish, stagnant, struggling liver and compensated by eating a healthy, low-fat diet, 50 percent bile production would be adequate to keep the digestion going while also allowing the liver to perform all its other important functions to sustain itself, giving your liver and you a longer life. Mind you: we're on high-fat diets in the United

States. We've been on them for a while now, and even more so in the present day. It's part of what contributes to weak livers. And because of this, so many people's bile production isn't enough to match their diets. The pancreas pays the price.

When you drink a whole bunch of olive oil, the liver goes into a frantic panic mode. It must stop all its other responsibilities immediately. That means hormone conversions, pathogen monitoring and killing, immune system functioning, red blood cell detoxing, and the other multitudes of chemical functions, including the ones you read about in Part I. All of this gets put on hold and the liver takes its every last reserve to create emergency bile, all because somebody once invented the concept that it would be good to purge some stones by drinking olive oil, and the idea sparked a trend. It's an example of a man-made protocol devised without a lot of understanding of what really happens in the body. During this drop-everything bile production, the liver knows that if we don't have enough bile to ward off those 4, 6, 8, 10, 12, or more ounces of olive oil we've downed in one shot, we could be facing a case of pancreatitis. It's a type of pancreatitis different from when the gland becomes inflamed by pathogens such as food-borne unproductive bacteria attacking it; the pancreatitis you're at risk for from a gallbladder flush occurs when the pancreas undergoes enormous stress and becomes inflamed from this form of injury.

That's the technical look at it. If the liver could speak, it wouldn't say, "I'm trying to ward off pancreatitis"; it would say, "Don't worry, I'm here to rescue you from damage." That's because the liver knows that the pancreas is at high risk from a fat-based gallbladder flush. Most people are unaware that the pancreas is already stressed from a standard diet, and even stressed from a normal, healthier, high-fat, high-protein diet or a radical ketogenic diet, all of which lead to low bile reserves. Add in a gallbladder flush and the liver is pushed to the extreme to try to protect the pancreas from becoming ill. This is why so many go through what they think are the symptoms of a cleanse or purge after a gallbladder flush. In reality, they became sickened from it, and then after a day or so, they naturally recovered.

Here's another problem: Much of the bile that the liver produces gets sent to the gallbladder, and when the gallbladder is filling with such high amounts of bile, it can dislodge a stone that was never supposed to be dislodged and sweep it away to the duodenum. If it's a large stone, it can get caught in the bile duct, causing immediate infection and requiring surgery. I've seen this many, many times over the years, when someone came to me after trying a gallbladder flush I'd never recommended.

You may feel better after a gallbladder flush, though that's only an illusion, because you were feeling so poorly during the flush itself. Anything after that protocol is going to feel like an improvement, and it will distract you from the reality that you're not doing as well as you were before the flush. That worsening is because if you have a sluggish liver to begin with, then after a gallbladder flush the liver will produce less bile than before. It will drop beneath that 50 percent threshold, down to more like 30 percent of your bile needs on a daily basis. This puts your pancreas at constant risk—unless your liver can get rejuvenated. Chances are, a person who tries a gallbladder flush will return to a trendy high-fat, high-protein diet afterward, unknowingly putting the pancreas in danger because there's not enough bile to adequately break down the fat they're consuming. You may realize after a little while that you're not feeling

as well as you'd like and decide that you need another flush. It becomes a vicious cycle, with the next flush weakening you further so that you think you need another, and so on, and you can experience a gradual decline. (The same thing happens with a liver stone flush.)

If, on the other hand, you had a strong liver and tremendous bile reserves before you tried a flush to try to get rid of gallstones, your liver's still going to have to work hard to produce a whole lot of bile during the "flush." At least you won't be up against that same risk as someone with a weakened liver and pancreas. The conundrum is that you don't know if you're someone who has a strong liver and pancreas. So it becomes a game of Russian roulette, a guessing game where you shouldn't be guessing. Because even if you have a perfectly healthy liver and pancreas, if you do have a gallstone, you put yourself at risk for dislodging it and getting yourself in trouble. You'll have less chance of that stone getting lodged in the bile duct because you'll have enough bile to keep pumping into the gallbladder to push it along, whereas someone with a weaker liver only has one big push of bile in them. Still, you don't know if you're the lucky one, and emergency gallbladder surgery is not how you want to find out.

TAPPING INTO YOUR BODY'S SECRETS

Why put yourself through all this? There are better ways to keep gallstones from growing, dissolve stones, and recover and restore the liver without going through the above. In today's world of big ideas, we get tricked into thinking something is bad when it's really good and good when it's bad. With all the advances in technology, we think we're smarter than ever, when the truth is that in areas like chronic illness, sometimes our society is dumber. That's why chronic illness is still such a mystery to the medical industry and why we try things that aren't necessarily right for us. Gallbladder flushes are one of them, and it's nobody's fault. It's just a case of not knowing how the liver really works and a lack of awareness of the mysteries inside our gallbladders.

One lifesaver we're fooled into thinking is bad is fruit. We shun fruit and tend to think of it as the enemy—when it's the very solution to free us. We carry around fruit fear, thinking we should be off every carb. Don't let that high-protein (translation: high-fat) diet with the green juices fool you. While it's better than the standard diet of fried and processed foods, don't think it's going to dissolve your gallstones. In fact, it can still create them (as well as kidney stones). While sodium-rich vegetables such as spinach, kale, radishes, mustard greens, celery, and asparagus can be great for getting rid of stones, if they're part of a high-protein diet, all they're going to do is fight against that high fat content that's giving the liver an extra load.

To dissolve stones, you need to lower your radical fat intake, and that means lowering your dense protein intake regardless of what diet you subscribe to, whether it's plant-based or includes animal products. Bring in plenty of fruits like cherries, berries, melons, lemons, limes, oranges, grapefruit (if they work for you), tomatoes, and a little bit of pineapple in addition to those greens. And don't fall into the fear that you need to deseed, peel, or tear apart your tomato. All that does is take away critical nutrients that help heal autoimmune conditions and other chronic illnesses as well as the liver, pancreas, and gallbladder. Regardless of how you've been conditioned to feel about fruit, stones won't dissolve without enough of it. A glass of lemon or lime water every morning and evening is a handy tool to enhance the stone-dissolution process (and cleanse your liver), as is juicing a handful of fresh, raw asparagus along with whatever else you're throwing into the juicer.

With every step you take to care for your liver and gallbladder, whether you've suffered from gallbladder infection, gallbladder stones, or another affliction—or if you've had your gallbladder removed, and this chapter has helped you finally understand and process what led to that—you're one step closer to tapping into your body's secrets. You're the one now saying, "Don't worry, I'm here to rescue you."

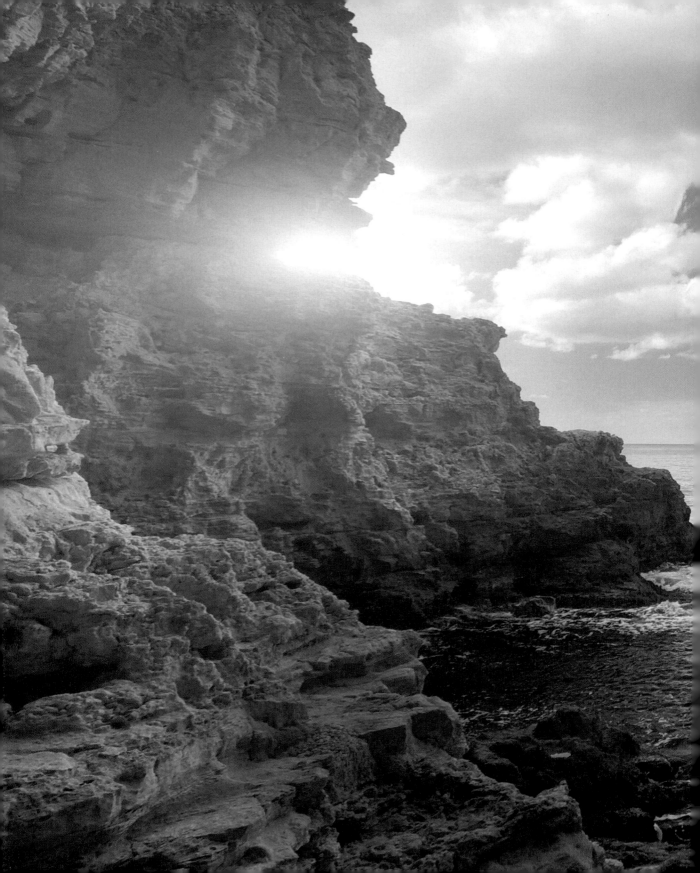

PART IV

LIVER SALVATION

HOW TO CARE FOR YOUR LIVER AND TRANSFORM YOUR LIFE

CHAPTER 33

Peace within Your Body

Your liver's unwavering, heroic fight for survival takes place because it has a baby to protect. That baby is you. From the time you were in the womb, your liver has taken responsibility for you. Like a newborn in a mother's arms, you're what your liver cares about more than anything else.

As your liver was developing in utero, it received precious directions and information directly from your mother's liver, messages sent via chemical communication about how to perform thousands of functions. One was paramount: to never give up on you. This blessing inherited from and ignited by our mothers' livers is the basis of survival. It's the foundational rock of the liver's over 2,000 chemical functions, and like many of the other functions, it is undiscovered by medical research and science.

This motherhood quality passed down from liver to liver is a never-giving-up mentality, one of the profound bonds between mother and child that exists beyond sight. Even when times are tough and an outside observer can't see what binds a mother to a child, deep in that mother's heart and deep in that child's soul, an unbreakable bond exists. It exists, too, between your liver and you: a whatever's-best-for-my-child

consciousness. Picture your liver as a parent saying, "What are the best schools?" "How am I going to put food on the table?" "Who's my child going to play with?" "Is my child safe? Happy? Warm?" You'll get a pretty accurate sense of how deeply your liver cares and wants to see you thrive. This is the source of your liver's willingness to persevere and keep you protected. Your liver learned, before you were born, never to surrender to weakness. It learned never to dodge a responsibility or opt out of a challenge before it. Your liver learned to take care of you as if you were its young for the rest of your life.

Regardless of how many obstacles in its path, your liver will try to climb them. It will do what's right for its baby: you. Your liver will fight to keep you young and safe even if this means that it's forced to grow old and sluggish in the process. It will even take bullets for you in the hopes that one day you may receive the message to rescue it, as it has done for you for all these years and as it will always try to do for you, no matter what.

Overworked and overtired, with an endless to-do list and not enough support, the liver is the organ with which we can most identify. It's the organ of our time, multitasking and adapting and forging ahead in the face of setbacks, just like we do. This also means we have unique insights into it. We can empathize with how it needs a moment's relief from the quicksand feeling of trying to keep up with each day. We can recognize its weariness from the pressure to be everything all at once. We can resonate with how after a lifetime of being a protector, it needs someone to have its back. Remember how at the beginning of this book, I called symptoms lifesaving? It's time to put that saving into action. After all these years of our livers coming to the rescue, we can finally be the heroes they need us to be.

SAVING YOUR LIVER

Here in Part IV, we'll explore what you can do to be that hero. When we think about taking care of our bodies, so often, it's about looks. In the quest for a lean physique and soft, glowing skin, we don't have an inkling of what really needs to be cared for: the liver. It's understandable. We can't forget about appearance, because it's plain to see. Meanwhile, unless we've just read over 30 chapters about the organ, we walk around without really thinking about our livers. Life keeps us busy and throws so many challenges at us that I even forget about mine unless Spirit reminds me. The liver sits out of sight, and we don't get Liver 101 to teach us about its invisible power. It's not part of a school's mission statement to look after children's livers. No one tells us, "Hey, don't let your liver get sluggish, dehydrated, and congested!" or, "Hey, cleanse your liver at least a couple times a year, just like you wash your car. And make sure you do it in a really safe, gentle manner. You've gotta look after that puppy!"

As I always say, we're a see-it-to-believe-it society, and that can hurt us along the way. If you see dirt on your car, you'll go to the carwash. If you can't see dirt on your liver, then it must not be there. If we can't see the toxins we inherited from the start, if we can't see the pathogens nesting, if we can't see the sticky film building . . . So the external occupies and consumes us. We focus on the right dress, skirt, shirt, socks, or pair of jeans, wanting them to make us look good while also being comfortable, and we never make sure that the liver is also comfortable. Is it girdled by a dress of fat? Is a scarf of toxins and other poisons suffocating it? Is there a too-tight hat of heavy metals on our liver's head?

When we focus inward, we don't have to abandon the hope of looking good. Ironically, by shifting focus to the liver, we de-age the skin, help slough off weight, enhance nutrient processing to build better muscles, look better in our clothes—all while freeing ourselves of symptoms and illness. The people who stay focused only on appearance may drink a martini or champagne while visiting the spa and then end the day with a steak dinner and a generous serving of butter, not realizing that they're burdening the liver and in doing so, fighting against the very goal they're trying to accomplish.

No matter what angle you're approaching liver care from—whether to look better, feel better, honor and repay the liver for all it's done, or help prevent problems down the road—it's a winning angle. It's one that helps clean up the blood and lymphatic system, loosen up fat cells in the liver, and give the adrenals a break. If you're gaining or holding on to weight despite your best efforts with diet and exercise, giving your liver the proper TLC will help change your direction. If you have liver damage from alcohol or prescription or recreational drugs, or if you have mystery scar tissue, you can work on bringing the organ back. It's not your fault. No matter what, since the liver is responsible for neutralizing harmful materials as well as flushing poisons and pathogens out of the body, getting the liver back up and functioning is critical for good health. If you've got to do it in baby steps, you can do it that way. You won't go it alone. Together, we'll all be working with you.

And you'll have tools—so many tools—laid out in the chapters ahead. In Chapter 34, we'll bust some liver myths. Steering clear of these fads, trends, mistakes, and misconceptions will give your liver critical protection. One of them, the high-fat trend, is overflowing with information, so Chapter 35 will get into more truths about why this one is not on your liver's side. Then it's on to Chapter 36, where we'll explore the liver troublemakers I've been referencing throughout this whole book; here you'll find more detail on what to avoid, why to avoid it, and how long different troublemaker types usually take to leave from your liver when you work on cleansing them. In Chapter 37, you'll find critical insights into how to fuel and heal your liver with powerful foods, herbs, and supplements.

And then it's the chapter that takes it all to a new level of life-changing: Chapter 38, "Liver Rescue 3:6:9." This nine-day cleanse will unburden your liver like nothing you've tried before, and the accompanying morning routine will give you a simple mini-cleanse to help work up to or maintain all that progress. In the following chapter, Chapter 39, "Liver Rescue Recipes," you'll get delicious snack and meal ideas, with full-color photos to get you excited about getting in the kitchen. And then comes Chapter 40, "Liver Rescue Meditations," where you'll find nine meditations tailored to your liver's different needs, such as releasing fat, reversing disease, and strengthening the organ's immune system.

With all you find in this how-to guide, between cleaning up your liver and being pro-active to guard against threats on the horizon, you'll finally have your liver's back. By the time you read my parting words for you in "The Storm Will Pass" and then turn the last page, you'll be fully equipped to transform both your liver and your life.

A WORLD OF PEACEFUL LIVERS

We look for peace in every form: in our minds, bodies, souls, and hearts; among neighbors; among family; and in the workplace. We seek world peace, wondering what our contribution can be to make this planet a better place. People even travel to the ends of the earth to find peace, never realizing that one of the greatest answers is this lowly organ inside all of us.

That can't be right, can it? Even after reading page after page about the liver, you must still be asking how a lump of tissue could change the world. Well, we all know that the brain is responsible for the advancements of society, even though you could call that a lump of tissue, too. Although it's only a hollow muscle, we revere the heart as our emotional and physical center. The lungs are just a couple of balloons, yet we know they give us the breath of life. So why don't we elevate the liver to its rightful place as peacekeeper? Simply because we haven't been shown how or why. Until now—now you know that your liver looks out for the rest of your body like a mother for a newborn, that it's your defense against countless health problems. It can't help that in its mission as peacekeeper, it gets pushed past its limits.

Imagine a world without chronic anger, without the suffering of babies and children, without aches and pains, without sleepless nights, without uncontrollable weight gain, without gnawing hunger, without out-of-rhythm hearts, without hot flashes and night sweats, without mood swings, without raging rashes, without roiling intestines, without backed-up bowels, without blood sugar spikes and drops, without strokes, without heart attacks, without cancer. That's a world of peaceful livers.

Peaceful livers mean peaceful minds and bodies. Our spirits, too, rely greatly on the strength of our livers. Imagine how much kinder we would all be to each other and ourselves if we didn't feel awful, or frightened of feeling awful, all the time. Now imagine how much more peaceful the world would be if we were all kinder. What *couldn't* we accomplish with that kind of power?

By working on the health of your liver, you're doing so much more. I'm so proud of you for diving into these next chapters. Together with the others reading this book, you're going to create a profound force for healing within your body and the world.

CHAPTER 34

Liver Myths Debunked

It's funny that our livers don't get enough credit these days, since the liver featured prominently in ancient thought. Our ancestors associated the liver with strong emotion, and as you saw in Chapter 27, "Emotional Liver: Mood Struggles and SAD," they weren't so far off. An ever-damaged and ever-regenerating liver was central to the myth of Prometheus, and as you'll read later in this chapter, that's not entirely different from its actual mechanics. Yet too often, we look back on this past fixation on the liver as silly. *Aren't we so much smarter now?* we tell ourselves.

The liver does still get some attention, although the liver myths out there in the present are far more outlandish. Sometimes they're merely fads, trends, and health flavors of the month that won't accomplish what they say they will. Sometimes they're more persistent theories and beliefs that we need to be aware won't help us. No matter what, it's important that we examine them so we don't unknowingly hold ourselves back with modern mythology.

COMPLETE CELL REGENERATION EVERY SEVEN YEARS

A lot of theories exist around how much time it takes for all of the cells in the body to be renewed, replaced, or re-created. There's no exact science out there to provide a true answer to how long it takes. It's one of those undiscovered mysteries of our bodies, similar to what happens to food when we eat, so far beyond the reach of modern medical tools that it can't be weighed or measured.

Many factors play a role in cell regeneration, and it's different for each person: nutrients, stress, pathogens, deficiencies, inherited and newly encountered toxins such as heavy metals, the environmental challenges someone's living with, even the emotional environmental challenges someone's living with and the resources available to that person. They can all influence the speed with which cells rejuvenate. It means that the exact timing of how many years it takes for cells to replace themselves in various organs, glands, tissues, and bones (when they *can* be replaced) can't be locked down by medical research and science, because there is no set timeline to lock down—except in the case of the liver. Let's take a glimpse of the liver's undiscovered rejuvenation process.

The liver is the rock of the body, the boulder in the middle of a meadow where dragonflies roost. That boulder is nearly impossible to roll, push, move along, or uproot with our own two hands, because a boulder has purpose in its placement. The power of Mother Nature's force and the hands of time have left it there in a finished state of being. Though it can change over the hours, days, years, and even centuries as the wind and rain and cold and sun affect it, for the most part, it's in its complete form. In its essence, this state of completion is true of your liver, too. While unlike the boulder, it does have the ability to renew, it has a boulder's steadfastness in a way that's unlike any other part of the body. A boulder is a timekeeper—ask a geologist. Tap into one, and a scientist can decipher the past. A boulder can never be wishy-washy. That's true of the liver, too. It's the body's clock. It can't run behind. Like the stopwatch holder in a race or the teacher timing a test, it must be dependable; it has a responsibility to uphold. With the body running in so many directions, between digestion, the central nervous system's functions, adrenal function, and so on, plus all we put the body through, someone has to be making sure it all runs according to schedule.

In order for the liver to be the peacekeeping timekeeper, it must hold a definitive cell renewal clock that tells what time it is no matter what else is happening inside or outside the body, including inside the liver itself. On a traditional clock, the number that holds it all together is twelve: "The clock strikes midnight," "Lunch is at twelve noon," the marker between morning and afternoon and then between the end of the day and the start of a fresh one. Twelve holds the spectrum of time together. For the liver, the number that holds it all together is nine. It's the number that resides in the core fabric of the liver's cells. The number nine contains within it the liver's responsibilities: cell renewal (which is the number three), the ability to sustain life (which is the number six), and a boulder's sense of completion (which is the nine itself). Beginning, middle, and end, the essence of human life, residing within the liver. Like the twelve on a clock face, nine is the number that unites the liver.

The liver carries information of the past in a way unlike any other organ, even the brain. Our livers hold intelligence from generations and generations past, and they pass this along to each new generation, which is a positive considering our livers also pass along poisons and pathogens. The livers of your children and grandchildren will contain stored-up information from your parents, grandparents, great-grandparents, and even further up the family tree. It means we can never outsmart the liver the way we can outsmart the brain or heart. The liver is immune to human folly because of the data it has on generations of mistakes. In essence, the liver lives forever.

The liver has an ability to renew that is more profound than any other part of the body—which balances the reality that it can't renew its entire self like some parts of the body can. That's because, as your ardent protector, your liver can become extremely scarred and damaged over time, with cells destroyed by pathogens and other troublemakers. As you've read, nobody's liver is running at 100 percent. The damage that occurs to the liver from neglect and misunderstanding is unlike the damage that occurs anywhere else in the body. Though some damaged liver tissue can still be in limited working order and able to be partially renewed, the liver can't renew much, if any, of the severely damaged tissue if someone's not actively working on it. This is what makes the number nine resonate and what gives the liver that heavy, boulder-like quality of standing still through time.

The profound part has to do with the liver's unique ability to renew the good parts of itself on a specific schedule in order to sustain life. Its responsible timekeeping in this area is unlike anything else in the body. The physical state that you're in, your body's resources, your toxic load, and so on—that list of factors from the beginning of this section: they make or break renewal in other body parts. With your liver, renewal happens, period. It's something you can rely on as surely as you can rely on your birthday rolling around on the same day each year: your liver renews all its healthy cells completely within each nine-year mark of your life.

It's not one big, continuous, everyday state of renewal, though some cell renewal can happen on an ongoing basis. The liver renews itself in thirds over those nine years. Usually, three months before a three-year mark is when renewal will pick up speed, and the liver will work on a fast, serious cell overhaul. Within just those few months, the liver can regenerate a third of its working cells. The same thing will happen again at the next three-year mark, renewing another third of the liver. And then, as it approaches nine years total, the liver will renew its final third for that cycle. It's the same timetable for everyone. It happened for us all as we approached our third birthday, our sixth birthday, and our ninth birthday, and then the cycle started over and continued and will continue for the rest of our lives. This means that any kindnesses you pay your liver around those special birthdays that are multiples of three will give it an extra boost as it works to bring new life to itself. (If you were born premature and underdeveloped, you have a few months to play with after each multiple-of-three birthday.)

Here's a really important point: just because they're new cells, that doesn't mean they're clean. If you're not pulling out troublemakers in between those birthdays, new cells can get contaminated by cells and poisons of the past. That's how toxins can stick around in your liver for decades. It's also why it's vital to cleanse troublemakers like viruses and heavy metals on an ongoing basis throughout your whole life. And, as we discussed, the cell renewal timetable doesn't mean that liver damage and disease and scar tissue go away after nine years if you're not actively working on healing them. If you create a great lifestyle for your liver, though, and do everything right for it using the resources in this book, you have hope of this renewal cycle reviving injured tissue.

As these special birthdays approach, think about letting them remind you to do a little more. In the lead-up to your 27th birthday or your 36th or your 48th or your 54th or your 60th or your 75th or your 81st or your 99th or any of the threes before, after, or in between, think about sipping some more green juices, eating a little less fat, getting more hydrated, and bringing in more antioxidant-rich foods such as fruit. And any time in between that you do the Liver Rescue 3:6:9 or the Liver Rescue Morning from Chapter 38, you help secure the possibility of your liver's cells replacing themselves properly so you can feel your best.

OX BILE

A fairly recent trend based on myth is to take the bile from an ox, encapsulate it, and use it as a supplement for people with digestive problems. The theory seems right, practically flawless. We have trouble breaking down fats and our own bile is potentially being underproduced, so the magic remedy must be some nice, strong ox bile, right? Wrong. Why is this a myth? Because the human liver doesn't like it. If your liver could speak aloud in our language, it would say, "Stop putting another creature's bile inside our body. Halt!"

Taking ox bile doesn't fix the problem of weak digestion. It doesn't fix the problem of your liver being stagnant or sluggish or underproducing its own bile. One of your liver's birthrights is to produce and control bile levels. This information is stored inside of it, and it keeps your liver programming and reprogramming itself to give you life for as long as it possibly can. Taking away that responsibility from your liver is like taking away your right to choose how much food you eat. What if you were completely stuffed, yet had no right to stop food from being put in your mouth? What if you were forced to chew and swallow even though your stomach's capacity was already past its limit and you could barely breathe anymore? It's very similar to what happens when the liver is weakened for the many reasons we've explored in this book, can't produce enough bile to efficiently break down radical fats from a variety of food sources, and then is force-fed foreign bile.

The ramifications of the liver being low on bile, as bad as you've read they can be, are not as problematic or damaging as adding bile from another source to the body is. To the liver, ox bile is like an alien creature source, not bioidentical, even if a lab has deemed it compatible enough and called it "bioidentical." That lab hasn't researched and discovered the hundreds of other chemical compounds that exist inside an ox's bile that are foreign to our stomach, the rest of our digestive system, and our body. We always have to remember that funding only goes as far as funding goes with any scientific endeavor. For any topic in science, if

there were more funding, so much more would be discovered. Space travel, for example, would be light-years ahead, so to speak, if there were infinite funding. The more resources allocated to a scientific project, the further along that project goes.

Bile is no exception. The reality is that no one is going to put hundreds of millions of dollars into the exploration of bile to find out what chemical compounds exist in another animal's bile that are damaging to the human body. What kind of undiscovered foreign enzymes exist in alien bile that can disrupt the human endocrine system or immune system or central nervous system, or that can be disease-producing, or that can hurt the human liver? That research to protect you isn't going to happen because the money isn't there. Instead, science knows that ox bile is at least the equivalent substance in that animal and that it contains similar mineral salts, and that's all they need to know to ship it off. What's good for the goose must be good for the gander.

In truth, ox bile's concentration is far different from our own bile's concentration—because an animal many times our size and weight is naturally going to produce much stronger bile—yet bile concentration remains completely unexplored. That alone would take millions of dollars to uncover. Ox bile also contains undiscovered chemical compounds that are different from the chemical compounds our own livers release, though they're not going to find that and focus on it, because medical research and science don't yet completely understand human bile, either.

A capsule of ox bile from a reputable source, as small as that pill may be, can shock the liver. If a swimming pool goes for a week with too many swimmers, too many people urinating in it, too much heat, too much rain that dilutes the pool chemicals, and not enough chlorine to begin with, it will grow slightly discolored and stale, definitely not safe to drink, and in need of refreshing. As soon as you throw some chlorine shock in the pool, an explosion occurs. That's kind of like the shock that the liver experiences from ox bile. When the liver has grown stagnant and sluggish, with loads of toxic heavy metals, pharmaceuticals, solvents, fragrance chemicals, hairspray, hair color, exhaust fumes from the diesel trucks that have been in front of you when you were driving down the highway, and more, and then you throw an ox bile pill in that mix, there's going to be a little shock.

It's not because the ox bile is killing anything off, the way the chlorine does. This shock happens because the foreign bile disrupts the balance that the liver is trying to calibrate nonstop for you. It's a critical balance to keep chaos from becoming chronic inside of a toxic liver. This shock is like when you're at work, trying to bring together five different parts of a project, and a new hire is directed to come in, grab your computer files, and start messing with them in an attempt to help you. When you know what you're doing and you're trying to put it all together, you don't need someone else's "help"; it throws off your balance, and it throws off the balance of the project. That's what it's like for your liver when ox bile enters the scene—here comes this invading entity to interrupt a process on which the real expert is at work. It breaks the liver's balance.

Taking ox bile brings back an old theory that goes back hundreds and hundreds of years, that if you have a kidney problem, eating kidney can cure it, that eating animal brain will cure your own brain, that eating heart will cure your heart, that eating liver will cure your liver, and so on. It's in that same category of Dark Ages conventional medicine. Even if the theory that

ox bile is an acceptable replacement for human bile proved true, there would be another stumbling block: figuring out how much ox bile a person should really take. There would be no way to know. It would be total guesswork, because medical research and science don't even know how much of our own human bile is necessary to do the job it needs to do. Again, our own bile and the role it plays are still under-researched.

Ox bile contains chemical compounds responsible for chemical functions that do not occur in our own human bodies. It also contains undiscovered amino acids that have no role inside of our own bodies. When you consume ox bile filled with all of these extras that your body can't use, the extras go from your stomach into and past the duodenum, absorb through the intestinal tract, and head directly through the bloodstream highway up to the liver, meaning that the liver must process this blood filled with foreign ox bile.

Why is this bad? Imagine it's like your best friend whom you care about and have trusted for years. You know each other's stories and secrets; you know everything about each other. Now say you're driving around together, and you decide to pull up in front of a café. While your friend runs inside to get you both coffee, you wait in the car. Say the person who walks back out, opens the door, jumps in your passenger seat, and hands you a cup of coffee is an entirely different person passing herself off as your friend. She looks very similar and says all the right things, and it seems like she could be your confidant until you realize she's really a stranger who knows nothing about who you are, nothing about your dreams and losses, your aspirations, your life story.

Along with this, the imposter smells really, really bad; it's an odor you can't put your finger on. It's not the body odor your friend sometimes gets after the gym. It's far worse, mysterious and terrible. It disturbs you so much that you lose your ability to function like you normally would, because you're too busy trying to figure out if this smell is a threat. Is it toxic? Harmful? Do you need to do something about it? You decide to throw your cup of coffee in the garbage, ask this person to leave the car, and speed away. As you drive down the road, the smell lingers and you begin to process what just happened.

Once you've had a chance to shake out of the confusion, you realize you need to go back to the coffee shop, where you find your real friend waiting at the curb. "Where have you been all this time?" she asks as she enters the car.

When it's forced to absorb ox bile and its chemical compounds that are foreign to the human body, your liver is in the same position you were in when an imposter came out of the coffee shop. When your liver takes on ox bile's extras so you don't get hurt, it's a major confusion to the organ. It has its own bile that it needs to reabsorb later to protect you. Ox bile can push the liver over the edge. The liver loses its focus on what it really needs to do: pick up its real friend, your own natural bile, that's been waiting on the curb.

When your liver is having trouble producing its own bile, what it really needs instead of ox bile is a glass of celery juice to help restore and heal itself. The liver identifies the proper mineral salts in celery juice and builds them up so it can step up to produce adequate levels of bile. The liver also needs lower dietary fat. When a physician identifies a patient as having minimal bile production, ox bile is usually offered with the goal of that patient continuing to eat plenty of dietary fat. Practically everybody has been on a high-fat diet their entire lives, between grilled cheese sandwiches and chicken Caesar salads and slices of pizza and so much more. The popular mistake is that by taking ox bile, you don't have to moderate that at all. The reality is that the millions of people with diminishing bile production are supposed to adopt low-fat diets more in keeping with the meal ideas in Chapter 38 and the recipes in Chapter 39 so that the liver gets some alleviation from the normal bombardment of fat that's often labeled as protein. With lower fat, the liver can get a chance to detox and restore its own bile production. Since high-protein eating is so trendy right now, with the world making the mistake that a diet high in fat is the healthiest option, people take the ox bile and eat more fat than ever, never realizing that it's making the problem worse.

EATING LIVER

The practice of eating liver is alive and well for two reasons: (1) many people truly love the taste of liver, and (2) there's a longstanding belief that eating liver is good for you, particularly beneficial for healing and strengthening the liver itself and for building the blood. People add turkey liver to stuffing, fry up cow and chicken livers for the family, and consider goose and duck livers delicacies, sometimes using them to make the popular dish foie gras.

That eating liver is good for your health is far from true. When we think about it in light of what your own liver does for your own body—what it does and what it's for—we can easily see that this is a sad, misled misconception.

First of all, it's rare to almost impossible to find a truly clean, healthy liver on Planet Earth, whether human or animal. If we did find a beautifully healthy liver from a creature raised in a pure, pristine environment, it would still be filled with toxins collected from that animal's own body. Normal bodily functions create toxins that the liver must process and store. While it's easy to think that a bear or a deer raised in a remote forest on wild game, grasses, or other plants would have the cleanest liver possible, that's not the case. Wild animals are constantly in fight-or-flight mode, which means they constantly release fear-based adrenaline. Just like us, their livers must act as sponges to absorb all of that excess stress hormone.

The liver isn't only a sponge for the toxic, though. What could seem like a great, healing benefit of eating liver is how incredible the liver is altogether. This amazing, powerful glandular organ holds and processes important enzymes, trace minerals, amino acids, antioxidants, and other phytochemicals—so it does make incredible logical sense to say that consuming liver could help you out. Reading this book, learning about all of its miraculous chemical functions and compounds, you may even be thinking now more than ever, *Would I benefit from eating liver? Would another liver's strength enter my own?* The answer is yes, you probably could benefit in some way, surprisingly or not. Yet this shouldn't automatically lead to the belief that people need liver, because there's another side to it. The precious nutrients that the liver holds are like a massive hoard of rare gold coins, emeralds, diamonds, and other priceless treasures buried deep within the earth. You have the tools to dig them up, only something lies on top: radioactive nuclear waste. Chances are, you'll get to the treasure trove just fine, though you'll live a very short life with those gems and jewels in your hands—you won't get to enjoy your invaluable finds because they came with poison. That's the reality of what the liver contains: both treasure and troublemakers. It's like being given a tonic that has the power to make you live forever mixed with poison that takes it all away.

We also run into the same issue raised by ox bile supplementation: what's contained in an animal's liver is not going to be compatible with the human body. The goodies stored in an animal liver will not match up with how our livers work. Animal livers produce and store animal enzymes and animal chemical compounds signature to their individual species' identities. Each one is tailored to the miraculous physical body of that specific creature. They can't be reidentified, tagged, reshaped, and used by our own human bodies. The exception is fat. If there's fat inside an animal liver, we can use that. Trouble is, that fat probably harbors plenty of poison, because fat cells in the liver store toxins. Out of everything else in that animal's liver, it's possible our liver can use some trace minerals or maybe, if we're lucky, a few antioxidants. They're not enough to balance the toxic load. Ultimately, your liver must process and store those poisons, as well as the unusable, animal-specific chemical compounds, and that contributes to your organ's overload.

If you wanted to receive the goodies a liver has the potential to offer, you'd have to eat a human liver. Of course, I wouldn't recommend it! Besides, any treasure in a human liver would be buried under waste, too: a plethora of toxic heavy metals, solvents, drugs (prescribed and recreational), plastics, mystery chemicals, viruses, bacteria, radiation, DDT and its cousins (that is, all pesticides, herbicides, and fungicides), and the like. The bad would far outweigh the good. Believe me: it wouldn't be worth cannibalism.

While we can laugh about cannibalism here, the truth is that a common practice in conventional medicine 150 years ago was to consume human body parts in various forms. Alternative medicine of the day was against this conventional theory, not to mention the secret black market practice of selling bodies, one of the darker sides of science in the past. One method of consumption was to soak human bones in water, creating a tonic much like today's animal bone broth. Another was to eat pieces of human skin to heal a skin condition and to eat parts of other human organs to strengthen those organs in a living person. This secret custom was born out of that Dark Ages theory we looked at in "Ox Bile" of healing a human body part with an animal's corresponding body part. It's why we still carry the belief that we can benefit the liver by eating liver. It's also why some supplements today contain little bits of animal organs and glands with the idea that they'll help your own organs and glands. This thought process is hundreds and hundreds of years old and has never healed anyone, and yet it has survived to this day.

For your own protection, take your cue from predators in the wild. When they eat an animal they've caught, they'll avoid eating the liver. It's the last-ditch organ that animals go for, usually left for scavengers and creatures pushed to starvation. Those animals forced to eat liver will end up eating more wild shoots and roots in the spring to cleanse their own livers of what intoxicated them. There's an instinctive, innate reason for these animal behaviors. We would do well to heed that instinct, too.

LIVER FLUSHES

Liver flushes always sound catchy. They seem like a perfect, easy answer to clean up and clear out. Well, they are catchy—in that there's a catch. Liver flushes are man-made theories of protocols that people think should work for the organ. Thinking for the liver is kind of like thinking for someone else. Do you like it if someone

puts words in your mouth? Probably not. Especially if it's about a specific, sensitive subject that could in some way alter the outcome of your life. When it comes down to it—I can't state this enough—forced liver cleansing comes with a price. If this gets you irritated, I understand. You could be someone who loves your liver flushes. I respect that. At the same time, I'm here to bring you guidance. That's my job, to look out for you.

It's not the end of the world if you've been doing liver flushes. What you need to know is that the liver has an existence of its own that we don't rule over. It runs on its own time. If your boss kept you at work until midnight when you were supposed to leave at five to pick up your daughter from band rehearsal, you wouldn't appreciate that infringement, would you? And if you were having a normal Sunday off when with no notice whatsoever, you were expected to drop your bagel on the plate, stop making pancakes for your kid, get dressed, and rush to work while watching other people in their cars getting to run their weekend errands—and then you were expected to stay as late as it took to finish the project, even if that meant not getting to leave until 2 A.M.—that wouldn't fit with your life either, right? And then say that at the same time that you were being forced to meet these extra scheduling demands, you were also expected to produce volumes of work every hour on the hour, more results than ever before in your career. Does this remind you of something? Is it anything like a liver flush, forcing it to cleanse on an unnatural schedule against its will while you check the toilet hourly for theoretical, make-believe liver stones? (More on liver stones in a moment.)

There are a lot of different liver cleanses out there. Some are for the liver only. Some are for the liver and gallbladder. Some are just aimed for the gallbladder. They're all liver pushers.

When you have a child and that child starts to grow up, what's one of the greatest threats you fear? That your child will run into a drug pusher? We never want a child's own will and potential to be overpowered by a force that doesn't have her or his best interests at heart. We should feel just as protective of our livers.

You get a lot more cleansing work done with your liver and gallbladder when you go with the grain, not against it. If you try to go against it with flushes and cleanses that aren't balanced, your liver will outsmart you every time. Think you're smarter than your liver? No way. You'll never be smarter than your liver. Not that you aren't an intelligent person—I'm not trying to break your confidence in who you are. It's just that none of us are going to outsmart our livers. They won't let us get away with anything. They cannot be controlled. The liver is a programmer, a think tank, all on its own. If you push it, it pushes back and performs less. If you push more, it performs even less. If you keep pushing hard, it throws itself into shutdown mode, running on backup battery, waiting for you to stop messing around with it. It stops cleansing altogether in order to try to normalize and seek homeostasis. Not until you finally stop does it take a breath and go back to actual, normal functioning. Does this remind you of anything in your life? You push it too hard, it resists, so you have to finesse it? This concept applies in so many situations.

Your liver holds ancient information from long before you were born. Remember: it also holds data about your life that you don't even remember. It senses all your crafty tricks because it's had to save your butt from one episode after another, like when you gobbled a greasy cheeseburger or chugged a quart of beer at a college party. It uses this memory in order to protect you. It knows if you've been bad or good, naughty or nice. It knows if you've

tried to flush a boatload of toxins all at once. In our human minds, we just think, *Get it all out at once.* We think these flushes send all the toxins out through the intestinal tract and kidneys, so that everything ends up in the toilet and we can say good-bye.

The liver knows better. When it's a flush done wrong, one that pushes the liver hard against its will, the bloodstream is where those toxins end up. The liver knows, even though we're not aware, that all these poisons entering the blood at once put the heart and brain under direct threat. An onslaught of toxic sludge and debris headed for our heart valves and ventricles is not the liver's idea of an ideal vacation method. It could cause erratic heartbeats, stress on the heart, inflammation, elevated adrenaline, and electrical confusion of the heart, all while we're busy looking for stones in the toilet.

By the way, those stones aren't stones at all. They're fatty globules from these oil-filled flushes. The excess olive oil in the colon coagulates and forms jelly balls, which are then expelled and, I'm sorry to say, in many cases mistaken for hundreds of stones. I hope this doesn't upset you as a reader. You deserve to know the truth: that they're evidence of your body trying to save you from all that oil. (See the next myth for more.)

Let's also touch on flushing the gallbladder for a moment. In Chapter 34, you saw that oil-based flushes aren't the best practice for removing gallstones, either. Over the years, I've seen too many cases of people pushing gallstones into the bile duct and requiring emergency surgery. There's a better way of getting rid of gallstones, and that's to dissolve them, which we already discussed.

And there's a better way to cleanse the liver, one that works with it, not against it, and ends up being more effective than any man-made protocol—we'll get to that in Chapter 38.

LIVER STONES

While you may hear that the liver can produce its own stones, it's not possible. There are cases where the duct leading from the gallbladder to the intestinal tract gets clogged with stones. Those are gallstones, and they're different from the mistaken theory of liver stones. There are no cases of the hepatic ducts inside the liver getting clogged with stones—so-called "liver stones"—because the liver does not pass already formed stones through the ducts that lead bile to the gallbladder. The liver is too hot for a stone to forge there; stones are forged in the gallbladder itself, through the process we examined in Chapter 32, with toxins and poisons moving from the hot liver into the cool gallbladder.

The liver's heat is actually a mechanism that protects you from stones forming there, whether hard or soft. If stones did form within it, the liver wouldn't be able to pass them through the bile. The hepatic ducts in the liver that carry bile are not as big as anybody believes. Only if you were a surgeon well versed in dissecting the bile duct system in human livers would you have a sense of how thin they are; they can't support stones passing through them, much less the very large liver stones that people believe they can eliminate during a cleanse. The liver can't send a stone out of a hepatic vein, either, because it would instantly cause a blood clot or heart attack. There's no way for your liver to get a stone safely to your feces to be eliminated. If stones really were forming inside the liver, they'd be getting stuck in the hepatic ducts, and people with sick, toxic livers would be in

total agony. Hospitals would be filled with millions of people requiring emergency liver stone removal surgery—and there would be a very popular surgery method for it, since surgery is one area where modern medicine excels. It would be just as common if not more so than kidney stone surgery.

If someone does a liver flush and sees "stones" in the toilet, it's really food and debris from the intestinal tract mixed with the oil from the concoctions that go with the cleanse. What about if someone is doing a liver cleanse that doesn't involve any olive oil flushing and is even entirely fat-free? There are still going to be bits and pieces of food waste coming off the walls of the intestinal linings, mixed with the large quantities of herbal mixtures someone is usually ingesting for a cleanse, and they can be expelled together with mucus from the digestive tract so that in the toilet, you think you're seeing liver stones when you're not.

The liver stone flushing trend has taken on a life of its own, even though many professionals in the field of healing are unaware of how the liver truly works. No one's perfect, not even practitioners and healers; we all make mistakes. The key now is to pick yourself up off the ground, dust yourself off, and get it right. Don't be afraid of moving past something that turned out to be wrong even though you once believed in it.

FRUCTOSE INTOLERANCE

If you buy into the fructose intolerance and malabsorption myth, you'll get cheated out of healing your liver. The confusion around fructose intolerance has everything to do with the liver. The more toxic your liver is, the more it may appear to someone that you're fructose intolerant, when in reality you're not fructose intolerant at all. Lactose (dairy sugar) and fructose are entirely different animals. For example, viruses and bacteria throughout the body feverishly feed off lactose from dairy—just as they do with gluten. When someone has a high bacterial or viral load that's going undiagnosed, and these pathogens feed off gluten, that person can wind up with an intestinal disorder diagnosis such as celiac. In reality, celiac isn't the body attacking itself; it's pathogens attacking the body. Dairy's lactose feeds pathogens as well, which can worsen symptoms and conditions of all kinds.

Just because bacterial or viral activity in your body can make you gluten or lactose intolerant, that doesn't mean you can be fructose intolerant. Fructose shouldn't be lumped in with lactose just because they're two forms of sugar. Fructose does not feed pathogens. It's impossible for any test in any lab or clinic to separate out fructose and know what it specifically does inside the body, whether negative or positive. Theoretical testing for fructose intolerance has never been accurate and most likely never will be, because it's backed by a belief system that is biased against fruit. The "fructose intolerant" label is part of the anti–healthy carb, anti-fruit movement that robs people of the very food that can help them heal from chronic conditions.

The liver desperately needs fruit sugar to restore itself and defend itself from pathogens. Because fruit is so purifying, someone who consumes fruit is going to cleanse and detox more than with any other food, and that leads to a common mistake when evaluating for fructose intolerance. Often people who are chronically sick and have sluggish, stagnant, sick livers react when they start detoxing, whether mildly or more heavily. One apple can cleanse your liver in more ways than anyone realizes, and all those poisons leaving can cause detox reactions and symptoms that confuse both patient and

practitioner, especially if the overall diet is not geared to cleansing.

Almost all practitioners who fall prey to the belief system of fructose intolerance also believe in high-fat diets, regardless of the fancy name or branding given to them. Even elimination diets—where certain foods are experimented with to see if they cause a reaction, making it feel for people like they're custom-made—remain high-fat diets. With a diet high in fat, the blood stays toxic and the liver stays toxic, and when someone eats fruit, which cleanses and detoxes the liver, those poisons have nowhere to go because the blood is so filled with fats and toxins. The resulting reactions are inevitably branded as fructose intolerance or malabsorption, keeping people away from what could really offer help. They only get to experience some relief of symptoms temporarily, not long-term healing.

Another big part of what people believe to be fructose intolerance is insulin resistance, which you read about in Chapter 2, "Your Adaptogenic Liver," and Chapter 15, "Diabetes and Blood Sugar Imbalance." When someone doesn't understand insulin resistance as having too much fat in the blood and a toxic, stagnant liver, fructose intolerance can get blamed.

Now, there's a distinction made between fructose intolerance, often called hereditary fructose intolerance (HFI), and fructose malabsorption. In neither case is the concept or the testing accurate. With HFI, it's not really genetic—the ALDOB gene and a deficiency of the aldolase B isoenzyme have nothing to do with the symptoms someone may experience from eating a piece of fruit. First of all, no one is completely missing the aldolase B isoenzyme. Secondly, when it is lowered, it's just one among dozens of other enzymes and hundreds of chemical functions that are not even on medical research and science's radar that diminish when the liver is dysfunctional. By focusing on aldolase B and attributing its deficiency to fructose issues, experts fall into the trap of not allowing you to eat the very food that would bring your stagnant, sluggish liver back to health, which would allow aldolase B and all those other enzymes and chemical functions to restore themselves. HFI is just a theory—which is why we're talking about it here in the myths chapter. (And by the way, a very small proportion of people actually react when eating fruit; it's more common to react to sweeteners such as table sugar.) Symptoms that seem to come from eating fruit have everything to do with fat intolerance, which comes from a dysfunctional liver. The HFI label is a bait and switch made to make you think fruit sugar is the problem while industries protect fats. Remember: everything that's not understood is blamed on genes, and if you go down that path you'll be cheated out of the very solution that will help heal your liver so you can become symptom-free.

With fructose malabsorption, experts believe that testing picks up on excess fructose in your system, meaning that you're not able to absorb it. What they don't understand is that you're really experiencing an intestinal tract filled with rancid fat that's not being broken down due to a weak, sluggish, stagnant, dysfunctional, sick, probably pre-fatty liver that needs attention. When you put a piece of fruit in your gut, it's going to trigger off a malabsorption test, both because the fruit sugar has nowhere to go—since the digestive tract is lined with hardened, putrid fats—and because the fruit is trying to cleanse your gut and heal your liver. Practitioners will see your test reaction as fruit not working for you, and they'll keep recommending lots of animal protein as your

main calorie source—the very factor that lowered your bile reserves over the years to begin with, causing fats to go rancid and stick to the linings of your small intestine and colon.

If people reduced their intake of fats, in turn minimizing their blood-fat ratio, they wouldn't be symptomatic anymore when eating fruit, nor would they trigger off tests for fructose issues—because there was never a fructose intolerance or malabsorption issue to begin with. Their livers would start healing, strengthening, and functioning better; fruit would be able to offer even more benefit; and they would start getting better, regardless of the HFI or fructose malabsorption diagnosis they'd received. Those who design high-fat diets are starting to wake up to the truth that incorporating more plant foods gets people better results, and these fancily named new diets are by default starting to contain lower fats. The next step in healing won't occur until people move past their fruit fear and start adding more than a green apple and a handful of berries to their day.

LECTIN CONCERN

Another popular trend that's on the rise is the concern that certain foods are high in lectins and therefore have a negative effect on health. You have to understand that for decades, there have been chronically sick people, and for decades to come, there will be chronically sick people. When someone knows what's wrong with her or his body, knows what's causing a symptom or condition, and knows how to heal it, she or he can heal it. Over dozens of years, I've witnessed tens of thousands of people do just this: recover their health, even from the most devastating conditions. These recoveries had nothing to do with lectin concern.

We can't live in a bubble, where we believe that nobody got better from what ailed them until the lectin trend came along. The promoters of lectin literature and studies have been completely in the dark about the thousands and thousands of people who've healed without their trendy misinformation—it's as if they've ignored people's healing because it didn't fit into their box of what they believed. They pretend that no one has ever healed from chronic illness so that they can build their lectins empire.

This is a prime example of entitled ignorance. The problem with lectin concern is that it removes foods that would actually stop the viruses and other pathogens in people's bodies that truly cause symptoms and disease. Lectin leaders don't know about these pathogens, or don't know their role in causing conditions and illnesses, such as EBV as the true cause of RA. They would rather think a potato is causing someone's RA than discover the truth that an amino acid in potatoes, L-lysine, stops EBV from causing RA. Instead, they believe that autoimmune is the immune system attacking the body's own cells and destroying itself. Since they don't understand that this autoimmune theory is inaccurate, they have nowhere else to turn besides blaming it all on lectins, believing in part that lectins are a problem because they supposedly confuse the body and cause it to turn against itself. Meanwhile, they remove the foods that can heal you, such as fruit and certain vegetables, roots, and tubers, leading you to eat more fats and hurt your liver.

The lectins in fruits and vegetables do not harm us. Please don't let any source confuse you into thinking that lectins are like the toxic alkaloids produced as a defense mechanism by some wild plants not fit for human consumption.

There are shoots and twigs and other plants that, if a deer takes a bite of them, surface alkaloids to repel that deer and other animals and insects from damaging them further. We already don't eat those foods because we know they're toxic to us—and lectins aren't even what makes them a problem. Garden-variety fruits and vegetables, and even the wild plants we know to be edible, are in a whole different category, yet they're being lumped together with problematic alkaloid-containing plants. Again, the lectins in the foods we eat do not cause harm.

There are certain proteins that aren't in fruits and vegetables and are in items such as dairy, eggs, and certain grains, including wheat, that do feed pathogens, creating inflammation. Lectins aren't one of them. As you'll read in Chapter 36, "Liver Troublemakers," dairy, eggs, and some grains are worth treating warily. There are dozens of proteins and compounds in dairy, eggs, and wheat for experts to hang dozens of hats on in their quest to alleviate chronic illness, and yet they try to hang their hat on the one that's not a problem: lectins. It's ironic. Yes, be concerned about gluten-rich foods. No, don't be afraid of potatoes and fresh, ripe tomatoes—I've watched them heal even the sickest people. I've even recently seen potatoes save some lives.

Look out for anti-lectin sentiment and be cautious about buying into it. This trendy mistake is going to continue to create confusion with healing into the future. It's another anti-fruit campaign, another biased design to stop you from eating the fruits that heal your liver and body, another excuse for medical research and science's lack of knowledge about what causes chronic illness. Please don't let it rob you and your children of what you need to heal along the way.

APPLE CIDER VINEGAR

Apple cider vinegar (ACV) has been getting extra acclaim these days for being good for the stomach and the rest of the digestive tract. With the gut, it's thought to create alkalinity, settle acid reflux, and help with bloating. It's getting even more acclaim for cleansing the gallbladder and liver.

Apples in themselves are miracles. They're amazing for digestion: They collect and rid bacteria, parasites, viruses, and mold from the entire gut. They create a stable alkaline environment wherever needed. They also help heal diverticulitis and reduce inflammation in the stomach and intestinal tract. Apples are incredibly cleansing and healing for the gallbladder and liver. Not only do they detoxify, carefully extracting sediment from these organs; they also help dissolve gallstones. Mind you, these are apples we're talking about, not apple cider vinegar. Apple cider is very helpful for all of the above, not apple cider *vinegar*. Apple juice is extremely helpful for everything I just mentioned, not ACV. Applesauce is great for all of it, too, though not ACV. Apple cider vinegar does not create alkalinity or cleanse your system—apples do.

You know that saying "You take the bad with the good"? Usually what we mean is that we know there are going to be some downsides to the positives in life. And whatever bad we end up going through, the good is enough to support it. It's half and half, give or take, or hopefully the good even outweighs the bad. That's why it's a somewhat positive viewpoint: whatever bad comes with the good, it's at least an equal exchange. With ACV, there's some good, there's a lot of bad, and it does not come out to an even 50/50. The good comes from amino acids, minerals, trace minerals, phytochemicals, and other nutrients from the apples used to make it—if the

vinegar was fermented and stored properly and contains "mother" in it, meaning living microorganisms. Then, at least, it provides some nutrition, although the living "mother" won't be alive much longer after entering the stomach. Even the mildest hydrochloric acid can knock the life out of these microorganisms.

Look, ACV is the healthiest vinegar to use if you're a vinegar lover. If you can't live without a little vinegar on your salad, ACV is the one to pick. So if I know it's the best vinegar and I love apples for what they do for us, why am I not a big advocate of ACV? The reason I have a problem with ACV is the same reason everyone has a problem with any vinegar, whether they know it or not: because if there's one thing our livers despise, it's vinegar. If your liver had a voice, it would shout that to the heavens. The liver hates vinegar as much as it hates alcohol. With alcohol, the liver gets slowly drunk and dysfunctional. With vinegar, the liver becomes disabled in a different way. The liver cells struggle to stay balanced and perform as they fight for oxygen, because vinegar steals oxygen from the bloodstream and the liver like a thief in the night.

Some people seem to heal a sore throat with ACV, and in truth, many more people *get* a sore throat from ACV. Some people relieve bloating with ACV, and many more people get extremely bloated from ACV. Some people relieve acid reflux from ACV, and many more people get the worst acid reflux attack they've ever had from ACV. Some people relieve gallbladder pain with ACV, and many more people get a really bad gallbladder attack from ACV. Still, the bad outweighs the good even when it seems like ACV is helping one problem. That's because, out of sight, the liver pays a price.

Basically, when we consume vinegar, the liver battles being pickled like a cucumber. Now, it takes salt and vinegar to make a pickle. Your raw, organic ACV with "mother" in it most likely doesn't come with added sodium. Salt ends up being added to the vinegar, though, as the ACV enters your bloodstream and liver. In order to survive, we need a level of sodium in the blood, so our blood is slightly salty, like a living ocean is salty. (Some of the sodium is from uncharted avenues, including the micro trace mineral salts we get from consuming the right foods, such as celery.) The liver also stores a certain amount of sodium; one of its chemical functions is to release sodium in times of dire need in order to keep enough sodium in the bloodstream. So even if we don't eat salt along with our vinegar, there's just enough salt in the organs, glands, and blood to mix with the vinegar as we consume it. As a result of the vinegar-sodium reaction, a pickling process occurs.

One could argue that this isn't the type of pickling that happens when someone is preserving a vegetable in a jar to last through the winter. Still, it is a variety of pickling that happens internally. Eating one salad with ACV dressing is not the worst thing that can happen to the liver. It can add up, though. If you're using ACV in a flush or taking tablespoons of it daily because it's supposed to be good for you, the liver will be affected by the long-term volume, and it will eventually retaliate.

Before an apple was turned into vinegar, it was neutral to alkaline. When you eat an apple, it can drive the stomach and intestinal tract to a higher level of alkalinity without disturbing the stomach's neutralization zone; that is, its balancing of everything that enters it before it moves on to the duodenum and the rest of the intestinal tract. (Your stomach can be alkaline and still have a very strong blend of hydrochloric acid; your stomach is not just one environment.) An apple is expected in the stomach. It was one of the very first foods bestowed upon humankind

for us to consume. It's a powerful, earned reward for the liver. Have you ever worked hard in your life, whether on a project, task, generosity, charity, or on the vital endeavor of keeping yourself afloat and rewarded yourself with an experience you knew you'd love? Maybe that was a day off, a drive to the beach, a walk in the park. An apple is the liver's great reward for all the work it's doing.

Unlike an apple, ACV (like any vinegar) comes into the stomach extremely acidic. The liver must put a halt to it immediately and use its every reserve to try to alkalize or at least neutralize it. The ACV fights back, and its acidic nature is so strong that the stomach loses the battle many times over. Instead of alkalizing your gut, it does the opposite. It weakens hydrochloric acid and breaks down gastric juices and heads down the pike still acidic. It's basically an assault on the stomach and intestinal tract. At first, as the vinegar pushes its way through the plumbing, the liver starts to become a little hysterical. Soon after, the liver gets a quick shot of acidosis. Although it's temporary, it's just long enough to stun it, like a friend smacking you across the face to snap you out of what he interprets to be a hysterical moment.

Is ACV all bad? No. There's much worse out there. Here's the important point: ACV is far from a liver cleansing or intestinal tonic. It's not a miracle food. Apple*sauce* is a healing miracle food for the liver and gallbladder. ACV? Along with other vinegar tonics, it's an insult to the liver. I know there's a big fermented foods movement out there, and people really enjoy them. The truth here has nothing to do with what you or I like, though. It's about what your liver would like. Your liver has needs. Do you write a needs list every day? "I need to do this," "I need to get that," "I need to have that." Well, the liver has a needs list, too, and fermented foods, ACV, and vinegar of any kind are not on it. Just as the liver is a storehouse, we can collect a lot of items in our lives. To keep our closets from overflowing, we'll try to turn down whatever we can before it ever enters our home: "I don't need a pair of skates right now"; "I've got plenty of beach towels, don't need a new one"; "No, thanks, I already have an electric toothbrush"; "I don't need those smelly candles. Thanks anyway." If your liver could opt out of ACV like this, it would. The liver doesn't need ACV.

At least with ACV's popularity, people are thinking apple. If your liver could speak, every visit to the natural foods store would be like a game of charades. As you walked toward the ACV aisle, your liver would be saying, "You're close, you're close, the word *apple* is on the bottle. That part is right . . ." When you picked up the bottle, it would shout, "No! Close, but no cigar. Try again." And when you were wandering past produce, skipping all the fruit because your trendy high-fat diet said to avoid it, your liver would be calling out to you, "Stop! Stop! Get the apples!" In every way other than fermented, the apple is a true powerhouse and miracle for well-being.

Everything being said, if you want to partake in some ACV, fine. It is the best out of all the vinegars. A little here and there as a dressing on a special dish if you really want it could be okay. Many people don't use much of it to begin with, and as a condiment it is healthier than most. It has those nutrients in it because of the apple, thank God. As far as using ACV in larger amounts to cleanse the liver goes, though, know that it's a myth. If it's liver healing you want, skip the shots of ACV and reach instead for some unfermented apples.

COFFEE ENEMAS

Coffee enemas are a popular, longstanding liver remedy, commonly used for pancreatic, colon, and other cancers as well as a general alternative healing avenue for just about any sickness. Coffee enemas are even hyped as a maintenance method for people who are already healthy to stay that way. They're not just a part of alternative medicine anymore, either; their popularity has spread to conventional medicine, as well. A coffee enema's theoretical function is to purge toxins from the liver, allowing the body to heal. It's a perfectly reasoned claim. Detoxing the liver does help you heal.

Here's where we start to run into trouble: to begin with, coffee is strong, harsh, extremely acidic, dehydrating, highly astringent, and over-stimulating. It's a drug. Remember: you can get addicted to it, and that's part of what has made people so attached to it as an enema tonic for healing. All of those challenges of coffee can be okay for the individual who likes to *drink* a cup of it. Coffee entering the stomach is a whole different story than coffee entering directly into the colon through an enema. Our stomachs are geared to handle a brew. It may not be perfect for our stomachs. Coffee does have the ability to challenge the stomach environment—its pH, its hydrochloric acid levels—though this can be fine for the people with stomach tolerance. It also has the potential to be hard on the nervous system for those with neurological-related sensitivities, symptoms, and conditions such as anxiety, tremors, tingles, numbness, brain fog, aches and pains, insomnia, and restless legs, to name just a few. Many people in these situations, as well as those with weak stomachs, acid reflux, pancreas issues, gallbladder problems, and digestive compromise and distress such as Crohn's, IBS, and colitis, have figured out that they feel best steering clear of coffee. People without these issues should be able to find enjoyment in coffee because their stomachs can take the hit as their first line of defense.

Coffee going to the stomach should be its only path. There's a controlled environment there, with built-in protective measures to safeguard you. When substances enter the stomach, alarm bells ring to prepare the pancreas, liver, and intestinal tract. Regardless of whether it's a can of soda, a glass of milk, a parasite picked up from eating out at a restaurant, or a cup of coffee, dispersal is delegated properly so that by the time it enters the bloodstream, it's already partially defused. It's part of the stomach's miraculous ability to balance and make neutral whatever enters it. Like a submarine deep down in the ocean of your body, its prime objective is to keep its systems untampered with. Everything must remain calm, cool, collected, and organized, or calamity will ensue. When it comes to any foods, liquids or fluids of any kind, medicines, parasites, or bacteria, whether good or bad, entering the intestinal tract through the rectum, however, the stomach's safeguard does not apply. When it's something gentle and mild entering this environment, it doesn't pose a threat. With a substance as strong as coffee, it's another story. Coffee's acidic nature and nervous system–assaulting effect is way too intense for the colon to handle on its own.

And when anything harsh or toxic comes in this way—when it doesn't go through the checkpoints that entering through the stomach provides—regardless of what it is, the liver becomes very vulnerable. For the liver, the stomach is like that friend who always has its back. The stomach knows that the liver is working for its needs, too, so it's a family-like relationship of mutual benefit. The liver is not made to handle a direct threat or hit. When one comes, it will instantly prompt the adrenals to release adrenaline as a defense mechanism, even though the liver despises excess adrenaline, since it needs to sponge it up to protect you. Still, in this situation, it employs adrenaline as an army of soldiers to do battle, armed with guns and knives.

Coffee enemas trigger these adrenaline surges. The adrenaline ordered by the general, the liver, is to warn the heart there may be trouble. This may sound extreme. A coffee enema seems so harmless. Logically, it doesn't seem like a threat; it seems like a safe protocol. When considered next to so many of the conventional protocols in medicine that are really, truly dangerous and unsafe, a coffee enema does pale in comparison. That's our assessment with our minds, though. Here, the liver calls the shots, and the liver sees the coffee enema as trouble.

There's a second adrenaline rush involved, and that's from the caffeine of the coffee itself. When coffee bypasses the usual stomach–duodenum–small intestine route—which would have delegated the caffeine properly and appropriately in the most delicate way possible so that it would be defused when it entered the bloodstream and in this way protect your heart from being assaulted by caffeine—and instead enters the intestinal tract through the rectum, the adrenals are triggered for another reason. That's because the caffeine itself is rogue. It finds its way into the bloodstream immediately, with no hydrochloric acid or other components of gastric juices or bile to slow it down.

This is something about which people with sensitive nervous systems and adrenal issues need to be aware. These are people who have trouble with caffeine to begin with. I'm sure there are people with high anxiety who don't know coffee makes it worse, so they're frequently in line at the coffee shop, ordering their favorite brew, meanwhile controlling their anxiety with antianxiety medication. There are also many who do know coffee puts them on edge. For people in both of these groups, when coffee is applied through an enema, it can really trigger or heighten a symptom like anxiety. Often, practitioners—loving, caring professionals who aren't at fault for the mistake—are taught to say that experiences like these are detox symptoms. The truth is that the adrenaline and caffeine of a coffee enema can be too much on the body because the digestive system is practically our second central nervous system.

For those who are still wondering: Putting everything else aside, does the liver really cleanse with a coffee enema? The answer is that while a coffee enema may force a little purging of the liver, a boomerang effect also occurs. Poisons that are leaving the liver, instead of being flushed out of the body, inevitably end up rerouted back to the liver because they're not being cleansed in a safe way; the liver sends chemical compounds into the bloodstream to try to round up and corral as many escaped toxins as possible to protect the brain and heart. The adrenaline that the liver calls out for and that the caffeine triggers quickly circulates and is sponged up by the liver, too. That is, the liver can end up more toxic from a coffee enema than when it started.

The liver does not like to be forced to cleanse, so when coffee enters the colon directly, the liver may nearly shut down, going on momentary low battery to prepare itself for enhanced functioning within a few seconds or minutes, when it will need to go into high gear to deal with the onslaught of adrenaline and poisons.

An enema can be extremely detoxing for the liver when instead of coffee, the enema solution is a little lemon freshly squeezed into pure distilled or reverse osmosis (RO) water. Distilled and RO water don't offer minerals when you drink them; in an enema, though, they drive out impurities, and the fresh lemon juice makes the water more effective. This type of enema is more effective than a coffee enema because it doesn't make the liver scream out for the release of adrenaline, and caffeine isn't present to release more adrenaline. If you're not a fan of enemas, you don't need to do one at all.

BEETS

The concept that beets are what the liver needs has been swimming out there for a long time. They're considered a liver-healing, blood-building food. Are beets really good for us? Yes, they're a powerful food indeed, and they do help the liver cleanse and heal a little bit—if they're organic and guaranteed to be non-GMO, which is hard to find these days what with cross-pollination. GMO contamination has made crops like corn problematic, and the same thing has happened with beets that are grown for sugar, canning, and industrial dyes. Cross-pollination is becoming such a problem that even many organic beets grown for fresh eating can be tainted at seed. That's not the greatest reason to stop eating beets for your health, though. The greatest reason is that you can do much better. For example, red pitaya, also called dragon fruit, which you can find in smoothie packs in the frozen food aisle of the grocery store or in pure powdered form, is much more liver-healing and blood-building than beets can ever be. After all, if you're going out of your way to grow or eat something for a specific reason, wouldn't you want to know what's really the best? Wild blueberries are far more cleansing for the liver than beets, as are asparagus and brussels sprouts. Even apples have beets beat by a landslide.

You don't have to stop eating beets if you like them. Just know you're not eating them for your liver. What organic, non-GMO beets offer are a variety of trace minerals, vitamins, antioxidants, and other phytochemicals, as well as valuable glucose that can be helpful for providing overall energy and healing throughout the whole body. (Do beware of GMO beets; they are destructive.)

At the same time, you've got to be aware of something. All normal cars have four wheels and an engine, and they can at least drive. Still, do you pick any old car? Or do you choose a car with fewer miles, better brakes, working air bags, and the modern conveniences we've come to expect? With the state of cars today, would you buy one that didn't have air conditioning and power windows? Not unless it were the only car available to you, or you were a vintage car collector—and the beet is not the equivalent of a classic. That ultimate classic beauty would be an apple. So if what you're after is liver healing, why not choose the miraculous apple, whose pectin outweighs beets' benefits? And if you're after an enhanced model—if you eat beets for the value of their rich coloring—why not go for the turbocharged pigments of red pitaya or wild blueberries? That beets are red and your blood is red and your liver is reddish— that's not a reason all on its own to eat beets for your liver. The miraculous, undiscovered antioxidants in pitaya and wild blueberries win. So do the blood-, lymph-, and liver-purifying properties of asparagus and brussels sprouts; for true liver cleansing, nothing can touch them. If you enjoy eating beets that you grow in your garden, don't stop. There are healing benefits to growing beets, plucking them out of the ground, knocking the dirt off, prepping the roots and the greens, and eating them—there's something inherently majestic about it, even.

With a greater sense of where beets stand in the grand scheme of healing foods, now you're fully informed, just as I'm sure you like to be fully informed when you're on the car lot, picking out a car. Ultimately, it's up to you: You only have so many meals left in this life. It's your choice what goes into them.

ALKALINE WATER

For quite a few years now, alkaline water has been touted as essential for maintaining health. Some experts claim a pH of 9.5 is most suitable for our needs. Is it? Suitable to what needs? The needs of a man-made digestive theory? The needs of a bottled water industry to keep ahead of competitors? Our mental need to feel like we're doing something for our health?

What about the needs of the liver? They're what we always bypass. So let's give the liver its due. What does the liver need? Will a higher and higher pH of ionized water cleanse our livers? No, I'm sorry to say it won't.

I'm not totally against highly alkalized water or ionized water in small dosages, because one thing's for certain: the water will most likely be pure and clean. Unless, that is, it's cheap tap water thrown into bottles with natural flavors (MSG) and cheap, industrialized vitamins and electrolytes (basically cheap road salt) and a fancy label slapped on for people to select as an after-workout restorative. This isn't an anti– alkaline water monologue, though. The bottlers of many waters do have their hearts in it, or at least did at one point. There are some great, high-quality water filtration systems and ionizers out there, and some great, high-quality bottled water. It's all needed.

What this is about is our livers. I've often seen and heard people using their high-alkalinity waters with the intention of healing their livers. Truth is, when very, very highly alkaline water enters the stomach, something happens of which medical research and science, medical communities, and the alkaline water industry are unaware. Here's the basis: Nothing liquid is supposed to leave the stomach unless it's been balanced, leveled out, neutralized, taken apart, and put together again. It's disassembled, reassembled, and reconstructed before it takes its journey into the intestinal tract and down the river of the bloodstream to the liver. As I always say, even hundreds of years from now, we as a society still won't know what happens to food and liquid when they enter our stomach. While we'll pretend we do, we won't know the half of it.

Your liver's best friend and first line of defense isn't you, I'm sad to say. Though our livers are our best friends, we are not our livers' best friends. As a human race, we have shown our livers that we call the shots. We eat what we want and do what we want, good or bad for our bodies. Someday in each of our lives, we're meant to recognize our liver's needs, trust the organ, and try to become its best friend, even if it doesn't trust us yet—because the human liver doesn't trust the human mind, not automatically. We have broken the liver's trust for centuries, and we've broken our livers' trust throughout our own lives. We need to earn the liver's respect. What your liver does trust is the stomach; that's its best friend.

When highly alkaline water enters the stomach, it must drop everything. Do you remember a time when you had to stop what you were doing and scramble—whether because of a phone call or a sudden deadline or when you realized you were running late for an appointment or you'd slept through your alarm? That's the position your stomach is in when it has to focus on bringing that highly alkaline water

down to the right pH before it can be of any use. We put things in our stomachs that we think are right, and then our stomachs adjust them to what we really need. The stomach must similarly adjust when we drink acidic water. Tap water is pretty acidic, as are some bottled waters that came out of reservoirs, were filtered, and that was it. No matter what the imbalance, even though it's just water, it takes the stomach's energy, reserves, and seven-acid blend, as well as pancreatic strength and enzymes, to change the water's structure and take it to a place where the stomach senses it can be safely dispersed to the rest of the body with the best results.

What does this have to do with the liver? For one, if someone drinks a large volume of high-pH, ionized, alkalized water at once, chances are that the stomach will have to default on its duty. It can't hold on to that much water for long, not long enough to straighten out the mess and reorganize it. Same if a large amount of acidic water is consumed at once. The stomach will need to let either type of water out of the floodgates, especially if someone is also dealing with any kind of gut issue—and a gut issue is already a low hydrochloric acid and liver issue to begin with. So as the overflow flows over, the liver is called into action. The liver doesn't blame the stomach for forfeiting; it knows who's responsible. To assist the digestive system, the liver releases a different batch of bile from normal, one not primarily geared to break down fats and instead made to trap water in the intestines until this special bile has raised acidity or lowered the alkalinity an acceptable amount. It's yet one more of the liver's undiscovered chemical functions.

This special variety of bile is made up of minerals, enzymes, and complex hormone blends that the liver has stored inside of it long term, along with a chemical compound that forms a sticky, mucus-y film. It takes liver reserves to produce this bile, and it's a costly slowdown process that doesn't help the liver or the stomach, though it does help you make up for the mistake you just unknowingly made. The extra work also means that your liver won't put energy into cleansing while it devotes its resources to neutralizing the water.

None of this means you can't partake in the benefits of highly alkaline water. It doesn't mean it's toxic or bad. If you enjoy and believe in it, then sure, I'm with you. You can play with your ionizer machine and create your alkaline water if you feel it holds true healing powers. Just know that it's not a liver healer or cleanser, and don't consume it in large volumes or use it as your regular drinking water. Use it as a medicine, in tiny amounts that won't force the stomach to let go of it before it's ready. Also learn to balance it with the water that your liver does like and use in higher volumes for cleansing: that with a 7.5 to 8.0 pH. This more neutral pH is perfect for the body and doesn't require extra reserves to process: It won't give your stomach extra work to neutralize or force the liver to employ specially made bile. It will allow your liver to go about its

business to keep you well in that moment. When you're throwing down highly alkaline water all the time, it's like tapping your liver on the back and interrupting and distracting it over and over when it's in the middle of an important project. Keep that in mind, and choose the moments when you're sure you want to interrupt your liver. Otherwise, stick with neutral water. If you want to be crafty, squeeze some fresh lemon or lime into water with a 7.5 or 8.0 pH; it will be its own ionization process, and the water will become more alkalizing for the body without putting your stomach or liver through anything. It will actually help properly cleanse your liver.

With this knowledge under your belt, you're that much closer to earning a place of trust with your liver. Free from unknowingly straining it, your power to heal is now exponentially greater. There's yet one more liver myth that we need to make sure we cover so you get all the knowledge you need, and it's one that I've mentioned more than a few times throughout this book: the high-fat trend. Since that's its own entity, we'll explore it more fully in the next chapter.

CHAPTER 35

The High-Fat Trend

The world has become so anti-sugar and anti-carb that it's become almost impossible to find experts in the field of health and wellness who don't shun fruits and starchy vegetables. How did this come to be? To begin with, a lot of trial and error by health-care professionals in the search for the best diet. Cutting out processed foods alone didn't seem to get most patients better from a myriad of symptoms and conditions. What to do next? How to feed people and keep them happy while also meeting their caloric needs and helping them heal or at least diminish their symptoms? Professionals couldn't lower protein in the diet because protein is what the entire medical model on Planet Earth is based upon; at least it has been since 1933, especially in Western cultures. Protein remains an untouchable topic, an untouchable aspect of our diets. It's ingrained in us that without protein, we'll diminish, die, disappear.

HOW WE GOT HERE

The food industry combined with the government in the early 1930s to indoctrinate children in grammar schools and then higher grades across the country in the protein act. It became a law of consciousness that can't be broken, like wearing socks. The world will never stop wearing socks. Although some people may stop wearing them with certain outfits to fit a style, or maybe there will be a decade when it's not hip to wear socks, in the end, socks will be back on people's feet. It's who we are: we wear socks. This practice holds its ground in a conventional sense, just as protein holds its ground in a conventional and now alternative medical sense.

In the old alternative medicine, protein was never a law. Alternative healers of the earlier days—for example, the 1920s—never held up protein as the highest source. They believed in vegetables, fruits, potatoes, other starchy vegetables, nuts, and seeds. They didn't pay particular mind to protein because they knew there was more than enough protein in these foods. Conventional medicine, on the other hand, became married to protein when we entered the animal industrial age of processing meat. The meatpacking industry worked with the government and made a contractual business decision, then joined forces with the pharmaceutical world, and ultimately indoctrinated the entire conventional medical industry in a decision that made sense momentarily and put monetary interest before people's physical interests. These grandfathered contracts still exist in vaults somewhere, not for public display. These were no cute secret cookie recipes. They were decisions made for us without any input from us—no votes allowed, no town meetings, none of our knowledge or say whatsoever in private business deals that still hinder our lives with confusion decades later.

By the 1970s, an awareness occurred in the conventional medical world that too much fat was not good. It was an awakening that was actually positive, a glimpse of light where they realized too much fat was bad for the heart—yet the discovery wasn't executed properly, so the potential for progress fell apart. It turned into a low-fat trend that made no sense. That's because the "low-fat" diets of the day were actually extremely high in fat. These diets increased portions of animal proteins of all kinds, including meats, while having the illusion of being low-fat because they stayed away from avocado, olives, coconut, oils, nuts, and seeds. These foods were practically banned. Coconut and avocado especially were considered poisonous, and if you were a professional in the medical field who suggested them to a patient, you were seen as grossly irresponsible. "Low-fat" and "fat-free" products lined the shelves. They weren't healthy products, mind you; they were just reportedly low-fat and fat-free. People thought they were triumphing by avoiding the lard and sugar of chocolate cake, only they replaced it with animal protein, which was filled with fats.

What made these the highest-in-fat diets ever without anyone realizing it was a mistake that was ignored then and is ignored now: they didn't realize that animal protein automatically translates to animal fat. We turn a blind eye to the reality that there's any fat in animal protein, and that was the goal to begin with in the early 1930s. That was the master plan: focus on protein, ignore the fat content—and it worked. When you grow up with parents and grandparents focused on protein, it's a rule you can't escape. Somehow, the word *protein* takes us over as if we've been bitten by a zombie, and now we've become zombies, too.

So in the early 1970s, everyone started buying their low-fat and no-fat products in the stores yet eating double or triple their amount of animal protein—which was loaded with fat—essentially doubling or tripling their fat intake despite shutting out old alternative medicine's healthy fats such as avocado, coconut, nuts, seeds, and olives. At the same time, they were keeping carbohydrates low and avoiding sugar at all costs while getting it in another way: through alcohol. In the early 1970s, alcohol use was at an all-time high. People were going through low-carb starvation on their diets, reacting emotionally, and needing to get their sugar somehow. It's a similar process to what we go through in today's trendy high-fat, high-protein, low-carb diets. People make sure they don't skip their wine or other alcoholic beverages, or they find themselves binge-eating sugar because the diets leave a gap. The "low-fat" diets of the '70s were one of the early mistakes with the right idea. They were well intentioned, realizing that high fat wasn't good for us, and done all wrong—because they forgot to fix one piece of the puzzle, which was that business marriage of the '30s made to convince us that protein was law. So even though observers had the right idea in the '70s when they realized that people were getting sick and that high dietary fat was causing problems, the execution failed instantly, with no one realizing that the protein law was the reason. Today's diets keep on making these well-intentioned mistakes. It's a little different now, which is what we're going to explore next.

TODAY'S HYBRID DIETS

There's a myriad of diet programs and food belief systems out there that have been renamed over and over again to repackage the same concept: a high-protein, low-carb diet. With a new name—for example, calling it an autoimmune diet—it seems like it's a different twist. It's not. It's just another anti-carb, anti-sugar, extremely high-fat eating plan—even if it incorporates "lean" proteins. Lately, some repackaged diets are proud to say that they are high in fat, as if high-fat is good for you. These are just slightly upgraded versions of the original high-protein diets of the '70s, '80s, and '90s. Today's high-protein diets have more greens thrown in, more green juices; many allow a green apple or some healthy berries in the door. They advocate eating a lot of salad and other vegetables. People suffered more from the early low-carb, high-protein, "low-fat" diets because they didn't get these healing foods that they needed.

As medical communities observed patients coming off standard diets, they observed many symptoms subsiding. "Eureka! We've struck gold!" physicians who were interested in foods said along the way. Sometimes long-term symptoms would fade, sometimes short-term ones, too, and even though some patients would experience no benefits at all and others' health would worsen over time, it felt like barriers were breaking down in the world of medicine— because conventional medicine was finally paying attention. Up until this point, conventional medicine hadn't generally oriented itself around diets and food; not much was known about them. For the most part, the conventional medical world believed that diet had nothing to do with disease or healing, with the exception of too much red meat not being good for the heart. Now offshoots of conventional medicine were

forming where doctors wanted to know more, learn more, get their hands in food more—they wanted more out of food—because they knew from their own experiences or watching others' experiences or hearing about alternative doctors' experiences that medical school wasn't teaching enough about healing foods. So they ventured past the usual strictures into alternative, holistic ways—ways that alternative doctors and herbalists had been balked at, laughed at, humiliated, discredited, or put in prison for teaching for years. Hundreds of alternative doctors in the U.S. alone were put in prison or their careers were destroyed through the 20th century, guilty only of doing something different. Today people take their advancements for granted as they freely and easily express personal views in alternative health; they don't realize where those rights came from or what had to occur in the past to be able to speak out in the present. As we moved into the 2000s, medical professionals who'd been brought up in conventional medicine and now finally saw what alternative medicine had to offer were creating hybrid medical models. Alternative medicine wasn't the lone wolf or the black sheep anymore. Now conventional medical professionals were blending the alternative wisdom of, for example, leafy greens and green juices into their conventional diets of less processed food and leaner proteins. They became the functional medicine and holistic and alternative medical doctors of our time.

At certain points along the way, they did start to realize there were limits. Turned out, outlawing bread and grains didn't solve life's mysteries or erase chronic illness. And too much meat and chicken and other animal protein in the diet weren't giving the results they needed. So they started to hybridize even more and bring in avocados and coconuts (once considered dangerously fattening) and high-quality nut and seed butters (which they themselves had similarly poo-pooed and shunned before). Today's popular diets are hybrid high-protein diets: high in quality "lean" protein, plant fat, leafy greens, green juices, and veggies, and incorporating just a handful of fruit. It's all formed by trial and error, mistakes made in the past, and stealing the hard-earned gems of success from the alternative health world. Healers have been ridiculed along the way for offering more sensible diets, bits and pieces of which are making their way into the mainstream today. No one knows this history, and you need to know it for any sort of perspective.

Is this better than the processed-food diets of the past? Yes. Is it giving people relief from their symptoms? Many people, yes. Is it curing chronic illness? No. Is there a special name for every new version of this hybrid diet? Yes. Are they all, underneath the names, the same? Pretty much. Although these diets may be a little different here and there, it's the same model, the same core. They are, no doubt, better than their old no-carb, high-protein, high-fat predecessor diets, and they do help people steer clear of junk food and fried food and cakes and cookies and most processed foods, when patients are committed. A patient will most likely see some results in overall inflammation. What we need to remember about that is that the medical model doesn't know why inflammation occurs in the first place or why it reduces on a given diet. The theory is that the inflammation is autoimmune, arising from the body attacking tissue, or they believe that a certain food itself is directly causing the inflammation or that the food is triggering an autoimmune response in the body.

It's still nothing like what it could be. For real healing food inspiration, doctors need to look back to the herbalists and naturopaths and holistic doctors who were getting results for patients long before the hybrid high-fat diets of today. These were physicians and other practitioners of the 1960s, '70s, and '80s and even going back 100 or more years who didn't have better technology, just better dietary sense, who were shunned and disgraced by the medical world and government for advising patients to focus on plant foods. Alternative communities were mostly plant-based in the old days, though they had to be careful, because practitioners could lose their livelihoods if word got out that they were advising patients likewise. Back in the 1800s, meat bars were the fast food establishments of the day, where you could go to drink ale and sink your teeth into a huge portion of meat. Alternative-minded doctors observed that these meals weren't good for the bowels or the heart, and that fueled their advice to lower animal sources and bring in more plant foods. As food became industrialized, the alternative minded also observed that boxed and canned food wasn't great. They knew they already had the ticket to alleviating ailments—many of which, whether they realized it or not, related back to the liver.

SUGAR, CARBS, PROTEIN, AND HIDDEN FAT

What has stayed a constant since the supposedly low-fat (and really high-fat) diets of the 1970s is that when a diet goes high-fat (what many call "high-protein," not realizing it automatically means high-fat), it goes no-carb or low-carb, too. You'll hear that it's because the sugar that carbohydrates break down into and sugar itself cause problems, in part by turning into fat. When low-quality carbs in a diet go up, doctors observe that patients' health declines, and they don't know why, though it's easy to blame the carbs. What no one realizes is that the problem is the combination of sugar *with fat*. Together, they clash.

Accidentally, people realized that eating chocolate mousse after a steak dinner might not be the best choice, so they kept the steak dinner and skipped the mousse with no idea that this isn't really a solution. They ended up attacking all forms of carbs and sugar. Since doctors think sugar is the problem, they take the sugar out of the diet and keep the fat, and it's true: A1C levels can drop, prediabetes can disappear, and diabetes can improve if someone's also exercising. No one knows the real reason why lowering carbohydrate intake makes a difference, though; they think it's because sugar is inherently problematic or plays tricks on the body. It's led to blaming the wrong culprit. Removing healthy sugar is not the answer. Reducing radical fat: that's where the answer lies for truly long-term healing, especially healing a chronic illness.

Fat and sugar: here in the U.S. and around the globe, the combination is everywhere. Sweet barbecue sauce on fatty ribs with buttered corn on the cob. Ketchup on hash browns. Pizza with sweet tomato sauce, a wheat crust, and fatty, oily cheese that's also filled with lactose (dairy sugar). Pork with rice. Fried chicken and mashed potatoes. Cheese and crackers. Grilled cheese dripping with butter. Bread and butter. A common sandwich—that is, bread with any kind of meat—because it combines the carbs of the bread, which break down into sugar, and the fat of the meat. And then add the works, and you've got a meal like a tuna sandwich (fat and sugar) with mayonnaise (fat), a bag of chips (fat and sugar), and a soda (sugar). It's what we've done all along, and it doesn't work for many health reasons, some that are known and some that are completely unknown by medical research and science. If you skipped over

Chapter 15, "Diabetes and Blood Sugar Imbalance," you may want to go back and take a look at the more in-depth information there.

What about protein? Doesn't the protein in the meals above overshadow everything else, since protein is king? And people on trendy diets often incorporate "lean" protein. So what's the problem? Here's the catch with protein: it comes with plenty of fat. It's how people on high-protein, no-carb diets survive—they're getting fat calories, whether they know it or not. Doctors in the older days knew that meat contained fat. For some reason, that's become a forgotten, hidden truth of medicine, so we need to be the ones who remember and see. People feared nuts and coconut because they knew they contained fat; now they're accepted more because fat is more accepted. People opt for chicken without knowing that chicken has more fat than nuts or coconut could ever have; we pretend that chicken breast has no fat and is just a protein source. If you were to take out fat from protein sources, people on high-protein, no-carb diets would literally starve to death . . . though at least they'd die thinking they were getting enough protein. Chapter 38, "Liver Rescue 3:6:9" will cover protein more.

As you read about in Chapter 2, "Your Adaptogenic Liver," we never really know how much fat is in a given food. There's so much hidden fat, even in what we think is lean. The nutrition labels we read are averages and estimates—because think about it: Do you have the same body-fat ratio as your neighbors? As everyone in your family? No, you're all different. The same goes for chickens in the coop and cows in the field and fish in the hatchery and game in the wild. They're individuals with different bodies, and each farm feeds the domesticated ones differently, so the grams of fat per serving are going to vary wildly. Same with nuts and seeds and other plant proteins: each tree or plant is going to be different. Since food companies need to standardize labeling, though—they can't separately test, measure, and weigh the fat content of every chicken's body and every walnut before they package it—we can never be sure how much fat we're truly consuming. It's frequently much more than we realize, so we're getting a lot more fat than we know. What we see on the label is not accurate; it can't be. There are diets out there that say they're low fat for the liver, and they still have hidden fat in them, because they incorporate, for example, lots of chicken breast. That's not what the liver really wants.

LOSING LONGEVITY

On a high-fat, strictly low- to no-carb diet, even most committed people will eventually break and binge to meet their sugar needs. What are sugar needs? Well, you know about blood sugar. It's what sustains us and keeps us alive: glucose. Beyond that, storage bins of glycogen keep your brain from atrophying, keep your liver strong, and keep other vital parts of your body going to keep you alive. On a high-fat, low-carb diet, the heart slowly becomes weary. It yearns for the person to eat the berries the diet permits them because it desperately needs and wants even the very little sugar they contain. While it won't really be adequate, it will be just enough to keep the heart going—because the heart is a muscle that needs that glucose for survival. At the same time, the heart struggles to pump blood through the body because of its high fat content. The brain and liver monitor their glycogen storage, and when it starts to get low their messages lead a person on a low-carb diet to binge and eat two slices of pizza at a friend's house, a bag of chips out at lunch, a candy bar from a hotel minibar, or a piece of organic chocolate calling out at the natural foods store. If you change the approach and bring in high-quality glucose from fruits and starchy vegetables—remember your CCC, critical clean carbohydrates, from Chapter 13—while lowering fat so the natural sugar can do its job, the brain and liver are no longer forced to sound the emergency sirens that lead you to grab the nearest dairy or coconut ice cream cone.

When you are eating radical fats, some of the best foods to eat with them are vegetables, leafy greens, lemons, limes, oranges, tomatoes, celery, cucumbers, and red bell peppers. A little bit of sweet fruit can be okay with fat—for example, if you want some mango on a salad with avocado, that's not the end of the world. An avocado-banana smoothie, on the other hand, isn't ideal, unless that's formula for a child. A great way to separate fats and sugars in your day is to snack on fruit (with some leafy greens, cucumber slices, or celery sticks, if you want) about 20 minutes before you eat a meal with radical fats. That gives the glucose time to disperse while filling you up so you don't need such large portions of radical fats. If you're looking for more guidance: when you can, consider avoiding the combination of radical fats with healthy carbohydrates such as potatoes, gluten-free grains, or beans, or unhealthy carbohydrates such as table sugar. It's also helpful to avoid adding more fats to animal proteins. Cooking animal proteins with oil, deep-frying them, or adding butter or an egg on top compounds the fats, which gives your liver more work.

If you keep carbs out for too long, your life can be shortened. I don't enjoy breaking this news. It's no fun, and it angers the high-fat, low-carb monarchy. It's like walking up to a beehive and rattling the branch; the bees become angry and start to sting. Rulers in the high-fat belief system who believe that high fat helps you live longer get extra angry. When people's life's work and resources are invested in a concept, the last thing they want is to be told they're wrong. It would be almost impossible to change course when they've dedicated everything they have to their endeavor. They also get angry because it's very possible that their livers are inundated with toxins and fats; they could have emotional, sluggish, cranky, and angry livers.

Low-carb is not a longevity diet; it's a *short-gevity* diet. This is part of why the hip, trending diets have been altered lately to bring in a little more carbohydrate to go along with the high fat and protein. Avocado, for example, has some natural sugar in it, not just fat, and that fructose is just enough to keep your heart from becoming injured or dying on a low-carb diet. Does the expert behind a diet know specifically that the sugar in the avocado is why people do better incorporating it into their meals? I doubt it. Regardless, they're bringing in avocados while also allowing a little more leeway for seeds and nut butters, which contain some natural sugars, too, and life-sustaining carbohydrates such as berries and apples, however sparingly. Somewhere inside, experts know that an all-animal protein diet with no carbs is not good for the long haul. So they reduce the animal proteins in trendy diets to some degree to make room for other fats, accidentally finding some more results.

Trial and error with low-carb, high-protein, high-fat diets of the past left a wake of sickness, remorse, and unproductive results. As each decade goes by, more and more mistakes get forgotten, and they're never really corrected or documented for all to learn from them. Instead of making progress by learning from the past, we're making random, accidental spurts of progress by stumbling in the dark until we finally get to a door that opens. It doesn't offer a foundation to explain why people are sick or why someone gets the result they do.

FEAR OF FRUIT

With hybrid diets, we're at a point in history when our best experts are the closest they've been in a long time to crafting food plans that make sense for our health. These diets still aren't anywhere to hang our hats. While it's great that people are cleaning up their diets overall of processed grains and other processed foods, junk food, and fast food—and because of this, starting to see improvements in some areas of their health—there's a limit. It's not the be-all, end-all. It's not the whole answer. In most cases of autoimmune and other viral-related illnesses—that is, hundreds of the most common chronic illnesses that plague the population today—these diets aren't enough to make the real healing happen.

Protein smoothies with nut butter and coconut oil for breakfast are better than bacon and eggs with hash browns. They're still not the best. I know the argument for these trendy diets is that they seem to help children with autism or assist people with losing weight. It's true that *some* children, *some* people see a difference in the moment. It doesn't mean the diets are healing anything at a base level. They may keep symptoms at bay and bring slight improvements, and yes, this is beneficial, and it matters. Any improvement counts. Still, we need to be aware of why we're getting any improvements at all, and then of how to get even more improvements—because the last thing you want is for your improvements to slip through your fingers like sand, disappearing without your ever knowing why. You need to know more. I've seen hundreds of people do high fat and stay the same with their symptoms and conditions or even worsen. The ones who do get some results at first end up worsening later. That said, these diets are a lot better than so much of what's out there, especially for someone who's not really sick, just experiencing a little symptom here or there. If someone just needs to lose a little weight and get the sniffles to improve, a trendy diet of today could get the weight to drop, clear the head a little, improve some focus and concentration, allow for more energy, reduce inflammation, and pick things up overall for many.

And yet, even with experts convinced there's nothing better than a high-fat diet, I'm here to tell you that there's much better out there for you. One of the biggest drawbacks to these trendy diets is that they shun fruit. That's because over the last decade or so, certain professionals in the field of medicine have put out information about certain foods that's false and misleading, and it spreads like poison ivy. It was a grave mistake for them to associate fruit with "bad carbs." (Read more in the "Fruit Fear" chapter in *Medical Medium*. Short version: If you ever hear the expression "Sugar is sugar," don't believe it. Fruit sugar is in a class of its own and should never be mistaken for a troublemaker.) With today's popular diets, if you're a kid suffering from any type of gut or cognitive issue, fruit will be taken away based on the false theory that the brain is made out of fat. The truth is that it's made out of glycogen (carbohydrate storage of glucose) solidified into highly active, electrically sustainable soft tissue, with small traces of omega-3s in and around it. The majority of the brain is carbohydrate.

When fruit is taken away on these diets, fat becomes the main calorie source, and that can hurt and even kill your liver over time. It may not hurt your liver as badly as if you were living on fast food; still, it could slow your liver down, make it more dysfunctional, and allow for the possibility of all the diseases and symptoms in this book. It's true even if you're an exercise instructor who works out all the time or you take walks religiously and you're thin, with low body-fat percentage—your liver can be stressed from a high-fat diet. These trendy diets, regardless, will lead you to a fatty liver, even if it takes 30 years. When you eat a lot of fat, the liver grows fat. If high fats in the diet are mostly from avocado, coconut, and nut butters and you're getting some natural sugars, that will at least allow for some improvement.

Don't let fruit scare you. There's misinformation out there that says eating sugar leads to a fatty liver and that eating fruit hurts the liver. It keeps people away from fruit, and that's misleading, deceiving, and devastating; it keeps them away from their true potential longevity.

A FALSE SUMMIT

Look: if you're on one of these high-fat, low-carb diets, you don't need to panic. It's better than fried food every night with a big chocolate cake afterward. At the same time, your liver wants more of what it needs. And it doesn't want to get fatty. What the experts who create pop theory lifestyle diets don't know is that your liver runs on glucose and stored glycogen to give you a healthy, long life, protecting your adrenals, heart, and brain. I know the image of ancient man foraging in the woods, eating only handfuls of berries and killing whatever he needed to survive. Times have changed. We have food that we can pick and choose now—we can pick and choose the outcome of our health, because we have options. And for what it's worth, whatever belief system you may hold, ancient humans ate very little to begin with and many times starved from going weeks on nothing more than a few mushrooms and some dirt. They ate wild game only as a survival tactic if it was even available in times of starvation. What ancient humans ate the most of were starchy tubers, rhizomes, shoots, and nuts because those were most accessible. When they could, essentially, they ate high-carb diets.

Since we think fat's the way to health and it's there at our fingertips, and we're not ancient man going from moment to moment of near starvation, we can decide to feed ourselves fat without a break. Since we're not being educated about how important healthy carbohydrates are for our health, we go through glucose deprivation and eat even more fats because we think that will satisfy us. It's the trend of the day. The label "science" can be used to put a spin on everything possible in conventional and alternative health. As long as that word is used, anything good can be spun to seem bad, and anything bad can be spun to seem good. Keep this in mind. And if you're concerned about what you're reading here, please turn to "A Note for You" at the beginning of this book and read it over and over again.

For the record, this chapter is not an attack on animal protein. It's when animal protein *defines a diet* that we need to take care and evaluate if that's best for that individual. All the popular diets include too much fat—vegan and vegetarian included. Vegans eat too many avocados, nuts, seeds, coconut, tofu, and oil. Vegetarians eat too much butter, cheese, eggs, and milk. (This applies even if it's from a cow in the backyard that you milked yourself.) Vegans and vegetarians alike indulge in bad carbs with bad fats: greasy foods like cheap falafel fried in cheap corn oil and French fries made in canola oil. Vegetarians enjoy baguettes with brie and grilled cheese sandwiches. With high-fat diets, whether they include carbs or not, whether they include animal products or not, things can go wrong with our health. I'm not here to pick a side in the food wars. My battle is to bring to light medical information that's from an independent source and undiscovered by research and science so you can protect yourself and your family. My job is to see through the fog and hear through the noise in the medical industry. It's not about picking one aisle or another in the food world—it's not about vegan versus paleo versus any new food belief system in between. It's about giving you the right information so you can make proper choices to heal.

The healthier vegan and vegetarian diets of today don't look all that different from the healthier diets that focus on animal proteins. The plant-based ones tend to lower carbs and incorporate gluten-free grains, with fewer fried options; better, higher-quality oil; higher-quality butter; more greens and other veggies; and more coconut, hempseeds, sunflower seeds, and avocado. The animal protein–focused ones often stay very low-carb and bring in lots of chicken, pasture-raised meat, eggs, and fish, as well as some avocado, nut butter, coconut oil, greens, and other veggies. Both versions stay high-fat and stick to low-sugar fruits. Through the hybridization of alternative and conventional medicine over the past 20 years, the different diets have grown together. As we saw in the beginning of the chapter, high fat from standard, conventional diets merged with greens and juices from past rivals and enemies, and we ended up with what you see on health shows, in other books, and in the latest articles. It's considered the best that it gets, the answer to all our problems, the pinnacle. Well, don't do your happy dance just yet. It's a false summit.

SEEING CLEARLY

Without knowing how we got here, we become prey to mistakes still happening that we cannot see. The system that's developing may or may not work in our favor; we can't tell if we turn a blind eye. That's why, here, we've needed to look back and understand how the high-fat trend came to be. You know how in life, you don't want to go into a meeting without being informed about why it's happening? How you don't want to eat a meal placed before you if you don't know anything about it? Somehow, a trend is all we need to feel like we've been fully informed. If others are filing into the meeting room, we'll follow. If there's hype, we'll eat the mystery meal. It's how we've arrived at this place where nearly everyone is on a high-fat diet. One has a little more meat, one has a lot less meat, one has fat three times a day, one has avocado and coconut sometimes. One only allows a handful of berries for carbs, one is focused on bacon and eggs, one brings in more green juices, one is focused on butter in everything. One says it's designed around your genes. A new diet is born every day. And then there are the people who like to decide for themselves what to eat, not follow a plan, and yet end up falling into the high-fat trap, too, even if they allow themselves more food groups. Whether we're conscious of their influence or not, ideologies and belief systems are what always stop or slow down progress in the medical world of chronic illness. And when it comes to food, that's one way to truly slow down results. One reason why alternative medicine was shunned and discredited for so long was because it did the opposite: it offered ways to slow down illness and disease that the conventional medical industry benefited from financially.

For decades before today's trendy diets, people—whether they ate animal protein, kept vegan or vegetarian, or did anything in between—benefited from the healing foods that they ate. No matter the food mythologies that come and go, healing foods always have been and always will be fruits, vegetables, leafy greens, nuts, seeds, herbs, and spices. They're like the originators of rock and roll. News flash: rock music's origin story did not begin with megahit British bands; it began as a birthright of African Americans' rich musical heritage that was then adopted by people from all walks of life. Conventional medicine now benefits from the alternative health field that was ostracized for so long—and in some respects, still is. From afar, conventional medicine watched as people saw differences result from consuming fresh fruits and juices and leafy greens; shots of wheatgrass juice; large salads with kale, sprouts, and pea shoots; and even bananas. And then, when the mainstream hybrid experts were starting on their paths, they decided to pick and choose what would fit into their high-fat belief systems.

Whatever they incorporated had to fit into a diet of largely animal protein, since that law of survival from the 1930s was still firmly institutionalized. Carbohydrates took the hit, which, when it comes to the bad carbs like breads and doughnuts and cookies and cakes and pastries and flours and other processed grains, has helped. Eliminating those was an accomplishment the medical world could have hung its hat on—if only they'd kept fruit in their popular diets. Instead, fruit got lumped in with bad carbs and cut out of diets.

The next decision that experts had to make when devising their diets was what type of animal protein to include. They landed on grass-fed and free-range, while minimizing dairy. Eggs were give or take with each diet rendition. They began to publicize their new high-fat diets with no fruits, along the way making those adjustments we looked at earlier, once again borrowing a different golden nugget after having once condemned it. This time, they brought in items such as vegetable juices that those in the alternative communities of the past had once broken their backs trying to bring to the world only to be deemed crazy for it.

Considering the degree to which high-fat diets are worshipped, with or without the protein label, it's easy to forget that millions of people are slipping through the cracks, still suffering, and that illness is on the rise like never before in history and not going to slow down anytime soon because these diets don't heal at the level so many people need. Especially for the people dealing with autoimmune conditions and other chronic illnesses and symptoms that are still completely misunderstood mysteries to medical research and science, it's time to lower the fat, I'm sorry to say. Getting better and lowering the fat means lowering the protein—remember, no matter how lean the animal protein source, there's a calorie, and that comes from fat. (Lowering fat doesn't mean no fat ever in your diet. Fats have their place; healthy fats in the right amounts do have value to offer.) Getting better means keeping those vital greens and vegetables in the mix. And one of the most critical parts of getting better and protecting yourself is bringing in some fruit. For 30 years, I've been able to help chronic illness sufferers live strong, healthy, robust lives by offering them these guidelines. They've been free from waffling back and forth or being swayed by new fads because they know better. I want you to know better, too, so you can see clearly along your journey.

If we rely on ideologies and belief systems, we won't see clearly. For true clarity, we need to ask ourselves, "What does my liver need?" because a happy liver is the key to health.

There's a trend that the key to life and health is our own happiness. I've known many fulfilled, happy people who got sick because they had an unhappy, unfulfilled liver inside of them. We get so self-involved, thinking all about what's going to make us happy, not saying, "Hey, is there a liver inside me that's completely unhappy? Maybe I should start focusing on that." The last thing our livers need is too much fat. You don't need me to tell you one more time what an overabundance of fat in the diet does to your liver. You've already seen how high-fat diets worsen all of the illnesses in this book. You don't need to hear about how with the liver weakening from too much fat, its bile production weakens, too, causing fats in the colon to putrefy and go rancid.

What you need are your own senses, your own mind, your own intelligence, your own logic, your own intuition, your own wits about you, and your own memory of what's real to protect yourself. No matter the new spins, the new hype, the new fear mongering, the new breathless praise for diets that enter the market, you'll be able to see a high-fat diet for what it is: one that won't end up helping your liver, which means it won't help you. It's not about animosity toward any belief system or what I believe versus what the inventor of a new food protocol believes. It's about what's right to support your liver and fend off disease, whether medical research and science have caught up yet or not. Have I said that enough? It's about your liver.

When you're not entangled in an old, institutionalized belief system, you can find its loopholes and climb through them, and do what's right for yourself. It's an opportunity to discover what your liver really needs to bring you abundant health.

CHAPTER 36

Liver Troublemakers

We're exposed every day to substances that threaten our health. Luckily, we're also blessed with miraculous, neutralizing, filtering livers. The liver does such a good job protecting us that much of the time, we're not even aware that anything potentially harmful ever entered our system. For the liver, though, these substances make mischief. That's why I call them liver troublemakers. They burden it, strain its resources, and put it under constant pressure to keep them contained for fear of what would happen to our health if they were let loose and became heart troublemakers or brain troublemakers or full-body troublemakers. You've read in detail about just what kinds of symptoms and conditions can result from liver troublemakers getting out of hand. Now we're going to examine the shocking full list of what most commonly crowds our livers—the unfriendly invaders that live rent free.

If you've been telling yourself that you're free and clear of troublemaker exposure, know that you're doing your liver an injustice with that belief. You're doing your health and well-being an injustice. You're doing your potential peace and happiness an injustice. The list later in this chapter will open your eyes to how much a part of our daily environment so many troublemakers are—they're literally at our fingertips and as close as the air we breathe. Only when you're conscious of what your liver has been exposed to throughout your life, and before you were even born, can you be ready to help your liver recover so you can finally feel better and guard yourself and your loved ones from illness for the future.

THE THREE DEPTHS OF THE LIVER

Each of the liver's two main lobes has three general levels: its perimeter surface, its subsurface, and its deep, inner core. While there are subtler layers within these levels, these three depths can form our basis for understanding how the liver stores and releases troublemakers.

You can think of the perimeter surface like the skin of an apple, where it's so integrated with the whole that if you peeled it off you might bring some flesh from underneath with it. The liver's subsurface has a good amount of room; it's like all that flesh of the apple. And the liver's deep, inner core, not surprisingly, is like the apple's core.

259

As you'll see in the list to come, some troublemakers stay in only one or two levels of the liver, and some can spread out across all three. Usually, if a troublemaker occupies more than one level, it's in different concentrations in each—for example, dioxins will settle in different strengths in each of the liver's three levels. The exceptions are chemical fertilizers, DDT and other pesticides, herbicides, and fungicides, which you'll see end up in equally high concentrations across all three of the liver's levels. Each level also contains a different combination of troublemakers. The "skin" of the liver can become saturated with materials that don't ever get into the liver itself. The "flesh" of the liver has its own mix of troublemakers. And the liver sends the worst of the troublemakers to its "core."

With as many dangerous substances as possible buried deep in its central core, the liver can protect you better. You can even walk around feeling good, because with these troublemakers tucked away, your liver can still function pretty well. What becomes problematic is when outside factors such as fat and adrenaline come to visit while the liver also has harmful materials buried within it—that combination can make you feel unwell. Think of it as a ship crossing the ocean. While your liver has both the capacity to handle a certain amount of cargo stored below deck and the courage of sailors facing rough seas, it also has limitations. When we pile extra cargo on top, or when we run into stormy weather, it has the potential to sink on us. That's why as a safeguard, we want to keep that cargo hold as clear of troublemakers as we can. Not to mention that your liver needs room to store all the good stuff like everyday provisions and emergency supplies, so we don't want to take up all its storage space with waste.

The deeper troublemakers go into the liver, the more it protects us in the moment and the more time it takes to pull them out later. It's one of the reasons that people's healing processes can vary so much in length. You might be following someone's healing path on social media, or maybe you're friends with someone who's taking the same steps you are, and you find yourself wondering why this person is bouncing back faster than you are. When you need more time to heal, it's because more troublemakers, and possibly more toxic troublemakers, are buried deeper within your liver.

In the list to come, you can read about where each type of troublemaker tends to settle in the liver, and you can use that as a guide to how long they take to cleanse. If a troublemaker sticks around in the liver's surface level, it will take less time to get out of your system, and if it goes into the liver's core, it will take more time and persistence to get it out. Times will also vary depending on the grade of toxin, poison, or pathogen, meaning that a more problematic liver troublemaker in, say, the subsurface level will take more time to get out than a less problematic one there.

Another huge factor in how long it takes to lose these troublemakers is what you're doing to cleanse and what you're eating. In the troublemakers list, you'll find general timelines of how long each takes to leave the liver—if you're actively working to get them out in a safe, effective manner. The timelines are based on someone who's cleansing properly, which means (1) keeping out the troublemaker foods (which you'll read about in a few pages), (2) lowering the amount of radical fat you eat, (3) incorporating some of the supplementation advice from the next chapter, (4) following the Liver Rescue Morning in Chapter 38 whenever you can, and (5) periodically bringing in the Liver Rescue 3:6:9

from that same chapter. If you suspect you're dealing with a decent amount of troublemakers based on what you're reading in this book, it's ideal to do the Liver Rescue 3:6:9 every two to three months. It will help you cleanse at a faster rate and get to deeper toxins than you can generally reach with the everyday measures. If that's too often, do the cleanse when you can, perhaps every six months.

THE TROUBLEMAKER LIST

Some of the troublemakers on this list are well known as taxing to the liver, such as alcohol and medication. You may be surprised to find that there are many more harmful substances that no one has warned you could hurt your liver, such as scented dryer sheets and plug-in air fresheners, of all things. You'll see the Unforgiving Four in this list and much more. Be prepared to see your world in a whole new light.

It's not that we need to live in fear or panic or wear hazmat suits to leave the house. Look, we have to live on Planet Earth. These troublemakers are part of life here, and many of them have been here since long before we were born. Some we can't avoid, so pick what you have control over. If you can't give up your hairspray, conventional makeup, perfume, or cologne; if you've got to cook with gas multiple times every day; or if you breathe in tons of exhaust as part of your job mowing lawns, maybe you can bring less fat into your diet and decide not to get your carpets cleaned with chemicals and opt not to drink a diet soda so your liver can still manage and cleanse while you're living your life. It's not about never pumping your own gas or never riding your bike in the rain (you'll see what I'm talking about soon). It's about taking care of your liver so you can live your life and do

everything you need to do. With the most dangerous items, like mercury, do everything you can to stay away. With the other troublemakers, if you can sidestep a few of the items on this list, you're doing well.

While the list may be surprising, shocking, or unnerving to some degree, it will also be enlightening. Do you want to step into a pothole, or do you want to know where the pothole is so you can avoid a sprained ankle? That said, being aware of what's around and inside of you doesn't mean becoming obsessive or afraid to live. You can't avoid every single pothole. What you can do is use the list to help light the way, so even when you hit a rough patch, you know what terrain you're navigating—where you are and where you're going.

Let this list be a window into how you might have been exposed to various substances that gave your liver extra work to do without you ever realizing. If you want to live well and protect your family, you can't keep the blinds shut, pretend the substances aren't there, and ignore your liver. That would be like pretending cavities don't exist and never visiting the dentist, only to be shocked later when there's a problem you can't ignore. Even if you weren't directly exposed to some of these troublemakers, you could have had secondary exposure—like secondhand smoke, secondhand troublemakers are around us. By understanding what could be inside our livers, we can understand how best to remedy them.

Petrochemicals Group

This group of troublemakers is extremely toxic to the central nervous system. Anybody with neurological sensitivities and symptoms will be especially sensitive to them. Many of these troublemakers settle deep in the liver's inner core, which means they take longer to come out of the liver. You don't need to be concerned about removing them from your liver all at once and immediately. Within the first two weeks of taking the steps I outlined in "The Three Depths of the Liver," you'll start getting the tip of the iceberg. After that, they'll continue to cleanse naturally in due time as you're caring for your liver.

- **Plastics:** We handle a lot of plastics each and every day. Anything plastic that you touch has the potential to leave residue on your skin. With too much lag time between touching plastic and washing our hands (or showering, if the plastic touched another part of the body), that residue has time to absorb into the skin and get into the system. It also enters our system when we ingest it from sources like plastic wrap, plastic food containers, plastic utensils and dishes, water bottles, the water supply, pharmaceuticals (they're filled with plastics), and packaged foods that were prepared using plastic assembly line parts. Some plastics such as high-end food processors, blenders, and juicers are of higher quality and less likely to leach, making them safe to use. Some plastics are low quality, and they leach instantly into the oils on your skin when you touch them. Plastics tend to settle in the subsurface level of the liver.

- **Gasoline:** In the old days, the petroleum exposure that comes from pumping gas was isolated to gas station attendants. With most states now pump-your-own, exposure has increased to virtually everyone, trickling right down to your teenage daughter putting gas in her new car. In the past, your teenage daughter or son never would have been exposed to raw gasoline outside of the rare occasion of mowing the lawn. It's a whole different ballgame today, with millions of teens pumping gas. People aren't very cautious at the pump, so teens aren't trained to be careful. It's not uncommon to get a little splash-back or drip of gas on your skin when you're filling your tank; the rubber guard on the nozzle doesn't stop this from occurring. Almost everyone gets an after-drop of gas on themselves in one way or another at the pump, plus if you stand too close to the spout you're breathing in the fumes. It's easy to catch a whiff from nearby pumps, too. Gasoline exposure like this at the service station is such a common occurrence that it's happened to almost everyone. Not to mention that some people handle gas for other reasons, like fueling lawn mowers, tractors, and weed whackers. Those gas cans sitting in the garage outgas, which means more inhalation exposure, plus it's easy to splash on yourself when handling them. Gasoline tends to settle in the subsurface and deep, inner core of the liver.

- **Diesel:** The exposure for this is the same as with gasoline. You get it from not being mindful when pumping diesel into your truck, car, tractor, or anything of the sort. Just like gas, it tends to settle in the subsurface and deep, inner core of the liver.

- **Engine oil and grease:** You often get grease on your hands just from popping your car's hood and checking the oil. And how many people have gotten oil on their fingers when wiping the oil stick? Even if you've only checked a car's oil stick once and it was ten years ago, any oil on your skin traveled into your liver, where it's still most likely sitting. While you might have long forgotten getting oil on your hands, your liver hasn't forgotten; it's well aware. It's easy to get oil on yourself when adding or changing the oil in your car, too. Engine oil and grease are even on nuts and bolts for brand-new manufactured items you buy such as tools. Roadways also have a thin layer of oil, grease, gasoline, and diesel on their surface. It means that when you're riding your bicycle or walking across the street in the rain, the splash-back you get from the pavement is filled with all four. Engine oil and grease tend to settle in the liver's deep, inner core.

- **Exhaust fumes:** This one speaks for itself, since it's everywhere. Exposure comes from walking down the street, grabbing a package at a delivery person's truck while the truck is still running, getting stuck in traffic on your way to work, passing a lawn that's being mowed or mowing your own, walking up to a restaurant for lunch just as someone fires up a car a few feet away, and so on. Although carbon monoxide is deadly if someone is poisoned by it when there isn't enough ventilation for exhaust fumes, it's not the poison in the liver. The petrochemical particles in the exhaust itself are what end up in the liver. These hundreds of types of exhaust chemicals settle in the liver's deep, inner core.

- **Kerosene:** While this one's not so everyday, and exposure is less now than it ever was, it doesn't mean you weren't exposed to kerosene heating devices back before portable heaters became more often electric. Plus there's still plenty of kerosene exposure to go around. For example, kerosene is often used to wash tools and paint brushes. It finds its way to the subsurface level and deep, inner core of the liver.

- **Lighter fluid:** Think you haven't been exposed to lighter fluid? Think again. Ever eaten a marshmallow roasted over a bonfire that was started with lighter fluid? Ever eaten food from a charcoal grill? The chemical residue sticks around on ignited wood, charcoal, and debris and lasts the whole fire—meaning that you get a marshmallow or hamburger with a hint of lighter fluid cooked into it. Not to mention that if you were the one squirting the fluid to begin with, you inhaled its fumes and likely got some on your hands, because we don't learn to be careful about exposure. I'm not trying to ruin your next cookout or bonfire meal of hot dogs on a stick and s'mores. You can still enjoy yourself; just make sure you're being proactive, so that if you absorb some of life's fun moments that are toxic, you also try to get some troublemakers out of your liver. The goal is to take care of your liver so you can live your life. Lighter fluid usually ends up in your liver's subsurface level and deep, inner core.

- **Gas grills, stoves, and ovens:** When you're lighting and using a grill, stove, or oven powered by natural gas, you inhale some of the gas, which gets into your body. While you're cooking, the gas is still burning. Although it's not raw gas, it's still a troublemaker that you're breathing as long as the appliance is running. Not that you have to avoid cooking; it's just a good idea to avoid cooking with gas excessively. Natural gas usually goes to the subsurface level of the liver and its deep, inner core.

- **Chemical solvents, solutions, and agents:** These include degreasers, lubricants for squeaky doors and drawers, jewelry cleaner, car cleaning products, and carpet cleaning products, and they instantly absorb through the skin in seconds, entering the bloodstream and invading the liver quickly. We're also exposed when we breathe in their fumes. They settle in the liver's subsurface level and deep, inner core.

- **Dioxins:** Imagine a world coated with a dust too fine to see that's inhaled and eaten by every creature on the planet. That's our world, and dioxins are the "dust." These pollutants, a byproduct of over 100 years of chemical factory malfeasance, find their way into air, water, and food. Modern life *is* generalized dioxin exposure. They settle in all three levels of the liver.

- **Lacquer:** When we use varnishes, sealants, or adhesives like epoxy, or when they're applied in our homes or we purchase items freshly lacquered, we're exposed to harsh chemicals that can settle in all three levels of the liver.

- **Paint:** Painting a piece of furniture, painting inside or outside the house, or working in a freshly painted office could have exposed you to this one. I always cringe when I see people frolic and play-fight with paint-filled brushes and rollers because I know the consequences upon the liver of these acts of lethal play. Paint chemicals tend to settle in the subsurface level and deep, inner core of the liver.

- **Paint thinner:** Sometimes used in paint and sometimes used to clean up paint, this strong brew usually goes to the liver's subsurface layer and deep, inner core.

- **Carpet chemicals:** These include the chemicals used to treat new carpets during manufacture, the chemicals released from old carpets when they're cleaned, and the carpet cleaning chemicals themselves (the last of which deserve to show up in this list twice, they're so affecting). We inhale carpet chemicals and also get them on our skin and clothes when we sit on carpets or walk on them in bare feet. They find their way into all three levels of the liver.

Chemical Neuroantagonists Group

The troublemakers in this group get into all three levels of the liver in equally high concentration. Their inheritance factor is also high, meaning they frequently end up in our livers as they're passed from generation to generation. Many of them are a downright disservice to humankind. As you can see from the group name, they're neuroantagonistic, too, making them particularly difficult for people with sensitive nervous systems and neurological conditions and symptoms. As with petrochemicals, the liver knows not to let these all go at once. Instead, it releases them carefully and cautiously, so they may take a longer time period to remove than some other troublemakers. Nevertheless,

the liver still releases them in small increments. If you're committed, you can start getting some of these out in as fast as a week or two, and then the liver will continue to dole them out in measured amounts over time so the body doesn't get flooded by them.

- **Chemical fertilizers:** These are around more than we know. It's easy to be exposed from lawns, gardens, parks, conventionally grown flowers, conventionally grown food, golf courses, country clubs, campus greens, town commons, and our own yards.

- **Insecticides, other pesticides, larvicides, and herbicides:** These include both the indoor and outdoor varieties. For example, exposure could come from cans of roach killer, ant killer, termite spray, and wasp killer used inside the home. It could also come from food and flowers that were treated with pesticides; from apartments, houses, offices, hotels, dorm rooms, and other buildings where pesticides were used inside or out; and from lawns, gardens, parks, country clubs, and campus greens. It's a common occurrence for people to care deeply about eating organic food and then spray the yard for ticks, mosquitos, and weeds—which is pesticide and herbicide exposure. Find out if you live in an area that's sprayed and stay indoors when it happens. Cities across the country spray for caterpillars when the gypsy moths come out around June, and it's extremely liver damaging. City-, town-, and statewide mosquito spraying is also very common in warm weather. It's often applied by helicopter, at any time of day or night without warning. If you like to spend time in your local park, find out its schedule, avoid it when it's freshly sprayed, and maybe even wait for a good rain before spending time there. If you're going to sit on chemically treated grass, make sure to put down a blanket first. Pregnant women should take special care; pesticide exposure can be enough to cause pregnancy complications.

- **DDT:** Although it fits within the category of pesticides, DDT is its own entity. Decades after being banned in the U.S., it's still in our environment, similar to how radiation and other nuclear waste affect generations. DDT has an extraordinarily long shelf life. It's the "gift" that will never stop giving. It remains in our oceans, lakes, streams, agricultural fields, and more. DDT from yesteryear is one of the most common troublemakers to inherit through the family line. It passes from liver to liver forever with ease until someone finally cleans it out of her or his liver so it can't be passed down to another generation. This is a prime example of why we need to cleanse and take care of our livers, so we can stop passing this "gift" down to our children. There

are also countries that still use DDT in high amounts, and when winds pick it up—wind can even carry it from continent to continent—we get fresh exposure through the air. It's still around, and it's not leaving our environment any time soon.

- **Fungicides:** They're being used more and more everywhere, sprayed on new clothing and manufactured goods, from jeans to dresses to underwear to outerwear to socks to shoes to furniture to mattresses to blankets. Originally created for mold remediation in applications such as fungus on crops and in hospitals, since hospitals are a breeding ground for fungus, fungicides now have a broad usage. Fungicide sales and marketing groups will go as far as they can to wheel and deal and convince businesses to find new ways to use it on their products. Fungicides are often used in new cars and in used cars that are being resold. They're regularly used on planes and in garbage cans and bags. Recently, some bottled water brands have been sold into using it on the outsides of their water bottles. Some foods are even treated with fungicides. They have a perfume-y scent to them that sizzles the nose if you pay attention. Whenever you can wash or wipe down an item after you've bought it, do so.

- **Smoke exposure of any kind:** Smoking draws a vast chemical industry compilation of hundreds to thousands of different chemicals into your lungs, bloodstream, and liver. Smoke inhalation from recreational sources such as fire pits, treated logs in the fireplace, and burning treated lumber also expose your liver to chemicals—though a regular smoker will face more chemicals than someone who visits a fire pit once in a while. It's also a common agricultural practice across the country to pile up and burn pesticide-laden plastic row covers from conventional crops. We all breathe in this white smoke; whether we like it or not and whether we can smell it or not, it's there.

- **Fluoride:** An aluminum byproduct that is highly toxic to the liver, causing liver cell damage.

- **Chlorine:** Highly toxic to the liver, it lowers the organ's immune function.

Problematic Food Chemicals Group

These tend to start leaving the liver fast when you're giving it what it needs to let go, and they don't take a long time to rid from your liver completely. With good liver care, you could eliminate all of these from the organ within six months to a year, with many of them beginning to release right out of the starting gate.

- **Aspartame:** You'll find this in diet sodas as well as hidden in flavoring. It goes to the liver's

deep, inner core and is unique in the way it's stored in the liver—it tends to injure small blood vessels inside the liver, causing them to atrophy or shrink.

- **Other artificial sweeteners:** These are highly toxic to the liver, too, and find their way to its deep, inner core.

- **MSG:** Sometimes listed overtly as *monosodium glutamate* and sometimes hidden as "natural flavors" in our food, this ingredient also goes to the deep, inner core of the liver.

- **Formaldehyde:** You can be exposed to this troublemaker from so many sources, everywhere from cosmetics to pharmaceuticals to carpets to food. It does what alcohol does to the liver, only much more extreme. It's also a viral fuel. Formaldehyde saturates all three levels of the liver.

- **Preservatives:** If you're already antipreservative and take care to buy foods that don't list them in the ingredients, it doesn't mean they're not sneaking into your food. Accountability is reckless as far as preservative labeling goes. Not to mention that there were all those years before you became aware, so your liver had plenty of time to collect different varieties of chemically created preservatives. Your liver could be holding on to preservatives from hot dogs you ate decades ago, cotton candy from a fair, a milkshake with imitation fruit flavoring, a purple ice cone . . . the list is never-ending. They tend to stay in the surface level of the liver.

Problematic Foods Group

This group of troublemakers is the first veil that comes off the liver when you start taking care of it. They all leave the liver fast, as long as you're staying away from consuming them while you're trying to cleanse them from the liver. (Keep reading for individual timelines.)

- **Eggs:** Keep pathogens thriving. Viruses and bacteria love eggs as their number-one food source, so when eggs are in the diet, pathogens can feed, causing harm to the liver. Egg whites don't get around the problem. When eggs are out of the diet, pathogens lose their favorite food and have to resort to other food sources in the liver. The particles from eggs can completely leave the cells of the liver within 90 days as long as you are avoiding them altogether during that time.

- **Dairy:** A pathogen food source. Also highly mucus forming, causing mucus to collect within the blood vessels and cells of the liver, which weakens the liver's personalized immune system. Like eggs, you can completely rid dairy particles from the liver's cells if you're avoiding it altogether.

- **Cheese:** Though it fits under the category of dairy, it deserves its own mention here because it has recently been reported as a longevity food. It's not; it doesn't protect you. This is an example of how science bends to certain interest groups. Cheese is another food source for pathogens that hinder and damage the liver. It's the ultimate diabetes-creating food, though often mistaken as a great food for diabetics. This is a disastrous misunderstanding that makes you wonder what other health advice out there is completely backward. Cheese is also responsible for creating stagnant, sluggish, fatty livers and like other dairy, weakens the liver's immune system by creating mucus within the blood vessels and cells of the liver. If you're a cheese lover, stick to enjoying it on special occasions while working to do positive things for your liver in between, or try nut cheese as an alternative.

- **Hormones from food:** These are extremely disruptive to the liver's ability to manage, produce, and organize the body's own hormones. The liver can make a positive out of the situation by neutralizing and storing some of these more-toxic hormones from food to later trap and defuse adrenaline, as we examined earlier in the book. That's not an endorsement for consuming them, since the liver can already do that with the body's own old hormones. Food hormones start leaving the liver quickly when you're looking after it, and after 90 days, you can get rid of all the poisonous hormones that the liver doesn't decide to hold on to as bait to neutralize fresh adrenaline.

- **High-fat foods:** A diet that's high in radical fat—regardless of whether it comes from a plant or animal source, whether healthy or unhealthy fat—is hard on the liver. You saw plenty of evidence of that throughout Part II, "The Unseen Storm," Part III, "The Call to Battle," and Chapter 35, "The High-Fat Trend." When you start tending to your liver, fats start breaking out of it immediately. The full process could take some time and will happen naturally; as all the other troublemakers are leaving your liver, it will keep getting less fatty and less fatty and less fatty.

- **Recreational alcohol:** Heavy drinking is known to create hangovers, and this has spawned a trend of diners, restaurants, and pubs offering hangover "cure" menus of waffles, pancakes, French toast, bacon, eggs, hash browns, mozzarella sticks, biscuits and gravy, cheese fries, French fries, grilled cheese, omelets, and the like. The thought is that after getting drunk, it's best to consume a lot of heavy, greasy food to "soak up" the alcohol.

This couldn't be further from the truth. The reason people have a hangover appetite is because during their alcohol binge, they starved their livers. Not only can the liver not function well when it's inundated with alcohol; it becomes starved of nutrients—so after recreational drinking, our livers need glucose replenishment. The problem with standard hangover meals is that they're a combination of fat plus sugar, which continues to inhibit the liver from restoring its glucose reserves. That prompts people to overeat, thinking more food will sop up the alcohol and satiate them, when what they really need to satiate their hunger and help their livers recover is the right *kind* of food, free from the interference of fat. For more on alcohol and the liver, see its entry in the Pharmaceuticals Group.

- **Excessive vinegar use:** Vinegar saturates the liver, causing a drunken effect, meaning that it slows down the liver's ability to function and operate properly. It's almost like vinegar should come with a warning that says the liver shouldn't operate heavy machinery when under the influence of it. While it's not as bad as what alcohol does to the liver, there is a similarity. Apple cider vinegar is the best out of all the vinegars to use; it has some positives to balance out the effects of fermentation, though you still don't want to overdo it. The cleansing process will start immediately when you start working on your liver. Within a month, you can rid all the vinegar from it.

- **Caffeine:** Causes a thinning effect on cell walls in the liver. Cells usually recover quickly from this, though the constant use of caffeine makes the liver's job of defending itself harder. Continually thinned cell walls make them more susceptible to pathogen invasion, such as from viruses, which can cause cell damage. Caffeine has a deeper saturation rate in the liver than many of the other problematic food troublemakers; it tends to go to all three layers of the liver. It has a very quick release from all three. You can get rid of all the caffeine stored in your liver in one week of caring for it.

- **Excessive salt use:** Is salt good or bad? Every decade in the health world, the trend seems to switch back and forth. The real answer is that a little healthy salt can be okay; sea salt or good mountain rock salt here and there is tolerable for your liver. A pinch of these salts in your life is not going to hurt it. It's when we overdo salt, particularly the wrong salt, and when we overdo salt within a high-fat diet that we need to be cautious. Fat cells tend to encapsulate salts, which in turn dehydrate the fat cells. When a fat

cell is forced to be dehydrated, it becomes denatured and not as easily removed from the body, bloodstream, or liver. Denatured fat cells tend to stick around and collect in the liver—so the more salt in the diet, the more fat tends to denature and stay there. Too much salt also dehydrates organs, muscles, and glands. The heart and liver, for example, need to sustain a certain amount of hydration, and excessive use of salt in its raw form conflicts with this. It's dehydrating to the brain, too. Even though the brain runs on sodium as a neurotransmitter chemical, that sodium needs to be derived from a food itself, not salt added to food. A common mistake in natural health right now is to add salt to water, thinking that it's healthy when it's really not. We should be adding celery and celery juice, coconut water, spinach, sea vegetables, lemons, and limes to our meals, because their naturally occurring sodium won't dehydrate our organs. It's actually very good for the liver, in part because this natural sodium clings to toxic, dangerous salts from poor-quality foods and helps bind onto and draw them out of the body while replacing them with a special subgroup of sodium the liver really needs. It also stabilizes blood pressure, bringing it down when it's too high and up when it's too low, and it doesn't denature fat cells. As with the other problematic foods, toxic salts and their residue start to leave the liver immediately when you're tending to it. They can exit the liver altogether within 90 days.

- **Gluten:** Feeds pathogens inside the liver. This is another troublemaker you can remove from the liver completely within 90 days.

- **Corn:** Another fuel for pathogens in the liver that can leave the liver in 90 days of caring for it.

- **Canola oil:** Contains undiscovered chemical compounds that are harsh to the liver, causing liver cell weakness. Takes six months to rid.

- **Pork products:** Their higher fat content and specific variety of fat slow down liver functions, which speeds up fat cell collection and weakens the liver's immune system. How long it takes to completely leave the liver depends on how much pork was consumed over a lifetime and how much pork fat has collected in the liver.

Pathogenic Group

This is the troublemakers group that's responsible for the misunderstanding of auto-immune disease. Pathogens are at the top of the food chain—they're the sharks of the liver, eating all the poisons in their path—so the key to getting rid of them is eliminating their fuel sources. When you take their food away, they either starve or leave the liver to eventually exit the body. Cleansing pathogenic fuel and waste

matter also makes room for the liver's immune system to go after pathogens, because these other troublemakers confuse it. Lifting that fog allows the liver's immune system to really identify, tag, and hunt down these pathogenic invaders. When you're working on your liver, viral toxins start leaving immediately and continue to cleanse out as you're doing what you need to do. The amount of time it takes to free the liver of pathogenic infection depends on how aggressive the pathogen is and how long it's been in the liver, what kind of supplements you take, and how regularly you follow that supplement protocol (see the next chapter for a suggested list). In addition to supplements, focus on taking away the fuel from these pathogens so they starve over time.

- **Viruses and viral waste matter:** Leading the way among troublemaking viruses is EBV with its over 60 varieties. EBV's viral waste (neurotoxins, dermatoxins, byproduct, and viral corpses) is toxic, too; these are the poisons responsible for hundreds of symptoms and conditions, ranging from fatigue to rashes to aches and pains to floaters in the eyes to tingles and numbness. Other viruses that make trouble for the liver include HHV-6 all the way up through the undiscovered HHV-9, HHV-10, HHV-11, HHV-12, HHV-13, HHV-14, HHV-15, and HHV-16; cytomegalovirus; and the over 30 varieties of shingles. To tame any viral presence in your liver, avoid the viral triggers you can read about in *Medical Medium* and *Thyroid Healing* (many of which overlap with the other troublemakers you'll find in this list) and keep your eye out for antivirals mentioned in the next chapter to help you with viruses and viral waste matter, which can end up in all three levels of the liver.

- **Bacteria:** *Streptococcus*, *E. coli*, *C. difficile*, *Staphylococcus*, and *Salmonella* are a few of the more common bacteria that can cause trouble for the liver, and you've especially read a lot about strep in earlier chapters. What you won't see in this list are the bacteria associated with Lyme disease—if you're interested in that topic, refer to *Medical Medium*. Bacteria go to all three levels of the liver.

- **Food-borne toxins:** We take great care to avoid coming down with trichinosis and food poisoning. The thousands of microorganisms, many of them uncatalogued and highly toxic, that live in raw fish, poultry, meat, and eggs (commonly on the outside of the shells) are usually killed off with proper cooking methods. What people don't realize is that once these living pathogens are killed, they don't just disappear. They become toxins. For example, when we cook a piece of chicken, we're concerned about killing off the *Salmonella*. We don't think about how the dead *Salmonella* could still cause harm. Most of the time, people don't feel the effects of these toxins because the liver

deals with them. They do build up, though, and in some cases can cause horrendous, acute sickness. These troublemakers tend to settle in the subsurface of the liver.

- **Mold:** If someone is exposed to toxic mold, whether inhaling it or eating it, it finds its way to the liver by way of the lungs or intestinal tract. There are different varieties of mold toxins, some more aggressive than others. Overall, mold is a *trigger* in that it lowers the liver's immune system (and other parts of the body's immune system), in some cases allowing a viral explosion to occur. It's not a *cause* of disease, even though illness is often blamed on mold. As *Thyroid Healing* examines, many different symptoms that are truly viral get blamed on mold, yet mold itself is not the problem. That's why one person can be exposed to mold and exhibit no symptoms while for another person, it's a potent trigger—the difference is whether or not someone has an underlying viral issue poised to wreak havoc. Mold mainly goes to the liver's subsurface level. While some mold cleanses immediately and the rest could take anywhere from three to six months, you could get rid of all the mold and still be dealing with symptoms, because they're really viral. They could stick around for another year or so as your body sends the virus packing and starts to recover.

Chemical Industry Domestic Invasion Group

When you make a choice for your own life, that's up to you. What's not right is when others' choices affect your life without your say-so. Smoking used to be a prime example of one person's choice affecting scores of others. With smoking now banned from many public buildings, that's gotten much better; you don't have to be subjected to cigarette smoke's toxins in the way you once did. With the troublemakers in this list, you don't get the same freedom. Unlike asking a friend to stub out a cigarette, you can't ask the person next to you on the train to wash off their perfume. You can't ask the dentist's office to extract the years of air freshener chemicals out of its walls. You can't ask the plane where you're about to spend six hours to purify its air for you. We live with these domestic invaders all around us, and what we can at least do to protect ourselves is limit their use in our own lives—and work on cleansing them. When you begin rescuing your liver, these troublemakers start leaving the liver within a week, and you could expel most of them within three to six months.

- **Plug-in air fresheners and scented candles:** Even if you don't use these in your own home, it doesn't mean you're not exposed in stores, doctors' offices, public restrooms, or friends' homes. Even if you find their smells pleasant, you can be guaranteed that your liver has a clothespin on its nose. When we inhale the scented, heated oil from these seemingly innocent units in the wall or the chemically saturated wax from fragranced candles, their chemicals end up in the surface and subsurface levels of our livers.

- **Aerosol can air fresheners:** Exposure to these comes from the same sources as above, and they can also settle in our livers' surface and subsurface levels.

- **Spray-bottle air fresheners and mists:** Commonly used to spray and deodorize furniture, these find their way to the surface and subsurface levels of the liver.

- **Cologne and aftershave:** Even if you avoid direct skin exposure by not using them, it's still possible to get inhalation exposure when you're close to someone wearing them. They end up in the surface and subsurface levels of the liver.

- **Perfumes and conventionally scented body lotions, creams, sprays, washes, shampoos, conditioners, gels, and other hair products:** Be careful what you purchase in the toiletry aisle. In your quest to smell fresh and clean, you could be washing yourself down with chemicals that will burden your liver by landing themselves in its surface and subsurface levels.

- **Hairspray:** While hairspray isn't as popular for everyday use as it once was, if you covered your hair with it back in the day, the chemicals that you breathed in and absorbed into your skin could still reside in your liver. As you've read, it's a myth that your cells completely renew every seven years. Though liver cells do replace themselves over time, old cells can contaminate new ones, which is how your liver could still be holding on to ancient hairspray. It tends to settle in the surface and subsurface levels of the liver.

- **Hair dye:** There's conventional hair dye and there's nonconventional hair dye. Whenever you can, opt for the more natural version; even though it can still have a toxic effect, it's much better. If you feel it doesn't "take" quite right, apply it twice to get the color. Conventional hair dye is very hard on the liver. This alone can be a trigger for perimenopause, menopause, and postmenopause symptoms. Usually around the time of this change, women are coloring their hair and using the most conventional, toxic dyes ever to cover their grays. They end up at the doctor, being told they have hormonal problems, when the problem was really the hair dye getting into their livers—hair dye seeps into your skin and bloodstream and travels directly down into the liver. For a woman who starts coloring her hair in her late 30s, it's the ultimate trigger for a perimenopause diagnosis, with no one realizing the truth: that hair dye chemicals are feeding EBV in her liver. Conventional hair dye goes to all three levels of the liver.

- **Talcum powder:** While it's easy to think of this one just on the skin, it's a fine dust that also gets

into the lungs and the intestinal tract by way of the mouth—when you pat talcum powder on your body, you're inhaling it and eating it at the same time. It finds its way to your liver, where it's toxic, settling in the subsurface and surface levels.

- **Conventional makeup:** If you're not used to reading the small print on cosmetics, the ingredients in some would shock you. The makeup industry also has secret proprietary blends and recipes that they don't include on the ingredients list—concoctions that they hide from the consumer—because revealing them would mean divulging them to the competition. That's been the case for over a century. The chemicals and even heavy metals in items like foundation can soak into your skin, and you end up ingesting a certain portion of whatever lipstick, lip gloss, or powders you use. Luckily, cosmetic companies came to realize lead wasn't safe along the way; it was a staple in cosmetics of yesteryear. Aluminum and copper, though, are still going strong as ingredients today. Makeup components find their way to the liver's surface and subsurface levels.

- **Spray tan:** When this covers every inch of the body, it can cause a particularly toxic situation for the liver; it actually suffocates the organ because the skin can't cleanse, and the skin is part of the liver's relief when getting rid of poisons. Spray tan itself goes to the subsurface of the liver. Since it prevents the skin's release of toxins, though, the application of spray tan makes it so that the deep, inner core of the liver gets oversaturated by other troublemakers that aren't able to get out through the skin.

- Nail chemicals: Nail polish, remover, and adhesive are notorious for their fumes, which is part of what makes them troublemakers. Nail polish contains paint thinner to keep it from hardening when it touches your skin—and it's very common to get nail polish on the cuticles and the skin next to the nails. Polish remover ends up all over the finger, which gives it a chance to soak into skin and get into the system. These chemicals end up in the liver's subsurface level and deep, inner core.

- Conventional cleaners: These traditional cleaning solutions, used in household, office, and industrial settings alike, contain ingredients that can burden the liver both when breathed in and when the skin absorbs them. This includes countertop sprays, all-purpose solutions, waxes, floor scrubs, and window cleaner. If you're not the one applying them, it doesn't mean you're free. Spending time in any area where they're used, though less potent when you're

not the one applying them, is still exposure. These settle in the liver's subsurface level and deep, inner core.

- Conventional laundry detergent, fabric softener, and dryer sheets: These products enter the lungs and skin easily and from there go straight into the bloodstream and find their way to the liver. Many conventional laundry products are created from petrochemicals. While they may seem clean, your liver feels dirty afterward; they leave a gift of toxicity behind. These troublemakers tend to stay in the surface and subsurface level of the liver. Depending on the brand and design of the chemical, it could find its way to the deep, inner core.

- Dry-cleaning chemicals: These end up in the lungs, especially when you've just picked them up from the cleaner's, as well as on the skin. It's expensive all around—dry-clean-only clothes usually have a high price tag, plus you pay the fee to have them laundered, and at the same time, your liver pays a high price. These chemicals usually end up in the subsurface and deep, inner core of the liver.

Pharmaceuticals Group

As I mentioned earlier in this book, some medications for certain circumstances can be lifesaving. There are times when they are truly necessary. The opposite occurs with many medications as well, with life-threatening situations arising. When we're not given answers from medical communities about how to heal chronic illness, then our illnesses can go on far too long, neglected due to lack of information from medical research and science, and we may find ourselves using medications to try to suppress symptoms. What we need to be is aware: aware that excessive use can burden the liver, aware that different prescriptions provided by different doctors who aren't all on the same page (or different self-prescribed over-the-counter medications) can create a cocktail your liver doesn't like, and aware that even without taking a single medication in your life, you can end up with them in your system. (When people who *are* on medications eliminate them, those pharmaceuticals end up in the water supply.) Once you've started to care for your liver, these can start coming out of the liver immediately. The total amount of time it takes depends on the pharmaceutical and how much you consumed over the years. It can take up to two years for the majority, provided you're not still using them—although if you are actively taking a medication, I respect that. It doesn't mean you can't work on healing your liver. There's so much poison that the liver has to work on ridding from so many sources; working on that, as well as working on feeding your liver so it can do what it needs to do, will help your liver be able to handle the pharmaceuticals you have to take.

- **Antibiotics:** Among other applications, prescribed regularly for cold and flu, childhood ear infections, sore throats, coughs, UTIs, acne, and also for sufferers of chronic illnesses such as Lyme disease. You could have been on antibiotics so early in life that you don't even remember. These troublemakers, which contain petroleum, tend to go to the liver's subsurface level and deep, inner core.

- **Antidepressants:** If you've been on one or more of these, you know it. They settle in the subsurface level and deep, inner core of the liver.

- **Anti-inflammatories:** Commonly taken by sufferers of injuries and chronic pain. They spread out among all three of the liver's levels.

- **Sleeping pills:** Medications for insomnia settle in the subsurface level of the liver.

- **Biologics:** These immune system suppressors commonly prescribed to sufferers of chronic illnesses such as MS and intestinal disorders such as Crohn's and colitis go to all three levels of the liver.

- **Regular immunosuppressants:** Often given to MS and other chronic illness patients, they go to all three levels of the liver.

- **Prescription amphetamines:** Prescribed for conditions such as ADHD and other focus and concentration issues as well as low energy. They settle in all three of the liver's levels.

- **Opioids:** Given to chronic pain sufferers, these drugs dive down to the liver's deep, inner core.

- **Statins:** Commonly taken for high cholesterol, when the irony is that cholesterol problems derive from the liver and statins worsen the liver's condition, elevating cholesterol even more, although the medication hides this. Statins easily hit the liver's deep, inner core and are highly toxic to the area.

- **Blood pressure medications:** You know if you've been on these. They stay in the subsurface level of the liver.

- **Hormone medications:** These include both conventional and bioidentical hormone therapy, human growth hormones, and human chorionic gonadotropin (HCG) diets. They go to the surface and subsurface levels of the liver.

- **Thyroid medications:** You'll know if you've been on these medications, though you may not know that they are not actually targeted to heal the thyroid or address the underlying thyroid condition and are instead another form of hormone medication. (More in *Thyroid Healing*.) Some of the top prescribed medications out there, these also go to the surface and subsurface levels of the liver.

- **Steroids:** Often prescribed for mystery symptoms and illnesses as well as following surgery and dental work, they go to all three levels of the liver.

- **The Pill:** Causing liver problems more often in women at younger and younger ages, this one lands them very early perimenopause or other hormonal diagnoses because it makes the liver so toxic so soon. One way it causes trouble is by restricting and atrophying blood vessels in the liver. This goes to the deep, inner core.

- **Alcohol:** This doesn't just apply to the alcohol in a bottle for recreational drinking. Alcohol is in virtually all toiletries, including hair care and skin care products and cosmetics. It's also manipulated in the pharmaceutical world and added to many over-the-counter and prescription medications, and not just the liquids; in dry medicines, it's often there in altered, dehydrated form. Alcohol is extremely hard on the liver, causing it to become sluggish and stagnant and injuring liver cells. It slows down the liver's ability to run its over 2,000 chemical functions for the body and makes liver lobule elves drunk so that Santa's helpers can't make toys. (Don't let this stop you from using hand sanitizer with alcohol in it. Killing off the flu virus or strep from a public bathroom or other germy spot outweighs what your liver's going to receive from that sanitizing wipe.) Alcohol saturates all three levels of the liver. Within 90 days of looking after your liver, you can get out all the alcohol residue.

- **Recreational drug abuse:** One of the few differences between recreational drugs and hardcore, more aggressive pharmaceuticals is that with these drugs, there are no prescribed dosages. You won't hear a dealer say, "Only do a half a gram every other day for a week." While you would think that quality control is far superior with pharmaceuticals synthesized in labs and that the dangerous, harmful chemicals from homemade street drugs make them a completely different beast, it's not that simple. No one knows how many mistakes are made in medication production. The reason drugs' impact on the liver is so much more severe goes back to dosages—there are no standards or regulations to keep them under control. Drugs go to the subsurface and deep, inner core of the liver.

Toxic Heavy Metals Group

Like the Chemical Neuroantagonists Group, toxic heavy metals spread out among all three levels of the liver and are also commonly passed down through the bloodline from generation to generation. In addition to the ones from yesteryear that we're born with (which, as you read about in Chapter 28, is how babies' livers can already be burdened), we get exposed to toxic heavy metals throughout life. Here's just a small

sampling of sources, some of them liver troublemakers in their own right: pharmaceuticals; city water; jet fuel falling from the sky; water pipes; restaurant food prepared with heavy scraping of metal pots, pans, and tools; nanosprays applied to manufactured items; and pesticides, herbicides, and fungicides. Find more below. When it comes to avoiding toxic heavy metals, question everything that's offered to you, including medical treatments. These troublemakers can start to leave your liver in your first week of caring for it. If you regularly apply the Medical Medium heavy metal detox described at the end of Chapter 38, you can get deeper layers of toxic heavy metals out of the liver within a year or two. This detox method is devised to kick metal out of the liver, among other spots in the body, in a way that your system can handle, so that they get eliminated, not recirculated. The Liver Rescue 3:6:9 also gets heavy metals out of the liver so they can't get reabsorbed. Plus it makes getting heavy metals out afterward much easier. These are responsible methods for getting heavy metals out of the body so a sensitive person does not react, unlike with other so-called heavy metal supplements, cleanses, and techniques out there.

- **Mercury:** Among other sources, we can get exposed when handling batteries in devices; getting metal amalgam dental fillings (or getting them removed); encountering pesticides, herbicides, and fungicides; eating fish; taking fish oil supplements (even the high-quality ones that claim to be mercury-free); and when spending time in lakes and other water sources. It's also the toxic heavy metal that's most easily passed down through generations, so the mercury in your liver could be truly ancient.

- **Lead:** Handling lead pencils as a child; getting exposed to lead paint (whether currently, when trying to remove it, or in the past, when it was fresh); using water that's flowed through lead pipes in old buildings or, in newer homes, pipes with lead sealers; and encountering pesticides, herbicides, and fungicides are a few of the ways you can end up with lead in your system. Also beware of growing a vegetable garden close to a house where lead paint was used on the exterior. The surrounding soil could now be saturated, and you could end up with lead-marinated vegetables.

- **Aluminum:** We come into contact with this one all the time, from cans to foil to takeout containers to kitchen tools to makeup to tap water to sunblock to pesticides, herbicides, and fungicides.

- **Copper:** The liver is really highly sensitive to copper. Since this metal is commonly used for pipes, copper particles can end up in our drinking and bathing water, plus it's frequently in pesticides, herbicides, and fungicides. There's a new trend of copper everything in the kitchen; try to be cautious about pots and pans and go with ceramic whenever you can; your liver will thank you.

- **Cadmium:** This one is in the air, falling from the sky, so it gets into our systems when we inhale it. It's in pesticides, herbicides, and fungicides, too.

- **Barium:** Another troublemaker we inhale when it falls from the sky. It also lands on our skin, plus it's in the water supply, so we ingest it. Often used in medical imaging treatments.

- **Nickel:** An ingredient in pesticides, herbicides, and fungicides.

- **Arsenic:** Another component of pesticides, herbicides, and fungicides.

Radiation

Your liver sponges up radiation you're exposed to from plane flights, X-rays, MRIs, CT scans, cell phones, food and water, and the continual atmospheric fallout from past nuclear disasters. Even if you haven't gotten an X-ray in your entire life, it doesn't mean your mom or dad didn't get one before you were conceived. That radiation is inherited and doesn't go away unless you work on getting rid of it mindfully. You can also absorb radiation from being near someone who just got an X-ray. It goes to all three levels of the liver. Within the first three to four weeks of looking after your liver, radiation particles can start to release. For the more penetrating radiation, it requires the right supplements and seaweeds as well as the heavy metal smoothie from *Thyroid Healing*, which is also a radiation yanker. It takes some time to get radiation cleaned up, usually about one to three years altogether. It could take longer, depending on your exposure.

Excess Adrenaline

- **Prolonged overabundance of adrenal stress:** Oversaturation with adrenal hormones can overload the liver's ability to perform its everyday responsibilities. It also provides extra fuel for viruses such as EBV as well as bacteria. When the liver is able to neutralize adrenaline, it stores it in its subsurface level. When the liver is forced to store caustic adrenaline because it is too overburdened for neutralization, it stores it in all three levels and usually takes one to three weeks to cleanse when you're working on it.

- **Adrenaline-based activities:** Bungee jumping, rollercoasters, sex, skydiving, surfing in large waves, snowboarding, BMX riding, car racing, and cliff climbing are a few examples of adrenaline-rush activities. They're better than being on drugs; adrenaline sports are big achievements. If you're engaging in them, you also want to make sure you're taking care of your liver, just like you make sure your bungee cord is maintained and your parachute packed just right. Instead, someone usually celebrates a successful jump from a plane or a win at the track with a good ale, giving the liver even

more to do. Not much of the corrosive adrenaline from one of these high-intensity activities can get neutralized, because it comes at the liver in such a rush. It usually saturates all three layers of the liver, the same way a sponge gets soaked when you sop up a spill, and takes one to three weeks to leave again when you're caring for your liver.

Rainfall Exposure

Rain is not clean like it once was. Rainfall is filled with toxins from the sky and air, from radioactive particles to barium to jet fuel to dust particles blowing off agricultural land, both domestically and from other countries, that contain residue of pesticides, herbicides, and fungicides. It's also filled with a tremendous amount of vaporized material that spews from chemical factories globally. These chemicals are not documented by any agency; they're rogue byproducts that fill the atmosphere by the hundreds of thousands. All of these toxins come down in the rain, and if it gets on us, our skin instantly absorbs it and the chemicals find their way to our livers, settling in the subsurface level.

This is where we should herald our livers as practically God for what they see and catalogue and understand about these thousands of different vaporized chemical agents in their most homeopathic, minute form. What the liver witnesses is beyond all of research and science's grasp and imagination. I'm not talking about acid rain here—that term doesn't even scratch the surface as far as what's actually in rain. There isn't a lab on the planet that can catalogue the contaminants in a raindrop. People who are sensitive, whether with neurological symptoms such as fatigue and joint pain or with chronic issues such as sinus problems, will tend to worsen for a couple of days after being soaked in rain.

I'm not trying to scare you here. Luckily, our livers are masters at cleaning up rain toxicity. The liver should get the Nobel Peace Prize for identifying and handling it. Enjoy your walks in the rain—and take care of your liver so that you *can* enjoy them. Past rainfall chemical exposure can leave the liver 100 percent within two weeks if you're taking all the right measures. Then the next time you get hit with rain, any toxicity from it can leave your liver within three days. This is partly because rainfall is active, living water with healing properties within it, which the liver can extract and use immediately. That living water codes and defuses any chemicals it contains to make them easier for the liver to work with.

———— CHAPTER 37 ————

Powerful Foods, Herbs, and Supplements for Your Liver

We've come a long way in how we think about our food. Today, we're more mindful than ever of junk food and additives and agricultural practices. We want to feed our families the best, so some parents who love animal products won't feed their children anything less than grass-fed or pasture-raised or free-range, and some parents who are plant-based won't feed their children anything less than organic produce. Now it's time to start thinking of our livers as part of the family. They need to eat, too, and they deserve the best liver fuel there is.

Our livers have the potential to come back from sluggishness and illness with tremendous power. When we see them for what they are—living, working organs—we get insight into how feeding them, and feeding them right, is the key to making the healing happen.

How does the liver eat? It has a lot to do with those little "elves," the liver lobules. Like us, they need fuel to do their jobs. If you'll recall from Part I, "Your Liver's True Calling," the liver is one of the busiest organs in the human body because it has a highway of blood running through it. Blood brings with it vitamins,

minerals, other nutrients and building blocks of our food, hormones, oxygen, and troublemakers such as prescription and recreational drugs; pesticides, herbicides, and fungicides; aluminum, lead, copper, mercury, and other toxic heavy metals; and disease-causing pathogens such as viruses and bacteria. The liver must be masterful at sorting the bad from the good, the poisons from the nutrients. The elves in the toy workshop, the liver lobules, are what do it. Because the highway of blood moves to the heart next, their task of deciphering what's useful, nonuseful, or even detrimental is particularly vital, so they can make sure to send only gifts—and no lumps of coal—to the precious heart.

There's also the liver's storage of helpful and harmful materials. As the helpful materials such as nutrients, hormones, biochemical agents, and chemical compounds are called for, the liver's intelligent system brilliantly dilutes, measures, balances, and releases just the right amounts of these items into the bloodstream. Then there are the harmful materials, the makeshift storage of which we addressed in Chapter 5, "Your Protective Liver," and in the previous chapter. To protect you, your liver tries to bury the most worrisome items in deeper pockets.

All of this work makes the liver hungry. In order to guard the doorways of the liver (blood vessels in and out), sort everything, strategically store the good, and drive the bad deep, the liver's cells, including the lobule elves, need to be fed. They need a breakfast time, a lunchtime, a dinnertime, and breaks with snacks, like a chance to eat a coffee and a doughnut—only the elves aren't asking for coffee and doughnuts. As I mentioned in Chapter 3, "Your Life-Giving Liver," your liver's most important requirements are oxygen, then water, then sugar, then mineral salts. Glucose—sugar—is the liver's fuel, along with the precious vitamins, minerals, antioxidants, and other nutrients that are delivered to the liver with the sugars from fruits and vegetables. The liver will only use nutrients that are surrounded by natural glucose and fructose. If someone's on a diet with no sugar, no carbohydrates, no sweet potato, no squash, no fruit whatsoever, the liver will slowly starve and the person will age rapidly. That's because the liver requires sugar to identify and hold on to the nutrients it needs to restore itself; it won't take them if they're not attached to food—sugar—for the elves. If the liver sees a nutrient come in that's not bonded to sugar, it won't draw in the nutrient; it will just let it roll on by in the bloodstream until it exits the organ. Natural sugar also keeps the liver's engine cool, which is vital, since it's the organ that runs hottest.

With the high-fat trend, people think that your liver needs fat to help break down fat. This is a massive blunder, taking the truth that your liver is responsible for breaking down fat and twisting that into the thought that your liver loves fat. It's almost like the trend-makers of today are experiencing depersonalization to what's happening in the body. Or it's like knowing someone you've worked with for years, hearing stories about their situation in life and passions and dreams, and never really listening to them or knowing who they are. If you did listen, you'd realize that asking them for a particular favor touched on one of their greatest injuries from over the years. Instead, you were just hearing the sounds of their words while thinking your own thoughts—and that's what's happening with the diets of today and how they treat the liver. You live with your body, pretend to understand, think you understand, assume you understand, and you're never actually taught how to listen or take the time to figure out what it needs. "If the liver breaks down fats, let's give it all the fat we can," the reasoning goes. The truth is that the liver's not hungry for fat calories. It's hungry for the right kind of sugar calories. It uses sugar to fuel itself to be able to produce bile to break down fat.

It takes the right balance in someone's blood to keep the liver fed properly so it can perform its adaptogenic bile functions and sorting and filtering process, as well as fulfill every other function, including storage and neutralization. Too much fat in the bloodstream is one element that can throw off the balance; it can create insulin resistance (which prevents cells' proper absorption of glucose), lower oxygen levels in the blood, and dehydrate the blood, which collectively deprives the liver of three of its critical requirements: glucose, oxygen, and water. I don't mean to scare you away from fats entirely. Some fats are healthy and great for you. As we've covered in this book, though, most people are unknowingly eating fats in excess.

Simply try knocking back your fat intake by 25 percent. If you're eating two avocados a day, get rid of one and bring in more spinach, tomatoes, oranges, mangoes, or potatoes in its place. If you're eating two servings of chicken a day, cut out one and replace it with roasted sweet potato. If you're eating two servings of olive oil or coconut oil daily, try cutting that in half and using lemon juice in place of one oil serving. If you're making a dressing with a half cup of cashews, try cutting it back to a quarter cup and blending in a quarter cup of celery to make up for it, or if you like to eat nuts out of hand, try replacing half with winter squash. Whatever the radical fat, whether plant-based or animal protein, such as meat, try to replace some of it with the healing foods in this chapter. By making these sorts of adjustments throughout the day, you can cut down your total radical fats by roughly a quarter. It doesn't have to be perfect. Another option is if you want to have a day where you indulge in the quantities of fats that your heart desires, you can do some fat-free days to make up for it. The Liver Rescue 3:6:9 and the recipes chapter will give you meal and snack ideas for getting through a day without radical fats. Either of these options—curbing a day's fat intake by 25 percent or giving your liver some fat-free days—will get you moving forward.

Alcohol is another imbalancer. Long before you feel its effects, it starts to get the liver lobules tipsy as it enters through the portal vein, and drunk elves can't do their jobs right. When someone drinks, it hinders the liver's ability to acknowledge, decipher, extract, and retain the vitamins, minerals, and other helpful materials that are also coming in through the blood. They end up bypassing the areas where they're needed. It also slows down the liver's ability to manage its over 2,000 chemical functions. It's like the power going out on a plane.

What can help a lot with balance is grazing. While your liver can store glucose and, in addition to feeding other organs with it, feed itself when needed, it requires as much glucose support as it can get. Especially when you're still building your liver back up, it's not going to

be in top shape to hop in with sugar supplies every time your blood sugar drops. Instead, your adrenals are going to step in to fill the gap. Since you want to save your adrenals from burnout and save the rest of your body from excess adrenaline, eating something every hour and a half to two hours is a really useful way to support both your liver and your adrenal glands. If you like your normal three meals a day, that's fine; just supplement with snacks in between.

And what about the best foods, herbs, and supplements to bring balance to your bloodstream and healing to your liver? Well, that is what the rest of this chapter is all about. Variously, the items you're about to read about help cleanse and oxygenate the blood; hydrate the blood with living water to expel, dissolve, and disperse fats and toxins from inside the liver; deliver critical natural sugars like glucose and fructose to the liver; and provide the blood with the highest-quality mineral salts around. And they do more: they're brimming with antioxidants to help restore liver cells, vitamins to feed your liver's immune system so it can kill off viruses and bacteria, minerals for the liver's critical chemical functions, and undiscovered phytochemical compounds that transfer information to your liver so it can strengthen and rise above the polluted environment in which we keep it. They're the most powerful way to feed your liver and bring it to a level of health you didn't know was possible.

HEALING FOODS

- **Apples:** Provide living water to support the liver's hydration capabilities, so it can store the water and then release it back into the bloodstream when dehydration or dirty blood syndrome occurs. The fruit acids in apples help cleanse the liver by dispersing toxic films that build up inside its storage banks. Apples starve out bacteria, yeast, mold, other funguses, and viruses from the intestinal tract and liver. Great for dissolving gallstones.

- **Apricots:** Offer easily assimilable vitamin A that does not overload the liver and instead protects it from cell damage. Also offer beneficial copper that can help bond to toxic coppers inside the liver and carry them out, a like-versus-like capability in your favor. Rich in antioxidants, many of them still undiscovered, apricots are medicine to your liver cells. Help prevent aging.

- **Artichokes:** Contain phytochemical compounds that stop the growth of tumors and cysts inside the liver. The liver relies on other chemical compounds found in artichokes for many of its own chemical functions—they work hand in hand to keep the liver's neutralization, screening, and filtering abilities strong.

- **Arugula:** Causes a gentle purging effect inside the liver, with undiscovered phytochemical compounds that allow the liver to decide the severity of the cleanse and what toxins it safely wants to release (versus a purge that would harm the liver).

- **Asparagus:** Provide a wealth of flavonoids, many of them undiscovered or unstudied, that are highly anti-inflammatory; they act as natural aspirin and soothe a hot, overburdened, struggling liver. The liver's ability to cleanse increases greatly from this calming effect. Asparagus brings order to a chaotic, sick liver. The liver's immune system strengthens instantly from asparagus. It increases bile production yet doesn't allow the liver to overwork itself in producing bile. Helps dislodge fat cells, expelling them from the liver. Helps rejuvenate the liver's deep, inner core. Asparagus is one of the most important liver-healing foods. Consider putting it on the menu at least a few times a week.

- **Atlantic sea vegetables (especially dulse and kelp):** Contain mineral salts that are pleasing to the liver and on which the liver depends. A very important one is iodine, a natural antiseptic to the liver that inhibits unproductive bacteria, viruses, and other unwanted microorganisms that can find their way to the liver and cause cell damage. Iodine at the proper level inside the liver can help prevent cancer and all manners of disease that occur within the liver and body. Atlantic sea vegetables strengthen bile salts as well, so that the liver's bile production is more potent (versus a large production of bile that may not be too potent).

- **Bananas:** The fructose in banana is liver's favorite source of food. It provides quick fuel to the liver and wakes up sleepy cells, increasing their ingenuity and work output. Soothes the linings of the intestinal tract and also soothes the nerves attached to the intestinal tract. Contrary to popular belief, bananas are one of the most antibacterial, anti-yeast, antifungal foods. A great food to combine with other nutrient-rich foods or to take with supplements, because they improve the liver's ability to absorb nutrients.

- **Berries:** A medicine chest for the liver. Loaded with antioxidants to keep a variety of liver cells, including hepatocytes and Kupffer cells, as well as liver lobules and capillaries, from becoming infected and affected by toxins and pathogens. Berries protect the liver from troublemakers causing damage; the many undiscovered antioxidants they contain help shield liver cells from harm. All berries, including raspberries, blackberries, and blueberries, stop the liver from oxidizing too easily when saturated with toxic heavy metals and poisons.

- **Broccoli:** The "trunks" of broccoli are rich in sulfur compounds, which are not researched to the extent needed—they're more

important than we realize. These phytochemical sulfur compounds act as harmful gas to unfriendly bacteria and other microorganisms inside the intestinal tract and also travel straight to the liver, where they saturate liver tissue, allowing the liver's immune system to have a fighting chance at controlling pathogens.

- **Brussels sprouts:** An ultimate liver-cleansing food, providing a vast array of chemical compounds and phytonutrients. The sulfur compounds found specifically in brussels sprouts are different from those in any other food in the cruciferous (that is, *Brassica*) family, as they're derived from the large mother stalk upon which the little baby brussels sprouts grow. This is some of the most powerful, beneficial sulfur for the liver; it has the ability to loosen hardened prison cells of poisons and inherited troublemaker toxins, because it has a greater reach for toxins that have been in your family line for generations, if not centuries. Once it loosens up the cell prisons, old poisons come out, though they don't go rogue. Brussels sprouts' sulfur has an ability unlike any other to cling to each poison and safely escort it out of the liver, whether through the kidneys, bile duct, or intestinal tract, staying bonded all the way until the troublemaker leaves the body. It's a food rarity.

- **Carrots:** A quick liver refueling source of glucose that's attached to minerals and vitamins. When carrots are eaten raw, they're higher in antiseptic phytochemical compounds that inhibit the growth of unfriendly microorganisms.

- **Celery:** Its undiscovered subgroups of sodium that I call *cluster salts* protect the liver's cell membranes and inhibit the growth of viruses, bacteria, and fungus. Celery restores the liver's bile production capability as well as the potency and complicated structure of the bile, which in most people is completely imbalanced. Its cluster salts bind onto free-floating poisons and toxins inside the liver and flush them into the bloodstream, remaining bonded so that the troublemakers leave the kidneys or intestinal tract safely. Celery purges the liver while bringing down liver heat to a safe level. It's the ultimate gallbladder rehabilitator, helping to dissolve gallstones over time, making them small enough either not to cause harm or to be able to pass through the bile duct. Celery's sodium also expands the bile duct so it's not restricted, in case a large stone does breach. Removes mucus out of the intestinal tract and liver and increases production of the undiscovered seven-acid blend of hydrochloric acid in the stomach. Disperses fat cells inside the liver. Without realizing it, we

get celery from different regions and different farms, even when we buy it from the same store. This is beneficial because different earth affects the mineral salt composition of celery grown in it, so we end up getting a variety of sodium compositions that help our immune systems. (Not that you should worry if you've eaten celery from the same farm your entire life. The soil has still changed over time, giving you variety over time.) Celery is a powerful herb we should never forget.

- **Cherries:** High in anthocyanins that bond to specific troublemakers from the petrochemical group that store deep inside our livers. Cherries' red color pigment acts as a degreaser, dispersing these sticky, gluey toxins and allowing them to gravitate out of the liver and into the gallbladder. The anthocyanins prevent the toxins from being reabsorbed back into the liver, and the rich fiber from the cherry fruit helps rush the poisons out of the small intestine and colon.

- **Cilantro:** Not only does this herb bind onto toxic heavy metals; its undiscovered phytochemical compounds also cling to other troublemakers—such as neurotoxins and dermatoxins that commonly end up inside our livers—and then expel them safely from our bodies. Cilantro is both a great liver cleansing and liver building herb. It helps regenerate nerve tissue in and around the liver—precious nerve tissue that sends messages from our brains to communicate with our livers.

- **Coconut:** Very helpful in lowering viral and bacterial loads inside your liver and lymphatic system—though only when it's used in small amounts. Too much coconut, including coconut oil, can slow down the liver, delaying its responses and rendering it incapable of performing its duties. That's true of any plant fats. While they have benefits, overdoing them takes away from what they have to offer.

- **Cranberries:** The anthocyanin in cranberries is multifaceted, as it does more than one job for your liver. Not only does it prevent oxidation in cells; it helps prevent cells from dying in general of toxic overload. It also removes and breaks free a variety of troublemakers, including those inherited from long past in the family line. The harsh fruit acid in cranberries that causes the mouth to pucker strips the cell membranes off pathogens, most especially bacteria. The vitamin C in cranberries holds similarities to the rare vitamin C in tomatoes in that it increases the liver's immune system strength.

- **Cruciferous vegetables:** These members of the *Brassica* family are always great for your liver;

they provide an abundance of vitamins, minerals, antioxidants, and rich phytochemical sulfur compounds that help the liver restore its nutrient storage banks. Cruciferous vegetables also help the liver convert nutrients, making them more bioavailable as they're released into the bloodstream to be delivered to other organs in your body. Some of the best crucifers to bring into your life are kale, radishes, arugula, brussels sprouts, red cabbage, broccoli, cauliflower, watercress, kohlrabi, collard greens, broccoli rabe, and mustard greens. You can read more about the first six throughout these pages.

- **Cucumbers:** Allies to the liver due to their ability to hydrate it. Your liver's always in need of living water that's filled with minerals and other nutrients, because your liver keeps your blood hydrated. It relies on sources such as cucumber for that living water. This minimizes dirty blood syndrome by helping reduce fats and toxins inside of dirty blood. Phytochemical compounds in cucumbers act as anti-inflammatories to the small intestines and colon. Cucumbers have a gentle blood-thinning ability, too, allowing for detox to occur naturally, without obstruction.

- **Dandelion greens:** The liver is practically a sponge, and if the right phytochemical compound approaches it, such as the bitter compounds of dandelion greens and stems, a purging effect occurs where the liver squeezes in reaction and loosens up prison cells filled with toxic debris. That bitterness also activates healthy histamines that encapsulate the freed poisons and pull them out of your body so you can detox. This can end up reducing liver spasms and increasing both bile production and potency. Never underestimate dandelion as one of the most beneficial liver-cleansing foods.

- **Dates:** The intestinal tract builds up mucus due to low hydrochloric acid and bile production, and that can slow down absorption of nutrients into the bloodstream. Dates expel and eliminate mucus, especially that produced by pathogens such as bacteria and fungus, from the colon. The sugars in dates feed the liver; they're a great source of glucose for recovery and restoration that allows the liver to maximize its over 2,000 chemical functions.

- **Eggplant:** Often shunned due to confused belief systems about nightshades, eggplant is more worthy than we are led to believe. It can help us more than anyone knows; the only reason it's avoided is because we don't understand it. In truth, eggplant has small quantities of an undiscovered astringent

phytochemical that improves blood flow to the liver, allows oxygen to be maximized inside the liver, and helps prevent all manner of disease. Eggplant also has phytochemical compounds that bind onto vitamin C, making it more bioavailable to the liver and the liver's personalized immune system. Eggplant thins out dirty blood filled with fats and poisons, which can help stop blood clots from occurring inside our veins and eases the heart, too, allowing it to not overwork as it pumps.

- **Figs:** All-around friends and allies to the liver, figs don't require a lot of hydrochloric acid or bile fluid to digest, so they give the liver a break. At the same time, figs bind onto and expel almost every variety of pathogen and toxin in their way in the intestinal tract—which means less poison heading up to the liver through the hepatic portal system. Figs are a win-win for your liver.

- **Garlic:** Since the liver deals with an onslaught of pathogens, it needs herbs and foods that help it fight its cause. Garlic is one such herbal food. The medicinal, pungent, astringent quality of garlic is a pathogen's worst nightmare. Phytochemical compounds from garlic seep through the walls of the intestinal tract into blood vessels that lead up through the hepatic portal vein into the liver. The liver's immune system welcomes these compounds because it knows they're like a relief army coming in so the immune system can find reprieve and retreat to build up its forces. These phytochemical compounds are like throwing sand in someone's eyes; they literally hit a variety of pathogens inside the liver, forcing them to back down and even killing off some of them. If you're sensitive to garlic, try onions; they have similar qualities. If you're not sensitive to garlic, don't be afraid to bring it in when you feel like it.

- **Grapes:** While grapes are shunned for their high sugar content, we ought to think twice. That very sugar content in grapes helps revitalize the liver. They're truly a longevity food, increasing the liver's performance in every one of its over 2,000 chemical functions. The fruit acid unique to grapes is a great dissolver of gallstones—think about that the next time you eat some rather than worrying if there's too much sugar or if they'll make you gain weight. Weight gain is the last thing grapes create.

- **Hot peppers (such as cayenne, Super Chili, habeñero, bird's eye, jalapeño, and poblano):** Hot peppers contain dozens of phytochemical compounds that are helpful for the liver. One such compound is capsaicin, which gives the liver license to heat itself without negative ramifications. The liver welcomes this food-initiated heat because it's a reset factor. Blood rushes oxygen through all the capillaries throughout the liver, and the heat caused by the capsaicin instantly draws fresh, clean blood into the liver through all avenues. It's like opening a window in your house to let out stale air and let in fresh air. This reset is beneficial for the liver's reaction to inflammation that's caused by pathogens and toxins. Try not to eat your peppers green; always eat them red and ripe. We have an obsession with eating green peppers, and certain people's reactions to these and other *unripe* nightshades are part of what unfairly gives all nightshades a bad name. Look to ripe hot peppers for a liver reset.

- **Jerusalem artichokes (also called sunchokes):** Hold phytochemical compounds that have the ability to halt quick-to-spread diseases. Some viruses, other pathogens, and cell-damaging troublemakers are more aggressive than others, and a phytochemical compound in Jerusalem artichokes can halt them. The same compound is involved in the growth process of the "artichokes" in the ground. These roots spread far, wide, and quickly in their growing season, and the compound responsible for that is the same that ends up protecting the liver from fast-spreading illnesses.

- **Kale:** A beneficial food for the entire intestinal tract because it starves unfriendly bacteria and microorganisms while feeding beneficial bacteria and microorganisms. Very helpful for improving the ileum environment, which in turn improves vitamin B_{12} production so the liver can receive this vital nutrient through the hepatic portal vein.

- **Kiwis:** Kiwis' fruit acid has a dissolving effect on gallstones unlike any other. It creates divots and pits inside the stones, weakening them so they can break apart. Kiwis also provide various nutrients upon which the liver relies.

- **Leafy greens (especially lettuces and their stems):** An extremely cleansing tool for your liver that you can apply on a daily basis. The leafy outer greens of lettuce provide dozens of micronutrients for the liver to stay healthy and balanced, while the core of the lettuce, down closer to the root, provides milky chemical compounds that act as a purging mechanism for it. When leafy greens are eaten with fruit, their medicinal qualities increase twofold.

- **Lemons and limes:** Improve hydrochloric acid production as well as bile production and potency. Contain micro mineral salts that break down pathogens such as unproductive bacteria, mold, yeast, and fungus to help protect your liver's immune system. The rich calcium levels in lemons and limes binds to the vitamin C within them, and both of these enter into the liver, where they waken a stagnant, sluggish, fatty liver, helping loosen and disperse fat cells. Lemons and limes clean up dirty blood syndrome, improve glucose absorption, and even protect the pancreas.

- **Mangoes:** Cool a toxic, overheated liver, soothing and calming it to prevent the organ from going into spasm. The yellow-to-orange pigment in mangoes feeds liver lobules and strengthens hepatocytes and Kupffer cells, allowing them to do the jobs they need to do. Mangoes also have a unique phytochemical compound that helps the liver's immune system destroy the pockets of bacteria that create liver abscesses. Help prevent your liver from aging and cells from dying while improving bile production.

- **Maple syrup:** The combination of sugars and high mineral content quickly travels to the liver and becomes instant fuel of phytonutrient composition. It's like an IV for the liver containing the best of both worlds: a vast array of vitamins, minerals, and other nutrients (many of them still undiscovered) coupled with high-quality sugar on which the liver thrives.

- **Melons:** A powerful liver-cleansing food because of melon's ability to hydrate blood all on its own and help alleviate your liver's overburdened state. The combination of melon's unique living water content with its nutrient content allows the heart to work less; melons thin out dirty, toxic, fat-filled blood, allowing the heart to not overwork itself in pumping blood. This reduces some of the liver's responsibility to protect the heart, which frees up the liver to focus on other important chemical functions that are needed in the moment. Melons also provide the liver with hydration to hold on to for when you're in a drought, living a lifestyle of chronic dehydration. They flush toxins out of the intestinal tract with ease and rebuild hydrochloric acid reserves in the stomach. And because bile is not needed to break down and digest melon, the liver can work on restoring its bile tank.

- **Mushrooms:** Contain hundreds of undiscovered phytochemical compounds, many of which are detoxifying for the liver without hurting it. Mushrooms are medicine for the liver. Many people fear mushrooms because they believe that their status as a type of fungus means they feed fungus within the body. It's just

the opposite. A mushroom is a fungus that destroys fungus, and the liver accepts mushrooms as allies—if the liver is dealing with unwanted microorganisms such as fungus, mushrooms are very helpful in pushing them out of the liver. Mushrooms also reduce fungus, bacteria, and viruses in the intestinal tract, allowing for cleaner nutrients and cleaner blood to arrive in the liver.

- **Onions and scallions:** Very similar to garlic, onions have antimicrobial sulfur compounds that expel unfriendly pathogens from the liver. Onions have a disinfecting quality for the liver, keeping it from becoming inflamed. They also improve the temperature control or "thermostat" of the liver so it can heat and cool itself properly.

- **Oranges and tangerines:** Provide a combination of calcium and vitamin C; when both are combined from the same food source, the liver can use both better than it could from separate sources. Another great fruit that allows for easy absorption and conversion of nutrients for your liver. While oranges and tangerines have a mild gallstone-dissolving capability, they have more of an ability to uproot and disperse sludge and sediment that can settle in the gallbladder after passing through the hepatic ducts from the liver.

- **Papayas:** When someone's intestinal tract is nervy from inflamed nerves caused by troublemakers all along the gut lining, papaya soothes those nerves, allowing inflammation to reduce. This improves the absorption of nutrients into the bloodstream to head up to the liver. The red-pigment phytochemicals in papayas allow liver cells to become more agile and versatile so the liver can function at its optimum.

- **Parsley:** Its phytochemicals have anti-troublemaker effects that dislodge poisons and catapult them out of your liver. The intense green pigment in parsley contains an alkaloid specifically for liver rejuvenation; tissue in the liver improves when exposed to these alkaloid compounds. Parsley has a purging effect on gallbladder sludge, though not on gallstones. Its phytochemical compounds settle at the bottom of the gallbladder, where the sludge lies, to do their good.

- **Peaches and nectarines:** The skin of peaches and nectarines has a quality that's sticky to toxins and poisons inside the intestinal tract. These skins cling to deep-seated pockets of debris; old, putrefied food; and mucus inside the small intestine and colon, driving them out to make room for friendly bacteria and microorganisms and allow for better nutrient absorption. The juicy nature of a peach or nectarine is unique in the sense that it's a combination of fruit acid along with mineral salts and sugars, with an astringent phytochemical compound close to the pit that allows for rejuvenation close to the liver's inner core.

- **Pears:** A calming, soothing, gently cleansing fruit that's incredible for agitated, inflamed, stagnant, sluggish, overburdened, or fatty livers. Pears also have a sedation effect upon busy parts of the liver that need to take breaks and cool down. They take the liver off autopilot when it's in constant crisis, allowing the organ to heal and rejuvenate.

- **Pineapple:** Dissolves gallstones. Its highly acidic fruit acid and chemical compounds also enter into your liver easily, acting as brushing mechanisms and dispersing degreasing agents to clean up and drive out sticky, mucus-y debris, gunk, and byproduct that can build up inside the liver from a multitude of troublemakers. Pineapple can be astringent, so I prefer the bottom two-thirds for the sweetest, most balanced part of the fruit. Even if you ripen it on its side, it's the bottom that's best. If the astringency doesn't bother you, you can eat the whole thing.

- **Pitaya (also called dragon fruit):** The red pigment in the red-fleshed variety of pitaya is a rejuvenator for your liver, bringing cells back to life. It helps your liver produce cells faster so regeneration of the liver can occur. It's a fountain of youth fruit for the liver that slows down and stops liver aging by caring for its deep, inner core, which in most cases succumbs to disease if left neglected for too long. Look for packs of frozen red pitaya in the frozen section of the grocery store or online, or you may find it fresh in your area. If neither is available where you live, seek out pure pitaya powder.

- **Pomegranates:** Contain anthocyanins to help rejuvenate liver cells at the same time that its astringent fruit acid helps dissolve gallstones. Excellent for cleaning the passageways of blood vessels and promoting better flow through the veins of the liver.

- **Potatoes:** Abundant in amino acids that specifically inhibit viral growth. Potatoes are high in glucose that provides substance to the liver, as it's precisely what the liver relies on to keep strong. It also helps build up glycogen storage, the very resource that protects us against blood sugar problems, weight gain, fatty liver, and dirty blood syndrome. Potatoes keep the liver grounded and stable, giving us a good constitution. They're also shunned for being a nightshade, when in truth they have the ability to reverse many varieties of chronic illness.

- **Radishes:** A strong medicine for our livers. The pungent, biting nature of radishes comes from a compilation of chemical compounds, many of them undiscovered, that act as disinfectants to the liver, stopping pathogen infection and boosting the liver's personalized immune system by increasing its white blood cells' ability to fight and destroy invaders.

- **Raw honey:** Contains a combination of sugar that the liver needs desperately and vitamins, minerals, and other nutrients—hundreds of which are not on the record with medical research and science. Honey is antimicrobial: antiviral, antibacterial, antifungal, all packaged into one. When it heads to the liver in its broken-down, assimilated state, it packs a punch, giving the liver everything it needs at once: the liver's immune system strengthens instantly. The liver lobules and cells get the fuel they need instantly. And hundreds of phytochemicals from the flowers that bees once harvested for pollen intoxicate the liver in a euphoric, healthy way, giving the liver the reprieve it needs to fight for us another day.

- **Red cabbage:** Helps your liver in more ways than one. Its greatest role is involved with the intestinal tract, where it minimizes pathogens, expels ammonia gas from the body, knocks down fungus and bacteria, and sweeps out old debris and putrefied food, making a better environment for the ileum so B_{12} can be produced. Red cabbage is the liver's secret weapon, as all these benefits to the intestinal tract benefit the liver, too. Just when you think red cabbage's duties are done, its sulfur compounds combined with its deep purple-red pigment head up to the liver, where they revitalize and regenerate injured tissue, including tissue in the liver's deep, inner core, making red cabbage an effective tool for liver recovery.

- **Spinach:** The mineral salts in a spinach leaf and especially its stem helps the liver with its over 2,000 chemical functions. Not only is spinach filled with lots of vitamins and other nutrients; they're nutrients that the liver can easily absorb. Spinach leaves release nutrients quickly into the intestinal tract, even when someone is experiencing weak hydrochloric acid or bile production levels. It massages the ileum, allowing for better B_{12} production, and helps the liver convert nutrients so the rest of the body can receive them once the liver releases them.

- **Sprouts and microgreens:** The liver appreciates sprouts and microgreens greatly, the way it appreciates any living fruit, vegetable, or leafy green from the farmers' market or your own

garden, or grown on your kitchen counter—because these foods harbor elevated biotics not found anywhere else. You can't buy elevated biotics packaged up in bottles at the store, and you can't even find them in fermented foods. They don't exist in any area of industry; they exist on a fresh sprout or microgreen or an organic apple you pick from a tree or on kale you pluck from your backyard plot. These elevated biotics create the strongest beneficial bacteria environment possible in the intestinal tract, and this greatly benefits the liver in ways undiscovered by medical research and science. Elevated biotics are the difference between true absorption of vitamins and minerals to benefit the liver versus the difficulty most people with conditions have absorbing nutrients due to the loads of troublemakers in the liver and intestinal tract.

- **Sweet potatoes:** An important glucose and glycogen storage food for the liver. All sweet potatoes and yams are beneficial, even white sweet potatoes. Similar to regular potatoes, they help support almost every function for which the liver is responsible inside our bodies. Sweet potatoes have phytochemical properties that calm heated, angry, stagnant, sluggish, and toxic livers and help prevent spasming. They also offer a range of hormone-balancing phytochemicals for the liver; the liver uses sweet potatoes and yams to regulate and control some of its hormone functions.

- **Tomatoes:** Harness critical micronutrients, phytochemicals, vitamins, and minerals to support many functions of the liver. Lycopene is a beloved nutrient that the liver admires: the liver uses it to shield itself from cell damage, plus lycopene helps the liver detox red blood cells safely, smoothly, and efficiently. The fruit acids in tomatoes help keep the gallbladder healthy, helping rid sludge from the gallbladder and even reduce gallstone size. Even poorly grown tomatoes have a high mineral content. These minerals often get to the deep, inner core of the liver, helping prevent disease where it commonly starts for people. Tomatoes grow at night, under the moonlight, and the liver also responds to moonlight—when it's a full moon, the liver tends to work harder at cleaning, filtering, and processing in the wee hours of the morning. When organic or heirloom tomatoes are in the diet, the full moon energy that they collected during their growing cycle works with the liver's ability to cleanse. If you're avoiding tomatoes due to trendy nightshade hatred that constantly recirculates over and over again, you're missing out on keeping your liver healthy and preventing disease.

- **Turmeric (fresh):** Fresh turmeric has two main responsibilities for your liver: it allows it to purge a host of different troublemakers, even from the liver's deep, inner core, and at the same time it protects liver cells from injury as these harmful toxins are being uprooted and leaving the body. Turmeric provides a renewal effect; it digs up deep, dark toxins and rids your liver of them, essentially erasing a part of your past you don't need.

- **Wild blueberries:** Contain dozens of undiscovered antioxidants, including anthocyanin varieties. There's not just one pigment inside a wild blueberry; there are dozens of pigments not yet researched or studied. The wild blueberry is to the liver as mother's milk is to a baby. Not only do wild blueberries have the ability to grab on to plenty of troublemakers, they also hold on to them as they leave the liver, in a way that most other healing foods cannot. The pigments in wild blueberries have the ability to saturate deep into liver cells and cross cell walls and membranes inside the liver, spreading their blue everywhere. Wild blueberries enhance the intestinal tract, feeding good bacteria there, which benefits the liver greatly.

- **Winter squash (including kabocha, acorn, delicata, and butternut):** Loaded with nutrients that our livers can easily store. High in carotenoids that protect liver cells from damage. The glucose in winter squash can stabilize the liver, allowing blood sugar to stabilize overall in the body.

- **Zucchini:** Very similar to cucumber in certain ways, as it is also a fruit that's helpful for liver hydration, which allows the liver to store micro pockets of water that it can later release back into the bloodstream during moments of chronic dehydration in your life. Zucchini have a mild liver-purging effect, allowing the liver to squeeze out poisonous troublemakers safely. It's also soothing to the intestinal tract walls, pushing out pathogens such as bacteria and fungus, allowing for better absorption of nutrients that can be sent up to the liver. Zucchini is a beneficial gallbladder food, containing phytochemicals that actually reduce gallbladder inflammation.

HEALING HERBS AND SUPPLEMENTS

You'll notice that the items to come are single herbs and supplements. What you won't find here are bottles and bottles of supplements with dozens of ingredients each—dozens of herbs, vitamins, amino acids, and more. There's a reason for this. When you fill a capsule with 20, 30, or 40 nutrients, it's only going to contain a speck of each one, and that's not going to help you heal. This is a practice some supplement companies employ so that they don't have to use up valuable nutrients in large amounts in each capsule. You end up getting ripped off.

At the same time, most people with chronic illness of any kind are highly sensitive. If you have a reaction to a pill filled with that many ingredients, you'll never know what's causing the reaction, so you'll never get to learn from it. Plus, a supplement with dozens of ingredients is a concoction thrown together according to what a so-called expert in the field of nutraceuticals believes, not what your liver needs.

Each one of the singles in these lists holds God-given powers to help your liver heal. Your liver can understand each one of these and knows how to use it. So if you see later in this chapter a list of 10 to 15 different single supplements to take for an illness or symptom, the healing benefits far surpass taking 10 to 15 different bottles of gimmicky supplements, even if they're supposedly high quality. What they really are is filled with dozens and dozens and dozens of guesses at what's good for you that end up confusing and overburdening your liver and other areas of your immune system.

What it boils down to is that chronic symptoms and conditions like the ones in this book remain mysteries to medical communities. How can an expert recommendation of a blended supplement help if no one knows what's really causing your ailment or disease? Only by knowing what really causes your health issue, as you can discover throughout the Medical Medium series, can you know what to take for it specifically. With the herbs and supplements here, the power is in your hands to take care of your liver and your specific symptoms and conditions.

Trying these supplements is an optional step beyond all the other recommendations here in Part IV. If you prefer to focus on foods for healing, you're more than welcome to do that. You don't have to play in Supplement Land if you don't want to—lowering fats and adding in healing foods is going to help with all your problems. This supplement guide is for people looking for something more, looking for options because their situations are perplexing to them. If that's you, then keep reading for a treasure trove of options. At the end of the chapter you'll even find specialized supplement lists for the individual symptoms and conditions in this book.

In the case of herbal tinctures, actively seek out alcohol-free versions (avoid the word *ethanol*, too). The alcohol in tinctures is normally corn grain alcohol, and therefore GMO-contaminated, even if it's organic, which (1) cancels out the herb's benefits and (2) soaks into the herb anyway and alters it. Not to mention that alcohol hurts your liver. If it's impossible to find an alcohol-free tincture, grape alcohol should be your first pick and brandy is the next-best preservative.

I'm continually asked, what is the most effective form of a given supplement, and does it really matter? Yes, it matters greatly. There are subtle and sometimes critical differences among the different supplement types available that can affect how quickly your viral or bacterial load dies off, if at all; whether your central nervous system repairs itself and how fast; how quickly your inflammation reduces; and how long it takes for your symptoms and conditions to heal. The supplement variety you choose can make or break your progress. To speed up healing, you need the right kinds of supplements. For these very important reasons, I offer a directory on my website (www.medicalmedium.com) of the best forms of each supplement listed below.

As you read through these supplements, which are listed in alphabetical order, keep in mind that the extent of what they do for your body and your liver specifically remains undiscovered by medical research and science. While a few are on their radar, many of them are completely unknown as liver rescuers and their benefits go far beyond what anyone realizes.

One powerful undiscovered tip is to consider taking your supplements with a piece of fruit such as a banana or even some potato, sweet potato, winter squash, raw honey, maple syrup, or coconut water. As you read earlier in the book, sugar is what carries vitamins, minerals, and nutrients through the bloodstream to help them find their way to where they need to go, and an organ won't accept vitamins, minerals, and other nutrients without sugar to assist it. Taking your supplements with natural sugars ensures that the liver and other parts of your body can actually use them.

- **5-MTHF (5-methyltetrahydrofolate):** Binds onto the B_{12} that elevated biotics create inside the ileum. Also enters the liver, igniting and bringing back to life storage bins of B_{12} that the liver keeps for emergencies while helping the liver convert it to a bioactive form that it can deliver into the bloodstream, coded with messages attached for specific organs. Chemical compounds that the liver produces attach themselves to the 5-MTHF and B_{12} so that other organs can identify and absorb the B_{12} easily.

- **ALA (alpha lipoic acid):** Easily enters into all liver cells, giving them added antioxidant protection from injury due to highly toxic troublemakers. Supports the nerves entering the liver and also improves glucose storage ability, increasing glycogen storage containment in deep levels of the liver. ALA perks up the liver and helps detoxify it at the same time.

- **Aloe vera:** The gel from a fresh aloe leaf binds onto toxic debris in the intestinal tract and carries it out of the colon during elimination. Reduces poisons and toxins in the intestinal tract so that they don't travel up to the liver. Also allows for cleaner blood flow through the hepatic portal system into the liver, bringing with it chemical compounds from aloe that specifically inhibit bacteria and certain viruses. Aloe expels and diminishes ammonia inside the intestinal tract that otherwise seeps into the liver when food is putrefying due to low hydrochloric acid and bile production.

- **Amla berry:** Contains a rich wealth of antioxidants that protect the liver from old, inherited toxins as well as from new, everyday exposure. Its high vitamin C content feeds the liver's personalized immune system, protecting the liver from infection and helping the immune system seek out and destroy pathogens that camp out and hide out inside our livers. Amla berry also improves the liver's

chemical functions and helps restore glucose.

- **Ashwagandha:** Strengthens the adrenals, keeping them from over- or underreacting, which is a pattern these glands assume as they weaken when under adrenal stress. Ashwagandha protects the liver from excess adrenaline exposure and helps the liver produce and store dozens of hormones.

- **Barley grass juice powder:** Contains phytonutrients that feed an undernourished liver while allowing it to detoxify dozens of toxins and poisons inherited from the past and exposed to in the present moment. It's a responsible detoxifier with take-and-give integrity, replacing the troublemakers it removes with vital nutrients.

- **B-complex:** The liver is the master at converting and storing B vitamins as more usable nutrients for all organs and tissues of the body. While the liver does have the ability to create a B vitamin if necessary in desperate times, through desperate measures, it's easier for the liver when B vitamins are present in foods and high-quality supplements so it can focus on its other, most important jobs. The liver tags a B vitamin with a chemical compound that assigns it to the organ in need; the high intelligence factor that the liver possesses works hand in hand with B vitamins. When the liver is cleaner and freer of toxins, the wonders of vitamin B-complex can really take effect.

- **Black walnut:** For rare occasions of certain parasites or worms, black walnut enters into the liver, injuring these unfriendly guests and sometimes only needing to smoke them out of the liver. Keep in mind that black walnut does not harm viruses or bacteria; what it's great for are those certain unfriendly parasitical guests.

- **Burdock root:** Filled with undiscovered anti-inflammatory compounds. The juice from fresh burdock root is extremely medicinal for the liver and versatile according to the liver's needs, improving liver functions from glucose storage to vitamin and mineral storage to screening and filtering blood. It purges the liver of deep, inherited toxins as well as newly encountered ones, helps expel old red blood cells that have congested the liver, and improves bile production. Dried burdock also makes a very medicinal tea. Burdock is essentially a root herb. It goes deep into the earth, so its phytochemical compounds hold a powerful grounding ability. The liver leans on burdock root, for it reminds the liver of its sole responsibility of being the rock for the body.

- **Cardamom:** Increases bile production and brings life and

beneficial, nontoxic heat back to stagnant, sluggish livers that have overheated for years and are now cooling down. Cardamom's heat ignites homeostasis.

- **Cat's claw:** Rather than detoxifying the liver, cat's claw destroys viruses, bacteria, and other unfriendly microorganisms that can camp out inside or invade the liver. Assists the liver's personalized immune system, giving it a chance to recoup its strength and restore itself for the next battle. Stabilizes the liver's environment.

- **Chaga mushroom:** Strengthens the liver while reducing toxic liver heat when the liver is under stress and burdened from troublemakers. Supports and strengthens the adrenals, which in turn assists in strengthening the liver, making it a more difficult environment for pathogens such as viruses and bacteria to survive in. Phytochemical compounds in chaga detoxify the liver in a steady, balanced manner.

- **Chicory root:** Reduces gallstone production by adding a phytochemical compound acid to bile that inhibits gallstone growth. Gently detoxifies the body in a manner that's acceptable to the body and easy on the adrenals. Contributes to many of the chemical functions for which the liver is responsible.

- **CoQ$_{10}$ (Coenzyme Q$_{10}$):** A gentle antioxidant that supports all functions of the liver and protects all liver cells from oxidative stress. One of the liver's chemical functions can alter, adjust, and customize specific antioxidants for its specific needs in the moment. CoQ$_{10}$ is one of them; the liver uses it as an antioxidant building block. Helps prevent extreme cell damage.

- **Curcumin:** This component of turmeric contains phytochemical compounds that calm the liver, resulting in fewer spasms. Helps prepare and purify blood before it enters the liver so that blood arrives with fewer toxins. Its healing properties ignite healing heat in a stagnant, sluggish liver, resulting in less disease.

- **Dandelion root:** Helps reset the filtering capabilities of the liver by expelling loose, rogue toxins inside it that haven't yet been compartmentalized in storage banks. Purges the liver so it can expel these free-floating troublemakers and essentially breathe and focus more on its filtration responsibilities. Also supports the liver's adaptation strength. The liver's ability to convert nutrients can restore while using dandelion root, plus bile strength increases.

- **D-mannose:** Binds on to bacteria in the urinary tract. Good for UTIs.

- **EPA and DHA (eicosapentaenoic acid and docosahexaenoic acid):** These omegas help improve the liver's personalized immune system by keeping toxic plaque and debris from sticking to the walls of the hepatic veins, hepatic artery, and hepatic portal vein. Keeping these vessels clear of obstructions allows for better blood flow into and out of the liver, which protects and eases the heart. Be sure to buy a plant-based (not fish-based) version.

- **Eyebright:** A great antibacterial, antiviral uprooter of liver antagonists. Also carries chemical compounds originally from its flowers and leaves that improve hundreds of the liver's chemical functions, specifically many involved with bile production. Strengthens the liver's white blood cells by arming them with a phytochemical compound that flushes out pathogens to be destroyed by other immune system cells.

- **Ginger:** Helps calm spasms in the liver and regulate liver heat—it can heat up the liver, perking it up out of stagnation, or cool a very hot liver, balancing it out, depending on what's needed. Helpful for a sluggish liver, stagnant liver, and dirty blood syndrome. Improves bile production and potency while improving the stomach's production of hydrochloric acid. Also feeds the liver with dozens of phytochemical compounds that it can use for many of its chemical functions. Some of ginger's phytochemical compounds expel ammonia and rotting, putrefying food, debris, and toxins from the small intestine and colon, allowing for cleaner nutrients to enter the liver from the intestinal tract. Ginger also dislodges fat cells inside the liver, allowing that fat to break free and exit through the bile and digestive tract, sometimes by way of the gallbladder.

- **Glutathione:** Saturates the liver quickly and easily, where it supports every single liver cell and its function. It's medicine to the liver, like someone coming along and making all your problems go away. Quickly leaves the liver, too, though the liver appreciates it greatly for its brief presence that assists the organ's over 2,000 chemical functions.

- **Goldenseal:** When goldenseal enters the liver, it quickly suffocates and destroys pathogens, both bacterial and viral. Also inhibits pathogens that are adjacent to the liver in the lymphatic system. Goldenseal has a gentle purging effect that expels bacterial debris, viral byproduct, neurotoxins, and other pathogenic waste matter.

- **Hibiscus:** The unique anthocyanin compound that gives hibiscus its red coloring helps rejuvenate the liver, bringing it back to life by cleaning mucus off cell

membrane walls and improving the liver's ability to perform its responsibilities. This herb is also a gallbladder rejuvenator—it cleans off gallbladder walls—and improves the liver's personalized immune system.

- **Lemon balm:** Kills viruses, bacteria, and other pathogenic microorganisms inside the liver. Makes a better environment in the intestinal tract, which supports the delivery of cleaner nutrients from the gut to the liver. Lemon balm calms the nerves of the liver, causing it to be less spasmodic, agitated, and angry, while also calming the nerves inside of the intestinal lining, which lowers toxic heat inside the liver. It also supports the adrenals, which makes the liver less toxic.

- **Licorice root:** Diminishes viruses inside the liver and brings down excessive liver heat due to a liver that's struggling and highly toxic. Calms liver spasms and helps eliminate toxic hormones stored inside it. Licorice also increases hydrochloric acid in the stomach, which helps ease the burden on the liver, and soothes an irritated, inflamed gallbladder and intestinal lining.

- **L-lysine:** Enters the liver and acts as a smokescreen to all of the viruses that are responsible for liver disease and autoimmune disorders. Viruses hate lysine. It's like the powder that comes out of a fire extinguisher—a viral retardant that deters viruses from proliferating. L-lysine strengthens the immune system in the liver and aids in some of the organ's most important functions.

- **Magnesium glycinate:** Supports blood vessels inside the liver, making them less restricted and more pliable and supple, allowing for easier blood flow throughout the liver. Magnesium gently flushes toxins out of the liver at the same time it calms liver spasms and agitation. It's responsible for dozens of the liver's chemical functions, including its adaptation skills. It also helps gently cleanse the intestinal tract, allowing the liver to receive cleaner, less-toxic blood.

- **Melatonin:** Helps reduce tumors and cysts inside the liver and helps prevent them from growing in the first place. A natural anti-inflammatory that doesn't confuse the liver's immune system, only strengthens it. If the liver is sluggish and stagnant and loses its ability to create melatonin, taking supplemental melatonin can reignite the liver's capacity to start up again. That's right: while medical research and science associate melatonin production with the brain, it's also one of the liver's hormone functions to create and secrete it. Always start with a small dosage.

- **Milk thistle:** Helps push out old red blood cells from the liver and detoxify any free-floating toxins, gunk, and debris that are in the hepatic veins. Improves bile production and helps cleanse bile pathways throughout the liver. Rejuvenates the liver and helps perk it up out of stagnation.

- **MSM (methylsulfonylmethane):** Loosens and helps expel fats from liver cells. Helps strengthen every cell inside the liver, making the organ less prone to attack from disease-causing bacteria and viruses. MSM wakes up a stagnant, sluggish liver, reduces toxic liver heat, and gently purges the liver of toxins in deep-seated areas. Also gently purges the gallbladder of small debris particles. Improves the immune system inside and around the liver.

- **Mullein leaf:** A great antiviral, antibacterial liver herb. Reduces inflammation, calming down liver spasms as well as toxic liver heat. Helps soothe an aggravated liver and decrease and expel mucus formation inside the liver's blood vessels and cells.

- **NAC (N-acetyl cysteine):** Provides building blocks for liver cells to regenerate. Helps the liver with its adaptation abilities and improves the liver's screening and filtering capabilities while contributing to hundreds of the liver's chemical functions. NAC also supports the adrenal glands, which in turn aids the liver.

- **Nascent iodine:** An antiseptic for the liver, preventing disease from viruses, bacteria, and other unfriendly microorganisms. Enters into every cell of the liver to aid hundreds of chemical functions for which the liver is responsible. Protects the gallbladder and even improves bile production. Helps the liver defend itself from cancerous growths.

- **Nettle leaf:** Increases hydrochloric acid in the stomach, which helps ease the burden on the liver. Also improves bile production inside the liver, calms an aggravated and inflamed gallbladder, inhibits gallstone growth, and supports the bile passageways throughout the liver. Nettle leaf enhances all liver cell functions, reduces liver heat from toxins, and even gently cleanses a variety of old, inherited toxins and troublemakers to which you've been newly exposed. It balances the adrenals, keeping them from being either over- or underactive, while improving the liver's adaptive abilities.

- **Olive leaf:** A great antiviral, antibacterial herb for the liver. It gently purges the liver of free-floating toxins, though not ones that are deeply rooted or stored in the liver. Olive leaf's phytochemical compounds provide various nutrients for some of the liver's chemical functions, too.

- **Oregon grape root:** Helps kill viruses and bacteria inside the liver and helps prevent them from going to the heart. Also improves bile production and reduces pathogenic activity inside the intestinal tract, allowing for better absorption of nutrients in the liver.

- **Peppermint:** Improves hydrochloric acid levels in the stomach and calms intestinal nerves and spasms, all of which makes for a reduction of toxins inside the intestinal tract so that the liver can better absorb nutrients. Peppermint calms a spasmodic liver, reduces liver heat from a toxic load, cleanses the liver, and helps the liver rebuild its glucose and glycogen storage reserves and abilities.

- **Raspberry leaf:** Helps remove toxic, unwanted hormones from the liver and improves the liver's ability to create and produce important hormones needed throughout the body. Gently purges the liver, detoxifying troublemakers stored inside of it. Acts as a tonic to the gallbladder, calming down gallbladder spasms, and improves hydrochloric acid in the stomach. Strengthens white blood cells in the liver, helping reduce liver disease.

- **Red clover:** Aids the liver with its screening and filtering functions by helping purify toxin-filled blood before it enters into the liver. Contains phytochemical compounds that bind to hundreds of toxins, helping drive them out of the body through the kidneys and intestinal tract. This allows the liver to cleanse on a deeper level because it's not being constantly burdened by toxic blood from every angle. At the same time, red clover has high mineral content that feeds the liver, making cells stronger, including red blood cells, while at the same time helping rid old red blood cells from the liver.

- **Rose hips:** Another grounding force for the liver. The roots of the rose bush can run deep and wide scouring for minerals and other nutrients, which they bring to the rose hips that form when the flowers fall away. The vitamin C in rose hips is another bioavailable source for the liver in fighting disease created by viruses and bacteria. The liver's personalized immune system uses the vitamin C from a rose hip more easily and aggressively than the vitamin C taken in a supplement on its own, so consider sipping rose hip tea on the days when you take vitamin C; the rose hip's vitamin C will activate the supplemental form of it, making it stronger.

- **Schisandra berry:** Helps increase the liver's adaptogenic abilities. Contains undiscovered antioxidants that protect liver cells from excess adrenaline damage and toxin overload. Helps increase oxygen to the liver and calms liver spasms by reducing toxic liver

heat. It's so filled with minerals and other nutrients that it bulks up the liver's nutrient storage banks.

- **Selenium:** Improves the liver's ability to process vitamins and other nutrients. Needed for the utilization and conversion of amino acids inside the liver. Increases the liver's cell strength and bolsters its personalized immune system of white blood cells throughout the entire liver. Helps maintain good levels of albumin in the liver.

- **Spirulina:** Provides an abundance of vitamins and minerals to reestablish the liver's storage banks of nutrients that it can easily convert into what it needs in the moment to release and deliver throughout the body. Stops viral and bacterial growth inside the liver, revitalizes the organ by binding onto hundreds of toxins and poisons and carrying them out of deep pockets of the liver, strengthens the liver's immune system, and helps in its over 2,000 chemical functions. Especially aids the liver's glucose storage and protein conversions. You'll see that Hawaiian spirulina was recommended in my previous books. I've since discovered a more beneficial product that's upgraded in quality. You can find it on my website directory.

- **Turmeric (supplement form):** Reduces liver swelling when a liver gets toxically hot. Helps squeeze out residuals of mucus from bile passageways and pockets inside the liver while it wakes up and stimulates liver cells, reigniting and rerouting energy throughout the liver. Helps with hormone production inside the liver while removing and cleaning out unwanted toxic hormones. Overall, increases liver performance.

- **Vitamin B$_{12}$ (as adenosylcobalamin with methylcobalamin):** Helps with liver cell communication, improving the ability of cells inside the liver to transfer information to one another with ease rather than resistance. Protects nerve tissue that enters and runs all through the liver. Vitamin B$_{12}$ is highly instrumental to all of the liver's over 2,000 chemical functions and highly instrumental in activating the liver's ability to utilize, process, and distribute all other vitamins and minerals that are stored inside of it. One of conventional medicine's most important discoveries was singling out B$_{12}$. It helps keep a liver out of stagnation, strengthens hepatocytes and all other liver cells as well as liver lobules, and prevents the liver's blood vessels from atrophying.

- **Vitamin C:** Strengthens all levels of the liver's personalized immune system. Speeds up white blood cell recuperation and recovery time in between wars with viruses and bacteria; also weakens pathogens exposed to it. The liver uses vitamin C in all of its over 2,000 chemical functions. It detoxifies and cleanses the liver, stops a sluggish liver, loosens and disperses fat cells stored inside the liver, strengthens the adrenal glands, and helps the liver recover after bouts of stress-related adrenaline surges. Helps stop and repair scar tissue deep in the liver's core.

- **Vitamin D$_3$:** The vitamin D stored inside the liver can grow inactive over time. It's unknown to medical research and science that supplementation with new vitamin D can ignite the activity of stored vitamin D when a liver is sluggish, stagnant, or highly toxic. (When the liver is in relatively good shape, the organ can activate its old storage bank of vitamin D without the help of the supplemental vitamin.) When taking vitamin D, do not take large dosages. Everyone has vitamin D storage inside the liver, even if it's from 15 years ago, through exposure from a food or the sun. If you take too much vitamin D, it may actually backfire, making the liver's main concern expelling, because too much of this vitamin is toxic to the liver. Rather than activating its storage bank of vitamin D, the liver may accidentally get rid of its stored vitamin D as it rushes to purge the new, supplemental vitamin. This is why I don't normally recommend vitamin D the way much of the health world does—I know the truth of how it works in the liver. In small amounts, vitamin D$_3$ can be helpful if your liver's not functioning properly. Don't take excessive dosages; you'll basically counter its effects.

- **Wild blueberry powder:** Powerfully speeds up healthy liver cell production, cleansing, and regeneration.

- **Yellow dock:** A great liver-cleansing herb to clean up toxins that are rogue and free-floating throughout the liver. Helps clear bile passageways and purge sediment from the gallbladder sac. Its extreme astringency and bitterness forces the liver to squeeze like a sponge, essentially squeezing out old blood while drawing in fresh, new blood through the hepatic portal vein and hepatic artery. Helps improve bile production and drive bad acids out of the body.

- **Zinc (as liquid zinc sulfate):** Responsible for all of the over 2,000 chemical functions of the liver, including the creation of your liver in the womb and the development of your liver as you grew and reached adulthood. The liver stores an abundance of zinc because it knows people are zinc-deficient, in part due to the lack of it in the food we eat. Without zinc, your liver can't perform its functions that protect your whole body, so despite its zinc storage, your liver always needs more, because the zinc output needed to respond to the mental and physical demands upon us is high.

The onslaught of viruses, bacteria, and other pathogens in particular drains our zinc reserves. One specific purpose of zinc reserves is to eliminate toxic forms of copper that are always high inside the liver and that can cause the organ harm. If someone is so zinc-deficient that even the liver's zinc reserves have dropped to a dangerous level, that person can develop a host of viral-related autoimmune diseases and illnesses, which you can read about throughout the Medical Medium series. Zinc helps the liver's immune system fend off every unfriendly microorganism that enters the liver. If zinc tastes too strong for you, feel free to minimize dosage to what's comfortable, even if it's just a few tiny drops.

INDIVIDUAL SUPPORT FOR YOU

If you're struggling with a specific symptom or condition that we covered in this book, or if you're looking for everyday liver and health maintenance, you may find it helpful to see a list of supplements that can offer specific support for you. In the pages to come, you'll find exactly that. You're welcome to start at a much lower dose with anything. Even with a smaller dose of one of these supplements, you will get more health benefits than if it's 1 tiny ingredient in an anti-inflammatory supplemental capsule with 20 others. If you're sensitive, talk to your practitioner about what dosage your body can handle. Alternatively, if you're not sensitive and you want to increase any dosages for your condition beyond what's listed on the supplement bottle, that's also a situation where you should talk to your practitioner about what's right for you. And with the exception of child liver and PANDAS, the dosages listed are for adults. If you're considering supplements for a child, consult with her or his practitioner about what's safe and appropriate.

If you're dealing with more than one symptom or condition at the same time, pick the one that looms largest in your life. For example, if you're plagued by eczema or psoriasis, focus on taking care of that and don't worry about bloating. Over time, you may find that working on one issue takes care of another, or you can switch off after a little while and focus on a different supplements list in these pages.

Once you've found your symptom or condition here, you don't need to take every supplement listed for it. If you're sensitive, you can try one a day. If not, you can put them all together as your daily regimen. As a middle ground, you can choose a couple to start off with, and then take it from there. Later on, if you're not experiencing what you want from a couple supplements, you can add a few more. You may already be taking other supplements you think are working for you. If so, talk to your practitioner about keeping those while adding these new ones.

Further, any supplement from the full liver supplements list that's not in your specific symptom or condition list is still an option to use, if your expert sense of what your body needs or your practitioner's recommendation tells you to do so. They're all helpful supplements for your liver and chronic illness.

Your practitioner can give you guidance on the length of time you may need to continue with supplements. The other measures you're taking to care for your liver—that is, adding in healing foods, lowering fats, avoiding troublemakers, and trying the Liver Rescue Morning and the Liver Rescue 3:6:9—will make a big difference to your healing timeline. How much your liver was struggling and how long you'd been suffering when you started on your healing path will make a big difference, too. Everyone has a different healing process and time frame.

Finally, a few notes on the supplement lists to come:

- When you see the term *dropperful*, that means as much liquid supplement as fills the bottle's eye dropper when you squeeze its rubber top. It may only fill up halfway; that's still considered a dropperful.

- There are also some supplements where dosages are given in drops. Make sure to check carefully whether it says *drops* or *dropperfuls*.

- Most of the liquid and powder supplements below are meant to be taken in water. Check the directions on the supplement's label.

- When you see multiple herbal tinctures in a list, you're welcome to combine them into one ounce or more of water and take them together.

- The same goes for teas. If multiple teas are listed for your symptom or condition, feel free to combine the herbs to make yourself a special tea blend or use a few different tea bags together.

- Some of the dosages are listed in milligrams. If you can't find capsules that line up with the exact suggestions, try to get ones that are close. Talk to your practitioner if you want to know how to adjust a dosage.

- Remember: almost all of these are adult dosages. Talk to a practitioner about what's right for a child.

- When you see the term *daily*, that means to take the given dosage of the supplement over the course of the day, and it's your choice how you do that. You're welcome to take the whole dose once a day. If you're sensitive, you may want to break it up into multiple servings. For example, if it says to take 2 teaspoons of barley grass juice powder daily, you may decide either to put both teaspoons together into a smoothie or have 1 teaspoon in a morning smoothie and 1 teaspoon in some water at night.

- Once you've figured out which items you're going to add to your life, go over the descriptions of the herbs and supplements from earlier in the chapter so you know all the wonderful benefits you're receiving.

Everyday Liver and Health Maintenance

If you're not experiencing any of the symptoms or conditions that follow, here's a list of herbs and supplements to help maintain your general health.

- **5-MTHF:** 1 capsule daily

- **Aloe vera:** 2 or more inches of fresh gel (skin removed) daily

- **Barley grass juice powder:** 2 teaspoons daily

- **Chaga mushroom:** 2 teaspoons daily

- **Curcumin:** 2 capsules daily

- **Lemon balm:** 3 dropperfuls daily

- **L-lysine:** 3 500-milligram capsules daily

- **Magnesium glycinate:** 2 capsules daily

- **Nettle leaf:** 2 cups of tea, 3 capsules, or 3 dropperfuls daily

- **Spirulina:** 2 teaspoons daily

- **Turmeric:** 2 capsules or freshly grated or juiced to taste daily

- **Vitamin B$_{12}$ (as adenosylcobalamin with methylcobalamin):** 1 dropperful daily

- **Vitamin C:** 4 500-milligram capsules Ester-C twice a day or 1 tablespoon of liquid liposomal daily

- **Zinc (as liquid zinc sulfate):** up to 1 dropperful daily

Acne

- Barley grass juice powder: 1 teaspoon twice a day
- Cat's claw: 1 dropperful twice a day
- Chaga mushroom: 1 teaspoon twice a day
- Curcumin: 2 capsules twice a day
- Goldenseal: 2 dropperfuls or 3 capsules twice a day (two weeks on, two weeks off)
- Lemon balm: 2 dropperfuls twice a day
- Mullein leaf: 2 dropperfuls twice a day
- Nascent iodine: 3 tiny drops twice a day
- Nettle leaf: 2 capsules or 2 dropperfuls twice a day
- Red clover: 1 cup of tea or 1 dropperful twice a day
- Spirulina: 1 teaspoon daily
- Vitamin B_{12} (as adenosylcobalamin with methylcobalamin): 1 dropperful daily
- Vitamin C: 2,000 milligrams Ester-C or 2 teaspoons liquid liposomal twice a day
- Zinc (as liquid zinc sulfate): up to 1 dropperful twice a day

Adrenal Problems

- Amla berry: 1 teaspoon or 2 capsules twice a day
- Ashwagandha: 1 dropperful or 2 capsules twice a day
- B-complex: 1 capsule daily
- Chicory root: 1 cup of tea daily
- Hibiscus: 1 cup of tea daily
- Lemon balm: 2 dropperfuls twice a day
- Licorice root: 10 small drops twice a day (two weeks on, two weeks off)
- Magnesium glycinate: 2 capsules twice a day
- Nettle leaf: 1 dropperful or 2 capsules twice a day
- Schisandra berry: 1 cup of tea daily
- Spirulina: 1 teaspoon twice a day
- Vitamin B_{12} (as adenosylcobalamin with methylcobalamin): 1 dropperful twice a day
- Vitamin C: 2,000 milligrams Ester-C or 2 teaspoons liquid liposomal twice a day
- Zinc (as liquid zinc sulfate): up to 1 dropperful twice a day

Autoimmune Liver (viral-caused autoimmune disorders and diseases)

- 5-MTHF: 1 capsule twice a day
- ALA: 1 500-milligram capsule daily
- Barley grass juice powder: 2 teaspoons twice a day
- Cat's claw: 2 dropperfuls twice a day
- Chaga mushroom: 2 teaspoons twice a day
- Curcumin: 2 capsules twice a day
- Glutathione: 1 capsule or 1 teaspoon of liquid twice a day
- Hibiscus: 1 cup of tea daily
- Lemon balm: 2 dropperfuls twice a day
- Licorice root: 1 dropperful daily (two weeks on, two weeks off)
- L-lysine: 4 500-milligram capsules twice a day
- MSM: 1 capsule twice a day
- Mullein leaf: 2 dropperfuls twice a day
- Nascent iodine: 3 tiny drops twice a day
- Nettle leaf: 2 dropperfuls or 2 capsules twice a day
- Oregon grape root: 1 dropperful or 1 capsule twice a day
- Selenium: 1 dropperful or 1 capsule daily
- Spirulina: 1 teaspoon twice a day
- Turmeric: 1 capsule twice a day
- Vitamin B_{12} (as adenosylcobalamin with methylcobalamin): 1 dropperful twice a day
- Vitamin C: 3,000 milligrams Ester-C or 1 tablespoon of liquid liposomal twice a day
- Zinc (as liquid zinc sulfate): up to 2 dropperfuls twice a day

Bloating

- 5-MTHF: 1 capsule daily
- Barley grass juice powder: 1 teaspoon daily
- Burdock root: 1 cup of tea or 1 root freshly juiced daily
- Cat's claw: 1 dropperful daily
- Chaga mushroom: 1 teaspoon daily
- Ginger: 1 cup of tea or 2 capsules twice a day or freshly grated or juiced to taste daily
- Hibiscus: 1 cup of tea daily
- Lemon balm: 1 dropperful daily
- Licorice root: 1 dropperful daily (two weeks on, two weeks off)
- Magnesium glycinate: 1 capsule daily
- Milk thistle: 1 capsule daily
- Peppermint: 1 cup of tea daily
- Raspberry leaf: 1 cup of tea daily
- Vitamin B_{12} (as adenosylcobalamin with methylcobalamin): 1 dropperful daily

Brain Fog

- 5-MTHF: 1 capsule twice a day

- Ashwagandha: 1 dropperful or 1 capsule twice a day

- Barley grass juice powder: 1 teaspoon twice a day

- B-complex: 1 capsule daily

- Cat's claw: 1 dropperful twice a day

- Chaga mushroom: 1 teaspoon twice a day

- Lemon balm: 1 dropperful twice a day

- Licorice root: 1 dropperful daily (two weeks on, two weeks off)

- L-lysine: 2 500-milligram capsules twice a day

- Nettle leaf: 1 dropperful or 1 capsule twice a day

- Spirulina: 1 teaspoon twice a day

- Vitamin B_{12} (as adenosylcobalamin with methylcobalamin): 1 dropperful twice a day

- Vitamin C: 2 500-milligram capsules Ester-C or one teaspoon liquid liposomal twice a day

- Zinc (as liquid zinc sulfate): up to 1 dropperful twice a day

Chemical and Food Sensitivities

Everyone with chemical and food sensitivities is different. You're welcome to explore any of the supplements here for your liver; this is just a starting point for some sensitive people. Take only one supplement one day, another the next, and so on, cycling through the full list of what you want to try over the course of several days instead of taking them all in one day. If you decide to take all of supplements in this list, it means you'll be on an eight-day cycle. A sensitivity is yet another reason to stay away from bottles of supplements with 50 ingredients.

- 5-MTHF: 1 capsule

- Barley grass juice powder: ½ teaspoon

- Lemon balm: 1 dropperful

- L-lysine: 500 milligrams

- Peppermint: 1 cup of tea

- Vitamin B_{12} (as adenosylcobalamin with methylcobalamin): 1 dropperful

- Vitamin C: 2 500-milligram capsules Ester-C

- Vitamin D_3: 1,000 IU

Child Liver

- **Amla berry:** ½ teaspoon daily
- **Barley grass juice powder:** ½ teaspoon daily
- **Ginger:** 1 cup of tea twice a day or freshly grated or juiced to taste daily
- **Lemon balm:** 1 dropperful daily
- **Magnesium glycinate:** 1 capsule or ¼ to ½ teaspoon daily
- **Milk thistle:** 6 tiny drops daily
- **Spirulina:** ½ teaspoon daily
- **Vitamin B$_{12}$ (as adenosylcobalamin with methylcobalamin):** 10 drops daily
- **Vitamin C:** 500 milligrams Ester-C or 1 teaspoon liquid liposomal daily
- **Zinc (as liquid zinc sulfate):** up to 6 small drops daily

Cirrhosis and Pericirrhosis

Taking supplements for cirrhosis depends on the severity of your case. Especially if you're in late-stage cirrhosis, consult with a physician before applying supplements.

- **Amla berry:** 2 teaspoons twice a day
- **Barley grass juice powder:** 2 teaspoons twice a day
- **Burdock root:** 1 cup of tea or 1 root freshly juiced twice a day
- **Chaga mushroom:** 1 teaspoon twice a day
- **Chicory root:** 1 cup of tea twice a day

- **CoQ$_{10}$:** 1 capsule twice a day
- **Glutathione:** 1 capsule or ½ teaspoon liquid daily
- **Hibiscus:** 1 cup of tea twice a day
- **Lemon balm:** 1 dropperful twice a day
- **MSM:** 1 capsule twice a day
- **NAC:** 1 capsule daily
- **Vitamin B$_{12}$ (as adenosylcobalamin with methylcobalamin):** 1 dropperful daily
- **Vitamin C:** 2,500 milligrams Ester-C or 1 tablespoon liquid liposomal twice a day

Constipation

- **Amla berry:** 2 teaspoons twice a day
- **Barley grass juice powder:** 1 teaspoon twice a day
- **Cat's claw:** 1 dropperful twice a day
- **Dandelion root tea:** 1 cup of tea twice a day
- **EPA and DHA (fish-free):** 1 capsule twice a day
- **Licorice root:** 1 dropperful daily or 1 cup of tea twice a day (two weeks on, two weeks off)
- **Magnesium glycinate:** 1 teaspoon of powder twice a day
- **Milk thistle:** 1 dropperful twice a day
- **Nettle leaf:** 1 dropperful or 1 cup of tea or 2 capsules twice a day

- **Peppermint:** 1 cup of tea twice a day
- **Rose hips:** 1 cup of tea twice a day
- **Vitamin C:** 4 500-milligram capsules Ester-C or 2 teaspoons liquid liposomal twice a day

Dark Under-Eye Circles

- **ALA:** 1 capsule daily
- **B-complex:** 1 teaspoon twice a day
- **Barley grass juice powder:** 1 teaspoon twice a day
- **Burdock root:** 1 cup of tea twice a day or 1 root freshly juiced daily
- **Dandelion root:** 1 cup of tea twice a day
- **Hibiscus:** 1 cup of tea twice a day
- **Licorice root:** 1 dropperful daily or 1 cup of tea twice a day (two weeks on, two weeks off)
- **Red clover:** 1 cup of tea or 1 dropperful twice a day
- **Spirulina:** 1 teaspoon twice a day
- **Turmeric:** 2 capsules twice a day
- **Vitamin B$_{12}$ (as adenosylcobalamin with methylcobalamin):** 1 dropperful twice a day
- **Vitamin C:** 4 500-milligram capsules Ester-C or 2 teaspoons liquid liposomal twice a day
- **Zinc (as liquid zinc sulfate):** up to 1 dropperful twice a day

Diabetes (Types 1, 1.5 [LADA], and 2) and Blood Sugar Imbalance

- **5-MTHF:** 1 capsule twice a day
- **Amla berry:** 2 teaspoons twice a day
- **Ashwagandha:** 1 dropperful twice a day
- **Barley grass juice powder:** 2 teaspoons twice a day
- **Chaga mushroom:** 2 teaspoons twice a day
- **Glutathione:** 1 capsule or 1 teaspoon liquid daily
- **Hibiscus:** 1 cup of tea twice a day
- **Lemon balm:** 2 dropperfuls or 1 cup of tea twice a day
- **L-lysine:** 2 500-milligram capsules twice a day
- **Nascent iodine:** 6 tiny drops daily
- **Nettle leaf:** 2 dropperfuls, 1 cup of tea, or 2 capsules twice a day
- **Rose hips:** 1 cup of tea twice a day
- **Schisandra berry:** 1 cup of tea twice a day
- **Turmeric:** 2 capsules twice a day
- **Spirulina:** 2 teaspoons twice a day
- **Vitamin C:** 4 500-milligram capsules Ester-C or 2 teaspoons liquid liposomal twice a day
- **Vitamin B$_{12}$ (as adenosylcobalamin with methylcobalamin):** 1 dropperful twice a day
- **Zinc (as liquid zinc sulfate):** up to 1 dropperful twice a day

Dirty Blood Syndrome

- **Amla berry:** 1 teaspoon twice a day

- **Barley grass juice powder:** 1 teaspoon twice a day

- **Burdock root:** 1 cup of tea or 1 root freshly juiced twice a day

- **Chicory root:** 1 cup of tea twice a day

- **Dandelion root:** 1 cup of tea twice a day

- **Milk thistle:** 1 dropperful twice a day

- **Nettle leaf:** 1 dropperful, 2 capsules, or 1 cup of tea twice a day

- **Red clover:** 1 cup of tea or 1 dropperful twice a day

- **Turmeric:** 2 capsules twice a day

- **Vitamin C:** 4 500-milligram capsules Ester-C or 2 teaspoons liquid liposomal twice a day

- **Yellow dock:** 1 cup of tea twice a day

Eczema and Psoriasis (including all skin conditions covered in Chapter 22)

- **5-MTHF:** 1 capsule daily

- **Barley grass juice powder:** 1 teaspoon twice a day

- **Cat's claw:** 1 dropperful twice a day

- **Chaga mushroom:** 1 teaspoon twice a day

- **Curcumin:** 1 capsule twice a day

- **EPA and DHA (fish-free):** 1 capsule twice a day

- **Lemon balm:** 2 dropperfuls twice a day or 1 cup of tea twice a day

- **Licorice root:** 1 dropperful daily (two weeks on, two weeks off)

- **L-lysine:** 4 500-milligram capsules twice a day

- **Mullein leaf:** 1 dropperful twice a day

- **Nettle leaf:** 1 dropperful, 1 cup of tea, or 2 capsules twice a day

- **Selenium:** 6 small drops or 1 capsule daily

- **Spirulina:** 1 teaspoon twice a day

- **Vitamin B$_{12}$ (as adenosylcobalamin with methylcobalamin):** 1 dropperful twice a day

- **Vitamin C:** 6 500-milligram capsules Ester-C or 1 tablespoon liquid liposomal twice a day

- **Zinc (as liquid zinc sulfate):** up to 1 dropperful twice a day

Emotional Liver and Mood Struggles

- Hibiscus: 1 cup of tea twice a day

- Lemon balm: 1 cup of tea or 2 dropperfuls twice a day

- Magnesium glycinate: 2 capsules twice a day

- Nettle leaf: 1 dropperful, 2 capsules, or 1 cup of tea twice a day

- Peppermint: 1 cup of tea twice a day

- Schisandra berry: 1 cup of tea twice a day

- Vitamin B_{12} (as adenosylcobalamin with methylcobalamin): 1 dropperful daily

- Vitamin C: 2 capsules or 1 teaspoon twice a day

- Vitamin D_3: 1,000 IU daily

- Zinc (as liquid zinc sulfate): up to 1 dropperful daily

Energy Issues and Fatigue

- 5-MTHF: 1 capsule daily

- Ashwagandha: 1 dropperful daily

- Barley grass juice powder: 2 teaspoons daily

- Chaga mushroom: 2 teaspoons daily

- Ginger: 1 cup of tea, 2 capsules, or freshly grated or juiced to taste daily

- Lemon balm: 2 dropperfuls daily

- Licorice root: 1 dropperful daily (two weeks on, two weeks off)

- Mullein leaf: 2 dropperfuls daily

- Nascent iodine: 6 tiny drops daily

- Oregon grape root: 1 dropperful daily

- Spirulina: 2 teaspoons daily

- Turmeric: 2 capsules daily

- Vitamin B_{12} (as adenosylcobalamin with methylcobalamin): 1 dropperful daily

- Vitamin C: 4 500-milligram capsules Ester-C or 2 teaspoons liquid liposomal daily

- Zinc (as liquid zinc sulfate): up to 1 dropperful daily

Fatty Liver and Sluggish Liver

- Aloe vera: 2 or more inches of fresh gel (skin removed) daily

- Amla berry: 2 teaspoons daily

- Burdock root: 1 cup of tea daily

- Cardamom: 1 dropperful daily

- Chicory root: 1 cup of tea daily

- Dandelion root: 1 cup of tea daily

- Ginger: 1 cup of tea, 2 capsules, or freshly grated or juiced to taste daily

- Milk thistle: 1 dropperful daily

- Spirulina: 3 teaspoons daily

- Yellow dock: 1 cup of tea daily

Gallbladder Infections

- **Cat's claw:** 2 dropperfuls twice a day
- **Ginger:** 1 cup of tea or 2 capsules twice a day or freshly grated or juiced to taste daily
- **Goldenseal:** 3 dropperfuls twice a day (two weeks on, two weeks off)
- **Lemon balm:** 3 dropperfuls or 1 cup of tea with 2 bags twice a day
- **Licorice root:** 1 dropperful twice a day (two weeks on, two weeks off)
- **Mullein leaf:** 2 dropperfuls twice a day
- **Oregon grape root:** 1 dropperful twice a day
- **Peppermint:** 1 cup of tea with 2 bags twice a day
- **Vitamin C:** 5 500-milligram capsules Ester-C twice a day or 1 tablespoon liquid liposomal daily
- **Zinc (as liquid zinc sulfate):** up to 1 dropperful twice a day

Gallstones

- **Cardamom:** 1 dropperful daily
- **Chicory root:** 1 cup of tea daily
- **Dandelion root:** 1 cup of tea daily
- **Ginger:** 1 cup of tea, 2 capsules, or freshly grated or juiced to taste daily
- **Hibiscus:** 1 cup of tea daily
- **Nettle leaf:** 1 cup of tea, 2 capsules, or 2 dropperfuls daily
- **Peppermint:** 1 cup of tea daily

- **Rose hips:** 1 cup of tea daily
- **Spirulina:** 2 teaspoons daily
- **Vitamin C:** 2 500-milligram capsules Ester-C or 1 teaspoon liquid liposomal twice a day

Gout

- **Amla berry:** 2 teaspoons daily
- **Barley grass juice powder:** 2 teaspoons daily
- **Cat's claw:** 1 dropperful twice a day
- **Chaga mushroom:** 2 teaspoons daily
- **Curcumin:** 2 capsules twice a day
- **EPA and DHA (fish-free):** 1 capsule daily
- **Lemon balm:** 2 dropperfuls or 1 cup of tea with 2 bags twice a day
- **L-lysine:** 3 500-milligram capsules twice a day
- **MSM:** 2 capsules twice a day
- **Nettle leaf:** 2 capsules, 2 dropperfuls, or 1 cup of tea with 2 bags twice day
- **Rose hips:** 1 cup of tea daily
- **Turmeric:** 2 capsules twice a day
- **Vitamin B$_{12}$ (as adenosylcobalamin with methylcobalamin):** 1 dropperful twice a day
- **Vitamin C:** 4 500-milligram capsules or 1 teaspoon liquid liposomal twice a day
- **Zinc (as liquid zinc sulfate):** up to 1 dropperful twice a day

Heart Palpitations

- 5-MTHF: 1 capsule daily
- Barley grass juice powder: 2 teaspoons daily
- Chaga mushroom: 2 teaspoons daily
- CoQ_{10}: 2 capsules daily
- Lemon balm: 3 dropperfuls daily
- Magnesium glycinate: 3 capsules daily
- Nascent iodine: 4 tiny drops daily
- Nettle leaf: 2 dropperfuls or 2 capsules daily
- Raspberry leaf: 1 cup of tea daily
- Spirulina: 2 teaspoons daily
- Vitamin B_{12} (as adenosylcobalamin with methylcobalamin): 1 dropperful daily
- Vitamin C: 4 500-milligram capsules Ester-C or 1 teaspoon liquid liposomal daily
- Zinc (as liquid zinc sulfate): up to 1 dropperful daily

Hepatitis

- Cat's claw: 1 dropperful twice a day
- Chaga: 1 teaspoon twice a day
- Eyebright: 1 dropperful twice a day
- Goldenseal: 2 dropperfuls twice a day (two weeks on, two weeks off)
- Lemon balm: 2 dropperfuls or 1 cup of tea with 2 bags twice a day

- Licorice root: 1 dropperful twice a day (two weeks on, two weeks off)
- Mullein leaf: 2 dropperfuls twice a day
- Vitamin C: 4 500-milligram capsules Ester-C or 1 teaspoon liquid liposomal twice a day
- Zinc (as liquid zinc sulfate): up to 2 dropperfuls twice a day

High Blood Pressure

- 5-MTHF: 1 capsule daily
- Ashwagandha: 1 dropperful daily
- B-complex: 1 capsule daily
- Barley grass juice powder: 2 teaspoons daily
- CoQ_{10}: 2 capsules daily
- EPA and DHA (fish-free): 1 capsule daily
- Lemon balm: 2 dropperfuls daily
- Milk thistle: 1 dropperful daily
- Magnesium glycinate: 4 capsules daily
- Spirulina: 2 teaspoons daily
- Turmeric: 2 capsules daily
- Vitamin B_{12} (as adenosylcobalamin with methylcobalamin): 1 dropperful daily
- Vitamin C: 6 500-milligram capsules Ester-C or 1 tablespoon liquid liposomal daily
- Zinc (as liquid zinc sulfate): up to 1 dropperful daily

High Cholesterol

- Aloe vera: 2 or more inches of fresh gel (skin removed) daily
- Amla berry: 2 teaspoons daily
- Barley grass juice powder: 2 teaspoons daily
- CoQ$_{10}$: 2 capsules daily
- Curcumin: 2 capsules daily
- EPA and DHA (fish-free): 1 capsule daily
- Ginger: 2 capsules, 1 cup of tea with 2 bags, or freshly grated or juiced to taste daily
- Milk thistle: 1 dropperful daily
- Peppermint: 1 cup of tea daily
- Spirulina: 2 teaspoons daily
- Vitamin B$_{12}$ (as adenosylcobalamin with methylcobalamin): 1 dropperful daily
- Vitamin C: 4 500-milligram capsules or 2 teaspoons liquid liposomal daily
- Zinc (as liquid zinc sulfate): up to 1 dropperful daily

Hormonal Problems

- Ashwagandha: 1 dropperful daily
- Barley grass juice powder: 2 teaspoons daily
- Hibiscus: 1 cup of tea with 2 bags daily
- Lemon balm: 2 dropperfuls daily
- Milk thistle: 1 dropperful daily
- Nascent iodine: 6 tiny drops daily
- Nettle leaf: 4 dropperfuls or 4 capsules daily
- Raspberry leaf: 1 cup of tea with 3 bags twice a day
- Schisandra berry: 1 cup of tea daily
- Spirulina: 2 teaspoons daily
- Vitamin B$_{12}$ (as adenosylcobalamin with methylcobalamin): 1 dropperful daily
- Vitamin C: 2 500-milligram capsules Ester-C or 1 teaspoon liquid liposomal daily

Hot Flashes

- Amla berry: 2 teaspoons daily

- Ashwagandha: 1 dropperful daily

- Chaga mushroom:
  2 teaspoons daily

- CoQ_{10}: 1 capsule daily

- Lemon balm: 2 dropperfuls or
  1 cup of tea with 2 bags daily

- Nascent iodine: 4 tiny drops daily

- Nettle leaf: 2 dropperfuls, 2
  capsules, or 1 cup of tea with
  2 bags daily

- Raspberry leaf: 1 cup of tea with
  2 bags or 2 dropperfuls daily

- Schisandra berry:
  2 dropperfuls daily

- Spirulina:
  2 teaspoons daily

- Vitamin B_{12} (as adenosylcobalamin
  with methylcobalamin):
  1 dropperful daily

- Vitamin C: 4 500-milligram
  capsules Ester-C or 1 teaspoon
  liquid liposomal daily

- Zinc (as liquid zinc sulfate):
  up to 1 dropperful daily

IBS

- Aloe vera: 2 or more inches of
  fresh gel (skin removed) daily

- Burdock root: 1 cup of tea daily

- Cat's claw: 1 dropperful daily

- Dandelion root: 1 cup of tea daily

- Ginger: 1 cup of tea, 2 capsules,
  or freshly grated or juiced to
  taste daily

- Hibiscus: 1 cup of tea daily

- Lemon balm: 1 dropperful or 1
  cup of tea daily

- Licorice root: 1 dropperful or 1
  cup of tea with 2 bags daily (two
  weeks on, two weeks off)

- Nettle leaf: 1 dropperful or 1 cup
  of tea daily

Inflammation

- 5-MTHF: 1 capsule daily

- Aloe vera: 2 or more inches of
  fresh gel (skin removed) daily

- Barley grass juice powder: 2
  teaspoons daily

- Cat's claw: 2 dropperfuls daily

- Chaga mushroom:
  2 teaspoons daily

- Curcumin: 3 capsules twice a day

- Lemon balm: 3 dropperfuls daily

- Licorice root: 1 dropperful daily
  (two weeks on, two weeks off)

- **L-lysine:** 4 500-milligram capsules twice a day

- **Magnesium glycinate:** 2 capsules daily

- **MSM:** 2 capsules daily

- **Mullein leaf:** 2 dropperfuls daily

- **Nascent iodine:** 4 tiny drops daily

- **Nettle leaf:** 3 capsules or 2 dropperfuls daily

- **Olive leaf:** 2 capsules or 1 dropperful daily

- **Spirulina:** 2 teaspoons daily

- **Turmeric:** 2 capsules daily

- **Vitamin B$_{12}$ (as adenosylcobalamin with methylcobalamin):** 1 dropperful twice a day

- **Vitamin C:** 6 500-milligram capsules Ester-C or 1 tablespoon liquid liposomal twice a day

- **Zinc (as liquid zinc sulfate):** up to 2 dropperfuls twice a day

Jaundice

Please note that while you read about babies' jaundice in Chapter 28, these are adult dosages.

- **Amla berry:** 1 teaspoon twice a day

- **Barley grass juice powder:** 1 teaspoon twice a day

- **Hibiscus:** 1 cup of tea twice a day

- **Lemon balm:** 1 dropperful twice a day

- **Nettle leaf:** 1 dropperful, 1 capsule, or 1 cup of tea twice a day

- **Peppermint:** 1 cup of tea twice a day

- **Red clover:** 1 cup of tea or 1 dropperful twice a day

- **Vitamin C:** 2 500-milligram capsules Ester-C or 1 teaspoon liquid liposomal twice a day

Liver Abscesses

- **Cat's claw:** 1 dropperful twice a day

- **Goldenseal:** 3 dropperfuls twice a day (three weeks on, two weeks off)

- **Lemon balm:** 4 dropperfuls twice a day

- **Mullein leaf:** 3 dropperfuls twice a day

- **Olive leaf:** 2 dropperfuls or 2 capsules twice a day

- **Oregon grape root:** 2 dropperfuls twice a day

- **Vitamin B$_{12}$ (as adenosylcobalamin with methylcobalamin):** 1 dropperful daily

- **Vitamin C:** 6 500-milligram capsules Ester-C or 1 tablespoon liquid liposomal twice a day

- **Zinc (as liquid zinc sulfate):** up to 2 dropperfuls twice a day

Liver Aging

All the supplements in this chapter help prevent liver aging. If it's a particular concern for you, consider these hand-picked ones:

- **Barley grass juice powder:** 1 teaspoon twice a day

- **Chaga mushroom:** 1 teaspoon twice a day

- **Curcumin:** 1 capsule twice a day

- **Glutathione:** 1 capsule daily

- **Nettle leaf:** 1 capsule or 1 dropperful twice a day

- **Spirulina:** 2 teaspoons twice a day

- **Vitamin B$_{12}$ (as adenosylcobalamin with methylcobalamin):** 1 dropperful twice a day

- **Vitamin C:** 1,000 milligrams Ester-C or 1 teaspoon liquid liposomal twice a day

- **Zinc (as liquid zinc sulfate):** up to 1 dropperful twice a day

Liver Cancer

- **ALA:** 1 capsule daily

- **Aloe vera:** 2 or more inches of fresh gel (skin removed) daily

- **Amla berry:** 2 teaspoons daily

- **Barley grass juice powder:** 2 teaspoons twice a day

- **Cat's claw:** 3 dropperfuls twice a day

- **Chaga mushroom:** 2 teaspoons twice a day

- **CoQ$_{10}$:** 1 capsule twice a day

- **Curcumin:** 3 capsules twice a day

- **Glutathione:** 1 capsule daily

- **Lemon balm:** 4 dropperfuls twice a day

- **Melatonin:** work up to 20 milligrams twice a day

- **Milk thistle:** 1 dropperful twice a day

- **Nascent iodine:** 6 tiny drops twice a day

- **Nettle leaf:** 4 capsules or 3 dropperfuls twice a day

- **Oregon grape root:** 1 dropperful twice a day

- **Rose hips:** 1 cup of tea twice a day

- **Selenium:** 1 dropperful or 1 capsule daily

- **Spirulina:** 2 teaspoons twice a day

- **Turmeric:** 3 capsules twice a day

- **Vitamin B$_{12}$ (as adenosylcobalamin with methylcobalamin):** 1 dropperful daily

- **Vitamin C:** 8 500-milligram capsules Ester-C or 1 ½ tablespoons liquid liposomal twice a day

- **Zinc (as liquid zinc sulfate):** up to 2 dropperfuls twice a day

Liver Insomnia

- **5-MTHF:** 1 capsule daily
- **Ashwagandha:** 1 dropperful daily
- **CoQ_{10}:** 1 capsule daily
- **Hibiscus:** 1 cup of tea with 2 bags daily
- **Lemon balm:** 4 dropperfuls or 2 cups of tea with 2 bags each daily
- **Licorice root:** 1 dropperful daily (two weeks on, two weeks off)
- **Magnesium glycinate:** 2 capsules daily
- **Melatonin:** work up to 20 milligrams daily
- **Vitamin B_{12} (as adenosylcobalamin with methylcobalamin):** 1 dropperful daily

Liver Scar Tissue

- **5-MTHF:** 1 capsule daily
- **ALA:** 1 capsule daily
- **Aloe vera:** 2 or more inches of fresh gel (skin removed) daily
- **B-complex:** 1 capsule daily
- **Barley grass juice powder:** 2 teaspoons daily
- **Cat's claw:** 2 dropperfuls daily
- **Chaga mushroom:** 2 teaspoons daily
- **Curcumin:** 3 capsules daily
- **L-lysine:** 4 500-milligram capsules daily
- **Milk thistle:** 1 dropperful daily
- **MSM:** 2 capsules daily
- **NAC:** 1 capsule daily

- **Nettle leaf:** 2 dropperfuls or 2 capsules daily
- **Spirulina:** 2 teaspoons daily
- **Turmeric:** 2 capsules daily
- **Vitamin B_{12} (as adenosylcobalamin with methylcobalamin):** 1 dropperful daily
- **Vitamin C:** 6 500-milligram capsules Ester-C or 1 tablespoon liquid liposomal twice a day
- **Zinc (as liquid zinc sulfate):** up to 1 dropperful twice a day

Liver Tumors and Cysts

- **ALA:** 1 capsule daily
- **Amla berry:** 2 teaspoons daily
- **Ashwagandha:** 2 dropperfuls daily
- **Barley grass juice powder:** 3 teaspoons daily
- **Burdock root:** 1 cup of tea twice a day or 1 root freshly juiced daily
- **Cat's claw:** 2 dropperfuls twice a day
- **Chaga mushroom:** 3 teaspoons daily
- **CoQ_{10}:** 2 capsules daily
- **Curcumin:** 2 capsules daily
- **EPA and DHA (fish-free):** 1 capsule daily
- **Glutathione:** 1 capsule or 1 teaspoon liquid daily
- **Hibiscus:** 1 cup of tea with 2 bags daily
- **Lemon balm:** 2 dropperfuls or 1 cup of tea with 2 bags daily

- **Melatonin:** work up to 20 milligrams daily

- **Nascent iodine:** 6 tiny drops daily

- **Raspberry leaf:** 1 cup of tea with 2 bags twice a day

- **Schisandra berry:** 1 cup of tea with 2 bags twice a day

- **Spirulina:** 2 teaspoons daily

- **Vitamin B$_{12}$ (as adenosylcobalamin with methylcobalamin):** 1 dropperful daily

- **Vitamin C:** 6 500-milligram capsules Ester-C or 1 tablespoon liquid liposomal twice a day

- **Vitamin D$_3$:** 2,000 IU daily

- **Zinc (as liquid zinc sulfate):** up to 2 dropperfuls daily

Liver Worms and Parasites

- **Black walnut:** 1 dropperful twice a day

- **Burdock root:** 1 cup of tea or 1 root freshly juiced twice a day

- **Cat's claw:** 3 dropperfuls twice a day

- **Chaga mushroom:** 2 teaspoons twice a day

- **Dandelion root:** 1 cup of tea twice a day

- **Eyebright:** 2 dropperfuls twice a day

- **Lemon balm:** 5 dropperfuls twice a day

- **Olive leaf:** 4 dropperfuls or 4 capsules twice a day

- **Oregon grape root:** 3 dropperfuls twice a day

- **Yellow dock:** 1 cup of tea twice a day

Methylation Problems

- **5-MTHF:** 1 capsule twice a day

- **B-complex:** 1 capsule twice a day

- **Barley grass juice powder:** 2 teaspoons twice a day

- **Glutathione:** 1 capsule or 1 teaspoon liquid twice a day

- **NAC:** 1 capsule daily

- **Selenium:** 1 capsule or 1 dropperful daily

- **Spirulina:** 2 teaspoons daily

- **Vitamin B$_{12}$ (as adenosylcobalamin with methylcobalamin):** 1 dropperful twice a day

- **Vitamin C:** 4 500-milligram capsules Ester-C or 2 teaspoons liquid liposomal twice a day

Mystery Hunger

- **5-MTHF:** 1 capsule daily
- **Barley grass juice powder:** 2 teaspoons daily
- **Cardamom:** 1 dropperful daily
- **Chicory root:** 1 cup of tea daily
- **Ginger:** 1 cup of tea, 2 capsules, or freshly grated or juiced to taste daily
- **Licorice root:** 1 dropperful daily (two weeks on, two weeks off)
- **Spirulina:** 1 tablespoon daily
- **Vitamin B$_{12}$ (as adenosylcobalamin with methylcobalamin):** 1 dropperful daily

PANDAS

- **Cat's claw:** 4 drops twice a day
- **Eyebright:** 4 drops twice a day
- **Goldenseal:** 10 drops twice a day (two weeks on, two weeks off)
- **Lemon balm:** 10 drops twice a day
- **Licorice root:** 10 drops twice a day (two weeks on, two weeks off)
- **Mullein leaf:** 10 drops twice day
- **Olive leaf:** 10 drops twice a day
- **Spirulina:** 1 teaspoon daily
- **Vitamin B$_{12}$ (as adenosylcobalamin with methylcobalamin):** 10 drops daily
- **Vitamin C:** 2 500-milligram capsules Ester-C or 1 teaspoon liquid liposomal twice a day
- **Zinc (as liquid zinc sulfate):** up to 6 small drops twice a day

Raynaud's Syndrome

- **5-MTHF:** 1 capsule daily
- **Amla berry:** 2 teaspoons daily
- **Ashwagandha:** 1 dropperful daily
- **Barley grass juice powder:** 2 teaspoons daily
- **Cat's claw:** 1 dropperful daily
- **Chaga mushroom:** 2 teaspoons daily
- **Lemon balm:** 2 dropperfuls daily
- **Licorice root:** 1 dropperful daily (two weeks on, two weeks off)
- **L-lysine:** 6 500-milligram capsules daily
- **Nettle leaf:** 2 dropperfuls or 2 capsules daily
- **Olive leaf:** 2 dropperfuls or 2 capsules daily
- **Spirulina:** 2 teaspoons daily
- **Vitamin B$_{12}$ (as adenosylcobalamin with methylcobalamin):** 1 dropperful daily
- **Vitamin C:** 6 500-milligram capsules Ester-C or 1 tablespoon liquid liposomal daily
- **Zinc (as liquid zinc sulfate):** up to 2 dropperfuls daily

SAD

- 5-MTHF: 1 capsule daily
- Ashwagandha: 1 dropperful daily
- B-complex: 1 capsule daily
- Barley grass juice powder: 2 teaspoons daily
- EPA and DHA (fish-free): 1 capsule daily
- Lemon balm: 2 dropperfuls daily
- Melatonin: 5 milligrams daily
- Nascent iodine: 6 tiny drops daily
- Red clover: 1 cup of tea daily
- Spirulina: 1 tablespoon daily
- Turmeric: 2 capsules daily
- Vitamin B$_{12}$ (as adenosylcobalamin with methylcobalamin): 2 dropperfuls daily
- Vitamin C: 6 500-milligram capsules Ester-C or 2 teaspoons liquid liposomal daily
- Vitamin D$_3$: 2,000 IU daily
- Zinc (as liquid zinc sulfate): up to 2 dropperfuls daily

SIBO

- Aloe vera: 2 or more inches of fresh gel (skin removed) daily
- Barley grass juice powder: 2 teaspoons daily
- Burdock root: 1 cup of tea twice a day or 1 root freshly juiced daily
- Cat's claw: 2 dropperfuls twice a day
- Chaga mushroom: 2 teaspoons daily
- Ginger: 2 capsules or 1 cup of tea twice a day or freshly grated or juiced to taste daily
- Goldenseal: 4 dropperfuls twice a day (two weeks on, two weeks off)
- Lemon balm: 4 dropperfuls twice a day
- Licorice root: 1 dropperful twice a day (two weeks on, two weeks off)
- Mullein leaf: 4 dropperfuls twice a day
- Olive leaf: 3 dropperfuls or 3 capsules twice a day
- Oregon grape root: 2 dropperfuls twice a day
- Spirulina: 2 teaspoons daily
- Turmeric: 2 capsules daily
- Vitamin B$_{12}$ (as adenosylcobalamin with methylcobalamin): 1 dropperful twice a day
- Vitamin C: 4 500-milligram capsules Ester-C or 2 teaspoons liquid liposomal twice a day
- Zinc (as liquid zinc sulfate): up to 1 dropperful twice a day

Sinus Infections

- Amla berry: 2 teaspoons twice a day
- Chaga mushroom: 2 teaspoons daily
- CoQ$_{10}$: 1 capsule daily
- Ginger: 2 cups of tea or 4 capsules twice a day or freshly grated or juiced to taste daily
- Goldenseal: 4 dropperfuls twice a day
- Hibiscus: 2 cups of tea daily
- Lemon balm: 4 dropperfuls twice a day
- L-lysine: 4 500-milligram capsules twice a day
- Mullein leaf: 4 dropperfuls twice a day
- NAC: 1 capsule twice a day
- Olive leaf: 3 dropperfuls twice a day
- Oregon grape root: 2 dropperfuls twice a day
- Peppermint: 1 cup of tea with 2 bags twice a day
- Rose hips: 2 cups of tea daily
- Turmeric: 3 capsules twice a day
- Vitamin C: 6 500-milligram capsules Ester-C or 1 tablespoon liquid liposomal twice a day
- Vitamin D$_3$: 1,000 IU daily
- Zinc (as liquid zinc sulfate): up to 3 dropperfuls twice a day

Strep Throat, Viral Sore Throat, and Mystery Sore Throat

- Eyebright: 2 dropperfuls twice a day
- Ginger: 2 cups of tea or 4 capsules twice a day or freshly grated or juiced to taste daily
- Goldenseal: 5 dropperfuls twice a day
- Lemon balm: 4 dropperfuls twice a day
- Licorice root: 1 dropperful twice a day (two weeks on, two weeks off)
- L-lysine: 4 500-milligram capsules twice a day
- Mullein leaf: 3 dropperfuls twice a day
- Olive leaf: 3 dropperfuls twice a day
- Rose hips: 2 cups of tea twice a day
- Vitamin C: 8 500-milligram capsules Ester-C or 1½ tablespoons liquid liposomal twice a day
- Zinc (as liquid zinc sulfate): up to 3 dropperfuls twice a day

UTIs, Yeast Infections, and BV

- **Aloe vera:** 2 or more inches of fresh gel (skin removed) daily

- **Amla berry:** 2 teaspoons twice a day

- **Cat's claw:** 2 dropperfuls twice a day

- **Chaga mushroom:** 2 teaspoons daily

- **D-mannose:** 1 teaspoon powder four times a day

- **Goldenseal:** 4 dropperfuls twice a day

- **Hibiscus:** 2 cups of tea daily

- **Lemon balm:** 4 dropperfuls twice a day

- **Mullein leaf:** 3 dropperfuls twice a day

- **Olive leaf:** 2 dropperfuls twice a day

- **Oregon grape root:** 1 dropperful twice a day

- **Rose hips:** 2 cups of tea daily

- **Vitamin C:** 6 500-milligram capsules Ester-C or 1 tablespoon liquid liposomal twice a day

- **Zinc (as liquid zinc sulfate):** up to 2 dropperfuls twice a day

Varicose and Spider Veins

- **ALA:** 1 capsule daily

- **Barley grass juice powder:** 2 teaspoons daily

- **Burdock root:** 1 cup of tea or 1 root freshly juiced daily

- **Dandelion root:** 1 cup of tea daily

- **EPA and DHA (fish-free):** 1 capsule daily

- **Lemon balm:** 2 dropperfuls daily

- **Milk thistle:** 1 dropperful daily

- **MSM:** 2 capsules daily

- **Nettle leaf:** 2 capsules or 2 dropperfuls daily

- **Red clover:** 1 cup of tea daily

- **Schisandra berry:** 1 cup of tea daily

- **Spirulina:** 1 teaspoon daily

- **Vitamin B$_{12}$ (as adenosylcobalamin with methylcobalamin):** 1 dropperful daily

- **Vitamin C:** 4 500-milligram capsules Ester-C or 2 teaspoons liquid liposomal daily

Weight Gain

- **5-MTHF:** 1 capsule daily
- **Aloe vera:** 2 or more inches of fresh gel (skin removed) daily
- **Ashwagandha:** 1 dropperful daily
- **Barley grass juice powder:** 2 teaspoons daily
- **Chaga mushroom:** 2 teaspoons daily
- **Lemon balm:** 2 dropperfuls daily
- **Nascent iodine:** 6 tiny drops daily
- **Nettle leaf:** 2 dropperfuls or 2 capsules daily
- **Raspberry leaf:** 1 cup of tea with 2 bags daily
- **Schisandra berry:** 1 cup of tea daily
- **Spirulina:** 2 teaspoons daily
- **Vitamin B$_{12}$ (as adenosylcobalamin with methylcobalamin):** 1 dropperful daily
- **Vitamin C:** 6 500-milligram capsules Ester-C or 1 tablespoon liquid liposomal daily
- **Zinc (as liquid zinc sulfate):** up to 1 dropperful daily

CHAPTER 38

Liver Rescue 3:6:9

Imagine a child standing on a diving board for the very first time. Feet gripping the plank, arms reaching out for balance, eyes fixed on the ripples beneath her, that child needs a chance to prepare herself before taking the plunge. While lingering forever won't help, neither will rushing it. Only after she's had a moment to acclimate to the challenge of letting go will she be ready to jump, on the count of three, into the water below.

Now, what would happen if some well-meaning adult, convinced the child was hesitating out of unhealthy fear, came along and gave her a shove? Tumbling off the board, the child wouldn't be able to brace herself or even hold her breath as she plummeted into the pool. She'd come up sputtering—water up her nose or even down her windpipe—struggling to figure out what had happened as she also struggled to keep her head above water and paddle to the edge. There, she'd have a coughing attack and maybe even an anxiety attack, having been robbed of the chance to prepare herself and adapt mentally, physically, and spiritually to the transition.

It's not just how a child would react; nobody of any age, the most accomplished diver included, would want to be pushed before they were ready. Anyone would climb out of the pool with a trust issue, from then on looking behind themselves every time they stepped on a diving board.

For the liver, embarking on a cleanse is like jumping off a diving board. Like any leap we take, it can be wonderfully freeing—a chance to lighten its load and almost fly—or, if it's not done right, the liver can nearly drown from being shoved into the deep end with no advance warning.

The liver doesn't like to be forced into anything. It doesn't like to be forced into processing rich foods; it doesn't like to be forced into dealing with an overload of toxins. Still, it soldiers on with these tasks in our daily lives. It draws a line at being forced to purge according to man-made ideals of how the organ should function. As much as your liver has been waiting for a moment of relief from its daily grind, it's much like cleaning out your home: If someone barged in your door and forced you to start throwing out your belongings nonstop for a week with no chance to get ready beforehand, you'd revolt. You'd purposely hide some items in order to spare the garbage collectors from picking up

500 pounds of trash. Or maybe you'd send all your junk down your building's trash chute only to bring much of it back up to your apartment when you realized that it had created an unsafe situation in the street when the dumpster downstairs overflowed. Either way, in the end, you'd be exhausted, disgruntled, and not at all happy with the week's results.

As I've mentioned, many cleanses put the liver in a position it doesn't like. They're the pushy diving instructors or the taskmaster cleaning specialists. They don't operate from a true understanding of how the liver works and what it needs. In response, the liver goes into shock or rebellion. In some cases, if it's forced to release toxins at a rate that's not healthy for you or itself, the liver will close its doors, purposely holding on to toxins to protect you—working harder than ever in the process, at the exact time it's meant to catch a break. If the liver must release an overabundance of toxins against its will because it doesn't have the strength to close certain floodgates, your blood can fill with so many toxins that the liver has to sponge them all back up feverishly to protect you, so they never actually get a chance to leave your body. Cleanses that operate from a harsh purge mentality often accomplish the opposite of what was intended. Not to mention that they often create very cranky, disgruntled cleansers, since their livers aren't truly releasing what's holding them back. Even if they don't realize it, that's affecting their mood.

The liver wants to let go. It wants relief from its daily overload of fats and from a lifetime of pathogenic activity and toxin exposure. Your liver wants you to get relief from your symptoms and conditions—and their underlying causes— so you can finally experience the clear skin or mood stabilization or weight loss or lifting of fatigue you've been seeking. It wants a chance

to scrub away its accumulated gunk and be shiny and new again—all so it can lead you to better health. What it doesn't want is to pursue any of this through unsafe or unnatural means.

If you've been reading through this book having realization after realization about how your liver functions and what it's up against, seeing how much of your overall health depends on the state of your liver, and wondering how on earth to take back years of unintentional damage to the organ, you've come to the right place. This, finally, is the answer.

It's all about working *with* your liver. To cleanse properly and effectively, your liver needs finesse and care. It needs a deep understanding of how it functions; it doesn't want to be treated like a machine. That's why this chapter's Liver Rescue Morning (a quick, easy cleanse you can try anytime) and the Liver Rescue 3:6:9 (a nine-day liver-healing plan like no other) are so powerful: they work with what the liver wants and needs, not an arbitrary guesstimation of how it should operate.

With the Liver Rescue Morning, you get a chance to give your liver the stability it's after in your day-to-day life. Try the plan for a few days on its own, a few weeks before or after the Liver Rescue 3:6:9, or incorporate it into your everyday routine, and your liver will be singing your praises. It's an incredible chance for your liver to keep up with its regular functions instead of always playing catch-up, so that it can help you stay healthy.

With the Liver Rescue 3:6:9, your liver finally gets the rejuvenation it deserves, freed up first to prepare itself, then to start to release at a measured pace, then to enter a deep cleaning mode that can offer you relief in so many ways. Like the child on the diving board, your liver needs compassion and support, and that's exactly what the Liver Rescue 3:6:9 has to offer.

Unlike some cleanses, the Liver Rescue Morning and the Liver Rescue 3:6:9 won't set your liver back. No other plan is this attuned to your liver's true needs: to press pause on the daily onslaught of modern life, to unburden itself of the debris that's weighed it down for so long, and to let go and reset on its own timetable. Combined, these two techniques, which you can turn to again and again when your liver needs relief, are the ultimate kindness to your liver—a kindness that your liver will repay a hundredfold with renewed health and vitality.

FOOD BELIEF SYSTEMS

Have you ever had an experience where you were trying to do a job and someone who was supposed to be on your team kept getting in the way? Whatever that job might have been, whether at school, work, home, or in the community, whatever you were trying to accomplish, were you up against a doubter, a Judas, someone who couldn't help but cause conflict? Did it interfere with your venture, task, or responsibility? Even if you could get some of your work done, did you feel hampered, limited, held back from finishing your real job? That's how the liver feels when we fight against it with methods that it doesn't like.

Your liver is a highly intuitive organ. As we've looked at in this book, it learns your patterns and anticipates your needs. It's also extremely responsive to what you think and how you feel. It can sense if you're at odds with it. So if you're trying to push it, the liver will pick up on that conflict between the job it knows you want it to perform and the way you're going about doing it. Not only does your liver need the physical chance to prepare for a cleanse; it also needs your thoughts and emotions aligned.

Part of what's limiting about many other approaches to liver cleansing is that they're built around theoretical food belief systems that take us out of alignment. When any sort of eating plan is developed within a rigid viewpoint about what fuels and heals the body, there's a good chance it fails to allow for the bigger picture. That's because it's a human viewpoint, and we all know how tough being human can be sometimes. We do our best to understand the world and make decisions based on what we think the facts are, and then more information comes along later—and we either shut it out to avoid discomfort, or we shift our perspective, only to readjust it again and again throughout our lives as more and more information comes to light. In any given moment, we can be guaranteed that we don't understand the situation as fully as possible. As human beings, we're in a constant state of discovery, which means we're in a constant state of not knowing for sure. There's always more on the horizon.

That's why I rely on Spirit for all of the health information I share. If it were me, Anthony, trying to figure out the best plan for my liver, I'd find every argument out there convincing. I'd be just as likely as the next guy to settle on what seems like the prevailing wisdom, only to find out later that I'd done my health a disservice by containing my thinking within that box. My life's purpose is to spare you from guessing about what's best for your health—so that you don't lose years to health belief systems that only hold you back. With Spirit's information, it's not about a belief system or viewpoint or opinion or theory or trend or any other earthly method of evaluating the world. Spirit only deals in truths: truths about how the body works, how symptoms and illness develop, and what it takes to heal—truths that, for the most part, haven't been weighed or measured by science yet. Spirit does not choose one belief system over another, ousting or elevating any particular mode of thinking. Spirit cuts straight to the heart of the matter: what's right for you.

Remember this if you're coming to this chapter married to a particular way of thinking about food, cleansing, or what the liver needs. Whether you believe that fasting until dinner and then eating a high-protein meal is the answer to resetting the body, that fruit sugar feeds fatty liver, or that detoxing is fake, you may find that you need to shed your belief system to move forward. If, on the other hand, you're wary of food rules, and you're worried that the Liver Rescue Morning and the Liver Rescue 3:6:9 form one more plan with an agenda, you can shed your concern. This is not a propaganda diet. This is not yet one more competing concept in the crowd, recycling and repackaging ideas you've heard a million times before.

Or maybe you're new to reading about health. You haven't been on the merry-go-round of repackaged information that leaves people on a continual search for more. If that's you, you have a unique opportunity to keep an open heart about what's right for you.

This is about you and your liver, period. What your liver needs is for you to be a cooperative member of the team. Your liver needs to know that you won't shove it off the diving board because you subscribe to a particular school of thought.

You're not supposed to feel like you've been brought down to the depths of hell on a cleanse. For one, that puts your adrenals—and, in turn, your liver—through too much. When you go through one of the super-intense cleanses out there, you're running on adrenaline: your adrenals flood your body with excess adrenaline to balance the chaos, which forces your liver to mop it all up to protect you—going against your very plan of detoxing, given that corrosive excess adrenaline was one of the factors that already caused some liver problems in the first place.

While fasting has its place, the Liver Rescue Morning and the Liver Rescue 3:6:9 are not fasts. That's because you don't need a fast to reset your liver. (You especially don't need a *dry* fast for your liver. If you're trying to get better from any sort of symptom or condition, eliminating both foods and liquids will not spur healing. Water and juice fasting have their place in the world of healing. Dry fasting doesn't.) Not only can fasts result in rapid detoxification that's overwhelming for many people; they're also impractical much of the time. You may need to be able to stay on the treadmill of life while also being able to flush out your liver and heal; not everyone can stop everything and take a break. A liver cleanse needs to both work and work for you.

Which is why the Liver Rescue Morning and the Liver Rescue 3:6:9 are here for you. Saving your adrenals, filling you up with delicious and nourishing fare, and cleansing your liver more effectively than any protocol you've ever tried, they'll take you outside the box of any food belief system that's held you back in the past. Finally able to work together with your liver, you'll be aligned and in harmony like never before.

LIVER RESCUE MORNING

At night, your liver goes to sleep at the same time you do. It gets in a few hours of rest, and then, around three or four in the morning (the precise time is different for everyone), it starts to wake up and get back to work. Your liver likes this period while you're still asleep; it's like being the first one up in the house before the chaos of the day begins. Your liver knows this peace means you won't be consuming heavy foods or drinking an espresso or experiencing adrenaline bursts from an emotional or dramatic event, any of which can force the organ to drop everything and deal with the situation at hand. (While your dreams may trigger adrenaline, dreams are also healing, and the spurts don't last long enough to harm the liver.) Instead, your morning sleep hours give your liver catch-up time: a chance to scrub up messes, collect any junk from the day, and take the trash to the curb. When you wake, you give yourself a huge healing advantage if you tap into the liver's normal, God-given cleansing functions—and that's what the Liver Rescue Morning is all about.

First of all, your liver wants you to get hydrated upon waking. When you get up, your blood is dirty with all those toxins and other waste that your liver has discarded during its early-morning shift. If you don't flush out the waste by getting hydrated, your liver is forced to reabsorb it and you can be prevented from making progress with your healing. If you're familiar with my work, then you've heard me recommend drinking lemon or lime water, celery juice, or cucumber juice on an empty stomach in the morning. Flushing out the bloodstream is one major reason why. Never underestimate the power of this. It's more potent than anyone knows.

There's more: hydrating when you wake also jumpstarts the liver to continue detoxifying—if you know how to safeguard the detox process. When your body is in need of healing, your liver wants you to give it that chance to keep cleaning up during the morning, rather than being forced to switch into fat-digesting mode. Do you ever say to yourself, "If only I could get up early and launch straight into work without interruptions, I'd really be on top of my life," whether that work is your job, your household to-do list, or your healing protocol? That's how your liver feels. It loves to get special morning focus time. The moment you consume radical fats (foods like nuts and nut butters, seeds, oil, avocado, coconut, eggs, bacon, milk, cheese, butter, yogurt, whey protein powder, turkey, chicken, sausage, ham, and more), it gets interrupted, and detoxing stops. Your liver switches over to producing bile to digest the fats, and from then on it's focused on its other business of the day. The detox window closes, and the moment of opportunity disappears.

With the Liver Rescue Morning, you keep the detox window open. You support your liver so it can stay in balance and keep up with daily life. Any time you incorporate this easy cleanse into your day, you help it renew its cells so that it—and you—can be healthier in the future.

What *is* the Liver Rescue Morning? How do you do it? When life gets busy and overwhelming, all you need to do is follow these two guidelines:

- Hydrate well, especially first thing in the morning

- Don't consume radical fats before lunchtime

That's it. You'll still eat—eat throughout the whole morning, if you want—just skip foods that contain fat, and also make sure you're getting plenty of liquids. There's a lot you can do to enhance the morning's health effects, which we'll discuss in a moment. The basis of the Liver Rescue Morning, though, is very simple, and it's those two bullet points you can come back to again and again. When you're having one of those days where your head is swimming from too much to take care of, know that getting through the morning accomplishing those two points—hydration and avoiding fats—is a triumph. A big triumph!

People don't get enough credit for taking care of their health. They're taught to put so much ahead of their own well-being, which means that when they take steps to heal, they can feel almost guilty about it, like it's not real work. They can feel like taking time to go to the farmers' market, or to make juice or cut up fruit or order their supplements, isn't as productive or important as if they were using that time to send e-mails or pay bills or check off other boxes on their to-do lists. Don't let yourself fall into the trap of thinking that caring for yourself doesn't matter. Know that every step you take to heal has great meaning. When you work on getting your liver in shape, even by doing something as simple as drinking lemon water first thing and skipping fats until lunchtime, it doesn't just make your life better. It matters on a larger scale: It heals your liver. It strengthens your liver's immune system. It helps rid you of the poisons that create the illnesses and symptoms in this book. It means you can live a better, more fulfilling life, which starts a chain reaction as others witness your healing. That's profound; it can change the world. So let any seemingly little thing you do for your liver feel like a big accomplishment in your life.

What if you want to supercharge your Liver Rescue Morning? Well, let's talk more about hydration. In *Life-Changing Foods*, I wrote about the two types of water contained in fruits and vegetables: *hydrobioactive water* and *cofactor water*. The first type holds life-giving nutrients to support your physical health and hydrate your cells better than any drink of plain water can. A squeeze of lime or some cucumber slices added to a glass of water can awaken and activate it, making the water that much more beneficial. Coconut water, aloe water, smoothies, and fresh fruit and vegetable juices are also enormously hydrating and therefore good for flushing out the bloodstream, as are water-rich foods such as melons, apples, cucumbers, celery, grapes, oranges, tangerines, berries, pears, cherries, apricots, peaches, nectarines, and papayas. Adding these types of foods and beverages to your morning is a very special way to assist your liver with its job.

There's an emotional advantage, too. The second type of living water in produce, cofactor water, has nutrients that specifically feed you on a soul level, so a morning of hydration helps you find mental and spiritual support at the same time it gives you physical relief. (You'll find more on living water in *Life-Changing Foods*.)

Now, what about protein? you may ask. With all these fruits and vegetables filling up your morning, isn't a key component missing? If you're not eating your almond butter smoothie or yogurt bowl or avocado toast or strips of bacon or egg-white omelet for breakfast, how are you supposed to power yourself through the morning? These are very valid questions, since so much food advice points to protein as the morning Holy Grail.

This is one of those times when we need to consider what your liver truly needs and shed any belief system that keeps us from taking care of it. First of all, fruits and vegetables do contain amino acids and protein that greatly aid us with our health—in fact, the best, most bioavailable and assimilable protein in the world comes from leafy greens. What we need to look out for during the Liver Rescue Morning are foods *high* in protein, because as we looked at in Chapter 35, the truth is that almost all high-protein sources are also high in fat. So if you're starting the day with egg whites, a nut-butter smoothie, or turkey sausage because you believe in protein above all else, you're also stopping your liver's detox process. That's okay; that's your choice.

You just need to know that's the choice you're making, so that if you run into trouble later with symptoms holding you back in life, you also know one of the changes you can make to help yourself heal: saving your servings of protein for later in the day. Nuts, seeds, avocado, coconut, whey protein powder, yogurt, kefir, milk, butter, eggs, cheese, smoked salmon, bacon, sausage—these common breakfast ingredients don't serve your liver during its morning cleanse phase. Even lean, grass-fed, pasture-raised, local proteins, because of their fat content, will hold back your healing if you eat them in the morning. Remember: high-protein foods have a calorie source, and that source is fat.

We think we're supposed to start the day with protein because that's supposed to help us feel full and fuel us for hours on end. Truth is, feeling full all morning can be deceptive. Regardless of how full your stomach is, regardless of whether you have an appetite or not, your blood sugar is going to drop an hour and a half to two hours after eating or even sooner. For many with weakened livers or other sensitivities such as neurological symptoms, blood sugar could drop after 45 minutes. That's why grazing is so critical to healing. If your blood sugar drops and your liver's glucose reserves are low to nonexistent like most people's are, your adrenals are going to be forced to produce excess adrenaline to compensate—corrosive adrenaline that wears out your adrenals and strains your liver and nervous system. So it can actually be helpful when you feel hungry every couple of hours because it's a signal to have a little snack and replenish your blood sugar.

Fullness is also not a guarantee of a high-protein morning. I've spoken to plenty of people who said they felt constantly hungry on a high-protein diet. As we looked at in Chapter 13, that nagging hunger happens when you're not getting enough glucose, either because you're not consuming enough of it in the first place or because the continually high levels of fats you're consuming are blocking your proper glucose absorption and storage. A morning that avoids radical fats and focuses on fresh, glucose-rich fruits, on the other hand, gives your liver a chance to collect and store the precious sugars it needs to keep your body running. For some, it may take time to fill the empty glucose and glycogen storage banks inside the liver and brain, so it's critical to have patience if fruit doesn't have you feeling full from the get-go.

If you're used to eating dense, rich, or heavy food in the mornings, don't fear the Liver Rescue Morning. Remember this: skipping fats does not mean skipping breakfast! You still get to eat, and you get to eat well as you're getting well. So many people have told me that switching over to a morning focused on hydration, mineral salts, and high-quality glucose has left them more satisfied than ever. The nutrients that you're delivering to your liver and nervous system with water-rich fruits and vegetables have a powerful effect. So does having license to eat more. When you're fueling yourself on green juices, smoothies, apples, melons, oranges, papayas, and other fruits, you don't need to limit your portions the way you do when bacon is your breakfast food—you get to eat to your heart's content and then eat again a couple hours later when your blood sugar needs another boost. In late morning, you can even go for some steamed potatoes, sweet potatoes, or winter squash for a really satisfying, glucose-rich, liver-healing snack. Chapter 39, "Liver Rescue Recipes," will give you more ideas for good Liver Rescue Morning breakfast items and snacks.

Finally, it's a good idea to avoid caffeine and processed foods during your Liver Rescue Morning. If you can skip these items on those mornings when you're trying to give your liver a break, you will be doing your health a huge favor.

The Liver Rescue Morning is not only the best first step you can take in transforming the health of your liver. It's the best next step and the step after that. As you'll see in the following section, every day of the Liver Rescue 3:6:9 includes the Liver Rescue Morning; it's that foundational. If you want, you can make this mini-cleanse a constant in your life, choosing to give your liver a vacation every morning, whether you're on the Liver Rescue 3:6:9 or not, after a lifetime of overloading it. If you prefer, you can use it like a maintenance tool in your back pocket, pulling it out whenever you feel your liver needs a tune-up. What you can count on, no matter how you choose to use it, is that it's not one of those fad ideas that will fall out of usefulness in 1 year or 10 or even 100. That's because the Liver Rescue Morning is not simply an idea. It's not a theory. It's not a trend. It's a certainty that taps into the true nature of how your liver works and what it needs to thrive. Turn to it when you're looking for a little help, or turn to it in your greatest hour of need. No matter what, for the rest of your life, this Liver Rescue Morning will be there for you.

MONO EATING

If you're really struggling digestively and you have serious hypersensitivities, you may not feel ready to try the Liver Rescue 3:6:9 that we're about to cover. Instead, you may want to try a technique I've recommended for decades called *mono eating*, in which you eat snacks and meals of only one food at a time. (The *mono* here refers to "one," not mononucleosis.) For example, a day or more of eating only bananas and celery juice can be extremely helpful for people who react very easily with food-related symptoms. You could do a day of only papaya and celery juice. I've seen steamed potatoes (though not sweet potatoes) and celery juice all day serve as one of the better options for people who have a lot of unfriendly bacteria in their guts or whose intestinal tracts have been injured by food poisoning or stomach flu. You can even extend your mono eating for weeks or months, until you recover your liver and intestinal tract.

Mono eating is not for everyone. It's for people who have had certain toxins created by certain viruses within the liver or who've gone through other digestive hardships that have given them unique intestinal and nervous system sensitivities. The nerves attached to the intestinal walls can become hypersensitive and contribute to symptoms such as anxiety, bloating, and cramping in addition to extreme discomfort when food passes through the digestive tract. For this group, mono eating can be tremendously helpful.

It even saved my own life when I was a child suffering from food poisoning. You may remember that story from *Medical Medium*. Spirit recommended that I mono-eat pears, and they brought me back to life. Ever since, as one of the original creators of the mono eating way many decades ago, I've recommended the approach and witnessed thousands recover from hypersensitivities with this technique.

Over the years, others have learned about this concept, though that doesn't mean they know why someone becomes sensitive in the first place. From this book, you've discovered that a viral issue in the liver can lead to neurotoxins inside the intestinal lining—which no one out there knows—and that excess adrenaline can make those nerves hypersensitive as well, plus you've read about how food sensitivities can develop. With that knowledge, you're not stuck mono eating forever. While it's a technique that can help you greatly right now, you also have a clear sense of your healing path—how you got here and how to move forward.

LIVER RESCUE 3:6:9

What do you get when you take all the benefits of the Liver Rescue Morning and raise them to a whole new level, and then the next level, and then the ultimate level? You get the Liver Rescue 3:6:9, a nine-day eating plan made up of three-day increments that gradually adjust your liver to letting go. Whereas the Liver Rescue Morning on its own is about keeping up with daily life, the Liver Rescue 3:6:9 is about digging deeper. It's the plan to turn to if you're struggling with your health, stuck with any of the symptoms or conditions we examined in Parts II and III, concerned with prevention, or want to make up for those times in your life when you didn't know how to care for your liver. It's the key that unlocks getting better.

The Liver Rescue 3:6:9 begins with a three-day preparation phase, which I call *The 3*, and this is integral. You won't serve yourself by skipping ahead to the plans for the later days because your liver needs this gear-up time to benefit from everything that's to follow.

During the next three days, when you're in *The 6*, the internal cleansing begins. This is when your liver gets to unpack some of its old "storage bins" of toxins, fats, and viral waste matter it's been holding for months or years, reaching more deeply than it gets to in your normal life.

And during the final three days, when you're in *The 9*, your liver gets to let go, sending multitudes of troublemakers into your bloodstream for delivery out of your body. It's the stage that completes the Liver Rescue 3:6:9 and the

stage that helps you finally move the needle on your health.

The number structure of this cleanse is not arbitrary. Anatomically and physiologically, the liver runs on threes, with many pockets of cells inside the liver grouped in round-pointed triangles. Liver lobules are in the shapes of hexagons, which medical research and science do know. (The six-sided lobule is a reminder of our mortal existence, because the liver is a key, critical aspect of a living, breathing human body. Lobules are not seven-sided, because the number seven represents everything outside the human body.) The liver also runs on an undiscovered nine-heartbeat cycle: with every nine beats, enough blood runs through the liver to bring in a fresh batch of nutrients and flush out a bundle of waste. All of this means that your liver communicates and resonates with threes, sixes, and nines on a larger scale, too, just as you read about in regard to cell renewal in Chapter 34, "Liver Myths Debunked." Similarly to how your liver anticipates your indulgence patterns (like cocktails and fried foods every Friday night) so that it can protect you and save your life, your liver also reads the signals of when you're offering it true assistance. When you give your liver relief for three days, for example, your liver tags it and logs it as a pattern of three, cautiously beginning to get itself ready to let go. With another three days, it registers that it's being given the chance to start the process of internal cleansing. And with a final three days, the liver really falls into rhythm and gets in tune with releasing toxins it's held on to in order to shield you. It reads the signals of when you're offering it assistance over three years, six years, and nine years, too.

Aligning yourself with these three-day liver-care increments that add up to nine put the organ into a deep cleanse state that can't be achieved with seven-day, twelve-day, fourteen-day, seventeen-day, or twenty-one day detoxes or other random number schemes based on man-made ideals. Nobody realizes that for cleansing that's all about honoring your liver, it needs to be constructed around threes in order to safely release the levels of toxins we've built up in this modern world. If you're wondering about the 28-Day Healing Cleanse from *Medical Medium*, that's geared for a mild cleanse state that helps the liver detox very, very gently while helping alleviate many health problems all at once on a flexible schedule. That protocol is not dependent upon a number of days, whereas the Liver Rescue 3:6:9 is—because it's about cracking the code of the liver, lining up with its true essence, and allowing for deep liver cleansing by opening the liver's floodgates in a safe, nonhazardous way. This is a whole different ballgame.

If you work Monday through Friday, a landmark way to approach this cleanse is to begin on a Saturday and end the next Sunday. That way you'll have the first weekend to ease into the eating plan as well as shop for ingredients and prepare food for the week ahead. Then you'll have the time and space of the second weekend to attend to the most potent days of the cleanse. If your week is structured differently, or if your preference is to begin on another day for any other reason, then go ahead and start your Liver Rescue 3:6:9 whenever you'd like. It's about fitting it into *your* life and supporting *you*.

Speaking of supporting you, one of the beauties of the Liver Rescue 3:6:9 is that it protects your adrenal glands. Unlike so many cleanses that make you go hungry, forcing your adrenals to squeeze out excess adrenaline and putting your liver through even more strain in the process of mopping it up, the Liver Rescue 3:6:9 doesn't wreck these precious glands because it doesn't starve you. If you're worried about hunger pangs on this plan, you can release your fear. You don't need to limit yourself to set portion sizes, and snacks are not only allowed; they're part of it. Even though the Liver Rescue 3:6:9 does lower dietary fat to take some burden off your liver, it does it a little at a time, and to balance that, you get to fill yourself up with other delicious flavors. Eat *plenty* on the Liver Rescue 3:6:9. Stock up so you have an abundance of fresh, healing foods at your fingertips. Feed yourself well. It's what will best serve your adrenals, your liver, and you.

Please note that during the Liver Rescue 3:6:9, you don't need to take the healing supplements from the previous chapter. If you're already on some of those supplements and you want to continue them, you're welcome to do so. Otherwise, know that the cleanse is almost like its own supplement for the liver, giving it the support it needs to do its full job, so you can skip the supplements during the nine days. If you're staying on supplements, you'll most likely find it best not to take them on Day 9, when you'll be enjoying mostly liquids. (If you're on medication, please consult with your doctor about its use.)

Your liver is very responsible and won't release a lifetime of toxins and accumulated fat in one cycle of the Liver Rescue 3:6:9. That would overwhelm your system and ultimately strain your liver, which would defeat the whole point. Rather, it releases as much as it possibly can safely and then holds on to the rest to let go of it in the future. If you're feeling very poorly and you want that future to be now, then after finishing one cycle of the Liver Rescue 3:6:9 you may find you want to roll directly into another, starting over again at Day 1 and cycling through the nine days as many times as you'd like until your symptoms have moved on. If you're seeking more gradual changes in your health, you may find that you want to try the Liver Rescue 3:6:9 once a month instead, with some Liver Rescue Mornings in between for maintenance. As I mentioned in the troublemakers chapter, it's ideal to try the Liver Rescue 3:6:9 at least once every two to three months if you suspect you're dealing with a decent amount of troublemakers in your liver. Or you may find that one go-round gave you just what you were looking for at this time in your life. The choice is yours.

Make the Liver Rescue 3:6:9 and the Liver Rescue Morning part of your life, and right away you'll start seeing and feeling the benefits. If you keep coming back to them you'll help secure the process of your cells renewing for the better over time. By the point when nine years have come around since you first started caring for your liver, you'll be remade—a healthier, more vital version of you.

——— THE 3 ———

	DAY 1	DAY 2	DAY 3
UPON WAKING	16 ounces lemon or lime water	16 ounces lemon or lime water	16 ounces lemon or lime water
MORNING	Breakfast and mid-morning snack of your choice (within guidelines)	Breakfast and mid-morning snack of your choice (within guidelines) One apple (or one serving applesauce)	Breakfast and mid-morning snack of your choice (within guidelines) Two apples (or two servings applesauce)
LUNCHTIME	Meal of your choice (within guidelines)	Meal of your choice (within guidelines)	Meal of your choice (within guidelines)
MID-AFTERNOON	Two apples (or two servings applesauce) with one to four dates (or substitutions below)	Two apples (or two servings applesauce) with one to four dates (or substitutions below)	Two apples (or two servings applesauce) with two to four dates (or substitutions below)
DINNERTIME	Meal of your choice (within guidelines)	Meal of your choice (within guidelines)	Meal of your choice (within guidelines)
EVENING	Apple (if desired) 16 ounces lemon or lime water Hibiscus or lemon balm tea	Apple (if desired) 16 ounces lemon or lime water Hibiscus or lemon balm tea	Apple (if desired) 16 ounces lemon or lime water Hibiscus or lemon balm tea
GUIDELINES	• Follow the Liver Rescue Morning • Avoid these foods: gluten, dairy, eggs, lamb, pork products, canola oil • Reduce your normal consumption of radical fats (nuts, seeds, oils, coconut, animal proteins, etc.) by 50 percent and wait to eat fats altogether until dinnertime • If you enjoy animal products, stick to one serving per day, eaten only at dinner • Substitutions for afternoon dates: mulberries (dried or fresh), raisins, grapes, or figs (dried or fresh) • Focus on bringing in more fruits, vegetables, and leafy greens every day		

This first phase is like the countdown you give to someone jumping off a diving board. It's not meant to be a drastic plunge. Rather, it's the beginning of a cycle. Without this adjustment period, the full cycle of the cleanse can't be as effective or successful.

Bypassing The 3 is like showing up for a test without studying. It's a mistake that many of the man-made trial-and-error cleanses out there make, putting the liver in the hot seat and forcing it to perform under pressure with no preparation phase. The liver can't operate with confidence in a situation like that. When it comes time to turn in the exam, it will be with hesitance, knowing the teacher will flip through the pages to find incomplete results. In order for that delivery to go well—for poisons and pathogens to be ushered out of the body effectively later on in the cleanse—the beginning especially needs to be kind to your liver. We can't give the liver too much to handle right away or put it in a position where it's forced to give your brain and heart too much to handle.

You'll start each of the three days simply: with 16 ounces of your choice of lemon or lime water to flush your liver's accumulated waste from the night before out of your system. (If you're a devoted fan of morning celery juice, you're welcome to enjoy that 30 minutes after the lemon or lime water.) The rest of each day is mostly up to you, as long as you follow the guidelines outlined below, make your morning a Liver Rescue Morning, and get in your hydrating, glucose-rich, liver-cleansing apple snacks.

Let's talk about those apple snacks. On Day 1, you'll incorporate two apples with one to four dates into your afternoon. On Day 2, you'll add an apple in the morning and continue with two apples and one to four dates in the afternoon. And on Day 3, you'll increase to two apples in the morning followed by the two afternoon apples with two to four dates this time. You don't

need to eat your dates and apples whole. You can blend them both into smoothies or enjoy them in the recipes Apples with "Caramel" Dip from *Life-Changing Foods*, Apple Porridge with Cinnamon and Raisins from *Thyroid Healing*, or the Caramel Apple Rings or Liver Rescue Applesauce recipes from the following chapter of this book. If you react to raw apples or find them difficult to chew, cooked applesauce is a perfect substitute. Just make sure that if it's not homemade, you select a high-quality organic applesauce with no additives such as sneaky citric acid, added sugar, or natural flavors.

We underestimate the power of the apple because it's so commonplace. If you were given an apple in your lunchbox as a kid, did you eat it? Or did you try to trade it or throw it away? When was the last time you ate a whole apple? It may feel more recent than it really was. With shiny piles of apples at the grocery store and apple imagery everywhere, we're so used to seeing them that we think they're more a part of our lives than we've really let them be. Like pouring a glass of water and then letting it sit on the desk and forgetting to drink it, we fool ourselves into thinking we're eating apples because of their constant proximity. Despite the "apple-a-day" saying, it's rare that someone eats one apple every day, never mind two, three, or four—so we don't get a chance to witness what this fruit can do. That will change when you've completed the Liver Rescue 3:6:9 and consumed 21 apples or more in nine days. Bringing apples into your life in quantity is transformative.

Dates have a special place as apples' afternoon sidekicks in this plan because they rev up the engine of the liver in a beneficial way. There are two types of liver heat: unproductive liver heat that's a result of a toxic, sluggish, overworked liver and unhealthy foods, and productive liver heat that gently warms up the organ, preparing it to detox. Dates create that second type of liver heat, the medicinal kind you want, which is why this food is part of both The 3 and The 6, those periods when you're giving your liver as much support as possible so it can go the distance when it reaches The 9. If it doesn't work to get your dates in at the same time you're eating your afternoon apples, that's fine. Just make sure to get them in you at some point. And if you don't enjoy dates, you don't have access to any, or you want to mix up the routine, mulberries (dried or fresh), raisins, grapes, and figs (dried or fresh), in that order, can all stand in for dates as beneficial liver warmers. You can swap in a handful of whichever you choose to substitute for the dates.

If you're hungry after dinner, turn to an apple or applesauce again. And an hour before you go to bed, make sure you get in another 16 ounces of lemon or lime water as well as a mug of hibiscus or lemon balm tea. These evening liquids may mean you need to visit the bathroom a few times in the night; it's worth it for the extra hydration and cleansing of your system.

Now let's cover the overall guidelines of The 3. To begin with, you'll be cutting down on dietary fat. Whatever amount of radical fat you eat on an average day, cut it by at least half. Much of this is already taken care of by following the Liver Rescue Morning. By skipping your usual morning radical fats such as yogurt, nutty granola, avocado toast, buttered toast, smoothie with coconut milk or whey protein powder, bacon, eggs, sausage, pancakes, waffles, or creamy coffee drinks, you'll already be reducing your fat intake by a lot. Plus, you're going to take it a step further by holding off on radical fats altogether until dinnertime. If cutting out radical fats in the morning and afternoon alone doesn't bring your fats down by 50 percent for the day, then think about halving some of your other usual portions of radical fats and increasing your helpings of fruits,

vegetables, potatoes, squash, leafy greens, lentils, quinoa, or millet to compensate. If you're used to adding olives to salads, for example, throw in half as many and add some chickpeas and chopped tomatoes instead. If you enjoy grilled salmon for dinner, serve yourself less than usual and heap your plate with Lentil Tacos or Ratatouille. Also be mindful of dressings, sauces, dips, and oils, which are often much higher in fat than we realize, and reduce them accordingly. For satisfying dishes and snacks that aren't high in dietary fat, turn to the Liver Rescue Recipes.

One major reason to cut down on fats during The 3 is to give your liver a breather from relentless bile production so it can restore bile reserves. Freed up from processing so many fats, it can put its energy into getting you ready to detox. Another reason is so you can get the glucose you need. As we've examined, eating less fat allows your liver to absorb glucose better, and building up your glucose and glycogen reserves is vital for the liver's hard work during The 9 of propelling poisons out of itself. As in the Liver Rescue Morning, potatoes, sweet potatoes, and winter squash are great, glucose-rich foods to eat during The 3 to build up fuel in your liver.

If you enjoy animal products, stick to one serving of them, eaten only at dinner. Make sure it's a serving of lean, organic, free-range, or wild meat, fowl, or fish so that it has the best chance of supporting your health during these transition days.

If you're raw- and plant-based, you can continue to eat raw for all nine days of this cleanse.

Finally, there are some foods you'll want to avoid altogether during the entire nine days: gluten, dairy, eggs, lamb, canola, and pork products. For more on why these will hold back your healing, revisit Chapter 36.

For some, following The 3 won't feel much different from the norm. For others, it will take a bit of adjustment. If eating a little differently from normal feels annoying, remember that it's only temporary. Find others online who are doing it at the same time, enlist your family and friends to try it with you, and whenever you start to get a craving for greasy pizza or mac and cheese, read over this section again to tap into the "why" of what you're doing. That why makes all the difference. Before you know it, all nine days will be over, and you'll be looking back on your Liver Rescue 3:6:9 remembering only how amazing it made you feel.

——— THE 6 ———

	DAY 4	DAY 5	DAY 6
UPON WAKING	16 ounces lemon or lime water	16 ounces lemon or lime water	16 ounces lemon or lime water
MORNING	16 ounces celery juice Liver Rescue Smoothie	16 ounces celery juice Liver Rescue Smoothie	16 ounces celery juice Liver Rescue Smoothie
LUNCHTIME	Steamed asparagus with Liver Rescue Salad	Steamed asparagus with Liver Rescue Salad	Steamed asparagus and brussels sprouts with Liver Rescue Salad
MID-AFTERNOON	At least two apples (or two servings applesauce) with one to four dates (or substitutions) plus celery sticks	At least two apples (or two servings applesauce) with one to four dates (or substitutions) plus celery sticks	At least two apples (or two servings applesauce) with one to four dates (or substitutions) plus celery sticks
DINNERTIME	Steamed asparagus with Liver Rescue Salad	Steamed brussels sprouts with Liver Rescue Salad	Steamed asparagus and brussels sprouts with Liver Rescue Salad
EVENING	Apple (if desired) 16 ounces lemon or lime water Hibiscus or lemon balm tea	Apple (if desired) 16 ounces lemon or lime water Hibiscus or lemon balm tea	Apple (if desired) 16 ounces lemon or lime water Hibiscus or lemon balm tea
GUIDELINES	• Avoid radical fats (nuts, seeds, oils, coconut, animal proteins, etc.) entirely • Stick to the foods outlined in the chart above • Eat as much as you need to feel full • If you're 100 percent raw, please see the full cleanse description for alternatives to the cooked meals		

Now we reach the middle, your liver's prime time to clean. You'll begin each day just like during The 3, with a big 16-ounce glass of lemon or lime water to flush your system. Half an hour later, you'll bring in 16 ounces of fresh, plain celery juice. (Unless, that is, you have an issue with celery juice, in which case, substitute fresh, plain cucumber juice.) Make it yourself, or order it fresh from your local juice bar.

Celery juice: How much can I praise this alkalizing, life-giving tonic? Taken on its own, with no fillers or add-ins, on an empty stomach, it strengthens your digestion of everything you eat for the rest of the day. Over time, it restores hydrochloric acid levels in the stomach for better long-term digestion. It helps balance blood pressure and blood sugar and provides your body with valuable vitamins, minerals, electrolytes, and digestive enzymes while it hydrates on a deep cellular level. It also starves pathogens and contains mineral salts with undiscovered disinfectant properties that make them actively antiviral and antibacterial to unproductive bugs in the body. For the liver in particular, celery juice contains cluster salts, subgroups of sodium, that bind onto neurotoxins, dermatoxins, and other viral waste, as well as troublemakers that are not pathogen-related, and draw them out of the liver. The white blood cells of the liver's personalized immune system also add the cluster salts to their cell membrane coatings, making them stronger, more durable, and toxic to viruses—basically, celery's cluster salts give them a field of armor against pathogens. That's why you want to start your day with this life-changing tonic for the remainder of the Liver Rescue 3:6:9.

Celery juice is a medicinal, not a caloric, drink, so you'll want to be sure to follow it up with breakfast: the Liver Rescue Smoothie. Make one serving or more, depending on how hungry you are, and have it whenever you'd like throughout the morning, as long as you've given the celery juice at least 20 minutes to work its magic beforehand. This delicious blend of red pitaya and other healing fruit will nourish your liver with bioavailable glucose and critical antioxidants. The liver thrives on the deep red of the pitaya (and the deep purplish-reddish-blue of the wild blueberries, if you go with Option A); the depth of those colors means they're abundant with undiscovered antioxidants to bring the liver back to life. Ready-to-use pitaya, also known as dragon fruit, and wild blueberries are both available in the frozen fruit section of many grocery stores, or you can order frozen pitaya, pitaya powder, or wild blueberry powder online.

If you're not a fan of banana, you can substitute papaya or leave out an extra fruit altogether and simply blend pitaya with the other ingredient(s) in the smoothie option you choose. If you have no access to pitaya or a strong aversion to it, you can resort to wild blueberries in its place or, in a pinch, blackberries, regular cultivated blueberries, or frozen cherries. In order to get the healing benefits your liver needs during The 6, you want to make sure you get those anthocyanins into your morning one way or another.

For lunch, you'll move on to a Liver Rescue Salad with steamed vegetables—specifically, steamed asparagus on Days 4 and 5, and steamed asparagus plus brussels sprouts on Day 6. Dinner will be very similar: salad with steamed asparagus on Day 4, steamed brussels sprouts on Day 5, and steamed asparagus plus brussels sprouts on Day 6. You're welcome to eat them raw if you prefer; just make sure that either raw or steamed, you don't prepare them with oil during the cleanse. As you read about in the previous chapter, asparagus and brussels sprouts are incredible liver-healing foods. Eating them in this kind of quantity allows for a deeper cleanse: the sulfur in brussels sprouts is a powerful liver-purging compound. Once you've eaten a brussels sprout, its sulfur leaves your intestinal tract and goes straight up to your liver to do its good. Asparagus contains a similar, though not identical, chemical compound that travels directly to the liver and triggers a purging effect.

If fresh asparagus and brussels sprouts aren't available, find them in the frozen food aisle and stock up so that you'll have plenty on hand. Don't worry if you can only find conventional; they're so beneficial to the liver that it outweighs any downsides to eating nonorganic asparagus and brussels sprouts. You can either steam the vegetables just before your meal or prepare them ahead of time and enjoy them cold on top of your salad. Again, you can enjoy them fresh and raw if you'd prefer, and you can even juice some of the raw asparagus if you'd like. We're not talking a little side dish of vegetables here; we're talking hearty portions. Make a nice, big Liver Rescue Salad and then heap on the asparagus and/or brussels sprouts and drizzle plenty of fresh-squeezed lemon, lime, or orange juice or Orange "Vinaigrette" Dressing on top. Fill up!

You may find yourself the most full and satisfied you've ever been on this cleanse. That's in part because asparagus and brussels sprouts are appetite suppressors. When you consume them, your liver is aware that you're doing something for it, since they send it the message to cleanse. Upon receiving that message, the liver releases an unknown hormone-based chemical compound into the bloodstream and drives it up to the brain to shut down appetite and also to the adrenals to calm them and stop them from becoming alarmed so the liver can cleanse appropriately. It's another of the over 2,000 undiscovered chemical functions of the liver. At no point in this cleanse should you force food down the hatch if you're overly full. Just don't hold back if you're hungry.

Between lunch and dinner, turn to apples (or applesauce) and dates (or their substitutes), this time adding celery for extra blood sugar support and liver-cleansing abilities. (If you make your own celery juice, you can give yourself a hand by setting aside these celery sticks when

you're prepping celery for juice in the morning.) Munch on additional fruits and vegetables if you're still hungry in the afternoon—find inspiration in the healing foods and snack ideas in this book.

After dinner, you have the same option as in The 3 of an apple or applesauce if you're hungry. Then an hour before bed, have another 16 ounces of lemon or lime water and a mug of hibiscus or lemon balm tea.

As in The 3, you'll follow the Liver Rescue Morning protocol during The 6 to give your liver that special, early support. This time, you'll continue that support by avoiding radical fats for the entire day and night. Nuts, seeds, oil, olives, coconut, avocado, animal products: save them for your post-cleanse life. At this point, if you consumed those fats it would break the cleanse. It would be as if you were scrubbing dishes and someone dumped grease into your sink—it would require starting over in order to truly get the plates clean. For your liver to navigate The 6 (and The 9) successfully, it needs to be free from the interruption of being forced to backtrack and process radical fats. Your liver will still produce bile to keep your body functioning during this time; it just won't need to produce the same strength bile for dissolving radical fats. By avoiding them, you allow your liver to use its energy to cleanse on a level it can't otherwise. Remember: it's very difficult for the liver to cleanse on a deep level on a diet that's high in fat.

Rather than relying on some of your usual favorite foods as you did in The 3, you'll stick to fruits and vegetables in The 6. The nutrient density of this healing fuel is exactly what your body needs at this point. Avoiding foods that take a little more effort to digest is well worth the effort of passing on them during this part of the cleanse.

To compensate, as I keep saying, you get to *eat*. Remember this: you're not going to be a hero by eating tiny portions, so don't skimp during The 6. You won't do yourself or anyone else any favors by getting through the whole morning on one little glass of smoothie. You won't save the world by proving that you can function on two brussels sprouts and a leaf of lettuce. Don't starve yourself! If you do, you'll starve your liver—and what your liver needs

desperately at this stage is fuel. Your liver needs the calories. In The 3, you increased your glucose intake in order to perk up your liver's functioning. Now it needs the foods from The 6 chart as diggers and cleaners so it can be ready for its time to shine: The 9.

THE 9

	DAY 7	DAY 8	DAY 9
UPON WAKING	16 ounces lemon or lime water	16 ounces lemon or lime water	16 ounces lemon or lime water
MORNING	16 ounces celery juice Liver Rescue Smoothie	16 ounces celery juice Liver Rescue Smoothie	Over the course of the day, consume: Two 16- to 20-ounce celery juices (one morning, one early evening)
LUNCHTIME	Spinach soup over cucumber noodles	Spinach soup over cucumber noodles	
MID-AFTERNOON	16 ounces celery juice At least two apples (or two servings applesauce) plus cucumber slices and celery sticks	16 ounces celery juice At least two apples (or two servings applesauce) plus cucumber slices and celery sticks	Two 16- to 20-ounce cucumber-apple juices (anytime) Blended melon, blended papaya, or fresh-squeezed orange juice (as many servings and as often as desired)
DINNERTIME	Steamed squash, sweet potatoes, or potatoes with steamed asparagus and/or brussels sprouts plus optional Liver Rescue Salad	Steamed asparagus and/or brussels sprouts plus optional Liver Rescue Salad	Water (sip at least 8 ounces every three hours)
EVENING	Apple (if desired) 16 ounces lemon or lime water Hibiscus or lemon balm tea	Apple (if desired) 16 ounces lemon or lime water Hibiscus or lemon balm tea	16 ounces lemon or lime water Hibiscus or lemon balm tea
GUIDELINES	• Continue to avoid radical fats (nuts, seeds, oils, coconut, animal proteins, etc.) entirely • Stick to the foods outlined in the chart above; eat or drink as much as you need to feel full • If you're 100 percent raw, please see the full cleanse description for alternatives to the cooked dinners		

Here we are: the moment your liver has been waiting for basically its whole life. That means it's the moment you've been waiting for, too, because what makes your liver happy makes you happy. When your liver unburdens itself at this stage, you'll be amazed at the positive influence it can have on both your body and your mood. The ripple effect from here on out—the people who see the change in you, the further changes you're inspired to make in your life—will be profound and far reaching. Who knows whose lives you're going to touch with your improved health? Who knows what you'll get to do now?

Over the past six days, you've been warming up your liver's engine and building its reserves, getting it ready so that here in The 9, it would have the power to drive out junk, garbage, and poison it's been holding on to for years. This goes far beyond the Liver Rescue Morning's ability to process out daily waste. These liquid-heavy three days are completely new territory.

Days 7 and 8 will follow the same morning routine as Days 4, 5, and 6: lemon or lime water, followed by celery juice, followed by Liver Rescue Smoothie. At lunch on Days 7 and 8, you'll go for delicious, nourishing spinach soup over cucumber noodles. While zucchini noodles are popular and a great alternative to wheat on other days, cucumber noodles are what you want at this stage because they're easier to digest. Raw zucchini can be a little tough on the stomach, and we want to go very easy on the gut during The 9 so the body's energy can be put into elimination. Over these three days, your liver is going to be excreting packages of waste for delivery

out of the body, so everything needs to be in service of that. Spinach soup over cucumber noodles is perfectly in service, as it supports your adrenals. You'll find the full soup recipe in *Thyroid Healing*. If you like to keep things simple, all you need to do is blend raw spinach, tomatoes, garlic, a chopped stick of celery, and some fresh-squeezed orange juice, along with any herbs you enjoy. It makes a remarkably rich and tasty meal.

Since the liver's engine is well warmed at this point, your afternoon snack will skip the dates. This time, instead, you'll focus on hydration and flushing toxins by sipping another 16-ounce glass of celery juice followed 20 minutes later by at least two apples (or two servings of applesauce) with sliced cucumbers and celery sticks. Feel free to make all your celery juice at once in the morning, setting aside this second serving in the fridge, if you don't have the time or inclination to fire up the juicer twice in one day. You can also get your celery juice from a juice bar, ordering both servings at once and saving the second one for now.

Dinner on Day 7 may take you by surprise: steamed potatoes, sweet potatoes, or winter squash accompanied by steamed asparagus and/or brussels sprouts and an optional Liver Rescue Salad. (If you're someone who likes to eat only raw, make your dinner a Liver Rescue Salad with plenty of sweet fruit, such as papaya, mango, or even banana. If you're going to put banana in your salad, leave out tomato; these foods need a little time apart to allow for better nutrient absorption.) We bring in these special comfort foods of potatoes, sweet potatoes, or winter squash to help moderate the cleanse. Here at the beginning of The 9, toxins are starting to be released, and this meal of cooked healing foods slows down that process just a bit so you don't get over-whelmed by detox symptoms. Remember: this isn't a reckless cleanse. We want to honor the load your liver has been bearing and not give it too much to handle by releasing everything at once. Dinner on Day 8 will pare back to asparagus and/or brussels sprouts, preferably both (steamed or raw), with an optional Liver Rescue Salad, to encourage more cleansing now that your body's had a chance to adjust.

The evening snack options for Days 7 and 8 continue to be more apple or applesauce, if you're not sick of it at this point. Then you want to get in that lemon balm or hibiscus tea an hour before bed again, along with an additional 16 ounces of lemon or lime water or even plain water.

And then you get to Day 9, a day of liquids to send on their way any remaining poisons that the liver unearthed during The 6. You'll start with 16 ounces of lemon or lime water, as usual. You'll follow that half an hour later with 16 to 20 ounces of celery juice. Then, over the course of the rest of the day, you'll want to get in two 16- to 20-ounce servings of cucumber-apple juice; as much blended melon, blended papaya, or fresh-squeezed orange juice as you'd like whenever you get hungry; and an early-evening 16- to 20-ounce serving of celery juice. Feel more than free to make or buy all the fresh juice at once in the morning and save your later servings in the fridge. And if you're very petite and can't get this much liquid in you, you can lower the serving sizes

of the juices, so long as you don't *underdo* it. You want to make sure you get enough of those precious nutrients to support your body as it does its hard work of elimination.

In between it all, make sure you're sipping water, ideally with a squeeze of lemon or lime in it, or plain if that's what you can handle. You don't want to go overboard with drinking water, since you're getting in so many other liquids; what you need is at least a good eight ounces every three hours. (A note on water: Avoid water with a high pH. Although this alkalized water is marketed as a cure-all, the truth is that it throws your body out of balance. Revisit Chapter 34 for more on this.)

For the cucumber-apple juice, make it a 50-50 blend, unless you don't like either cucumber or apple, in which case you can increase the amount of whichever one of those you prefer so that you end up with a 25-75 or 75-25 blend. Go with the apples of your choice; don't be afraid that you need to stick with Granny Smiths. While that's a good type of apple, there are so many other great ones that offer the medicinal benefits of their red skins: Braeburn, Gala, Red Delicious, Fuji, Honeycrisp, Pink Lady, and more. Explore what's available in your area and have fun trying different types. And don't be afraid of those skins; keep them on when you juice the apples for maximum benefit. If raw apple doesn't work for you, it's not the end of the world if you do straight cucumber juice instead. While it will be lacking in calories, you can get glucose and calories from the blended fruit.

One important distinction that makes this day of fluids different from juice fasts or cleanses you might have tried before is that the blend of the celery, cucumber, and apple that you're getting throughout Day 9 has the right balance of mineral salts, potassium, and natural sugar to stabilize your glucose levels as your body cleanses itself of toxins. On this final day, when your body's working so hard to make you better, it's as important as ever to safeguard your adrenals—and that's just what Day 9's special tonics do.

If you can, take it easy today. Think about saving certain commitments for another time. Maybe you can schedule Day 9 as a sacred rest day, or a day with at least some rest in it. At minimum, be mindful of all your liver's doing for you during this period. Take a moment to pause and think about your liver and try the hands-on liver flushing technique at the end of the chapter. This is the end of your liver's great big plunge into the depths of purification, and it's doing beautifully. So are you.

You'll be finishing the day as you have the previous eight: lemon or lime water plus hibiscus or lemon balm tea for that nourishing, hydrating flush of your system. Every time it has you running to relieve yourself in the night, remember: you're saying good-bye to that much more of what doesn't serve you.

That's it. Nine days—just a little over a week—and you'll be in a very different place in your life. Physically, yes, as well as emotionally and spiritually. In tune now with your liver's healing secrets, you'll finally get to move forward.

Transition Time

Because the Liver Rescue 3:6:9 protected your adrenals, you can get back to life afterward without feeling like all the energy's been squeezed out of you. In fact, you may be feeling so great that it will be easy to forget your liver still likes TLC.

If you're able, take a couple of extra steps to honor everything your liver has just done for you. For your first post-cleanse day, begin with the Liver Rescue Morning. You don't want to put your liver in shock by breaking your cleanse with chocolate cake, pork, chicken, or even an egg-white omelet; liquids and high-quality glucose are more in line with what your liver needs at this point. In addition, see if you can avoid radical fats such as coconut, avocado, oil, nuts, seeds, and animal products; instead focus on fruits and vegetables from Chapter 37 and Liver Rescue Recipes for your entire first day back. It's a great chance to use up any leftover potatoes, sweet potatoes, winter squash, brussels sprouts, asparagus, and the like. If you can get one celery juice and at least one apple into your day, all the better. These measures will help stabilize your system as it adjusts to coming out of the cleanse.

On your second post-cleanse day, see if you can try the Liver Rescue Morning again. Later in the day is a good time to reintroduce radical fats. Stick to one serving, either of animal protein or plant-based fats; if you're a big fan of both, go with one little serving of each. Again, this is a great day to turn to those Liver Rescue Recipes in the next chapter for meal and snack ideas.

As we covered, you may decide to keep going through some more cycles of the Liver Rescue 3:6:9 rather than transitioning out right away. If you're dealing with serious symptoms or illness, for example, or if you have a lot of weight to lose, you can take this longer term. When you eventually come out of it, remember the tips above.

Your liver will be so relieved by these kindnesses that you pay it during reentry that you'll serve your long-term health that much more. As you continue on your way, you're also welcome to keep any habits you enjoyed from the Liver Rescue 3:6:9. The Liver Rescue Smoothie for breakfast, apples in the afternoon, hibiscus tea before bed, or any other idea from the past nine days . . . if you liked it, it's yours to use again and again.

Now pat yourself on the back. Give yourself a "congratulations." You're a Liver Rescue 3:6:9-er now, and that means more than you'll ever know.

HEAVY METAL DETOX

If heavy metals are a concern for you, focus on getting those out once you've been through a cycle of the Liver Rescue 3:6:9. At that point, your heavy metal detox efforts will be more effective than ever. The Liver Rescue 3:6:9 is about addressing the broad group of troublemakers that limit the liver. As part of that, the liver will eliminate some heavy metals during the cleanse—and not just any cleanse would do that. Most importantly, this cleanse gets other poisons and toxins out of the liver so that you can more successfully detoxify toxic heavy metals afterward. Freed up from other troublemakers following the cleanse, your liver and other parts of your body will be able to deliver deeper pockets of metals for extraction—pockets that you couldn't have gotten to before.

It does take the right measure to detox heavy metals in your post-cleanse life: consuming wild blueberries, cilantro, barley grass juice powder, spirulina, and Atlantic dulse every day. This combination is a responsible, effective way to drive heavy metals out of the body, as these foods work as a special team unlike any other. The Heavy Metal Detox Smoothie recipe in *Thyroid Healing* is an efficient, delicious way to get all five foods in one go. It's not only the liver that's held back by heavy metals; metals are also present in people's brains, holding them back in life. What's great about the smoothie is that it's effective at extracting heavy metals from both places. You can use this heavy metal detox technique long term after you've tried the Liver Rescue 3:6:9 to help free yourself of these pernicious troublemakers.

HANDS-ON LIVER FLUSHING TECHNIQUE

Here's a way to heighten the effects of the Liver Rescue 3:6:9. For each of the nine days, take five minutes to lie down with your hand over your liver. If you can do this at home, in a moment of peace, that's great. If all you can grab is 10 seconds sitting at your desk or in a parking lot, that works, too.

Rest your hand on the front, right-hand side of your upper abdomen, around the area of your lower ribcage. You can even gently walk your fingers along your last rib, going across your abdomen. All along there are wakeup pressure points for your liver. Now very gently, press (don't poke!) the liver area with your whole hand. Find an anatomy illustration if you need a good visual of what your liver looks like and where in your abdomen it's situated. Let yourself connect with your liver. If you'd like, envision that you're breathing white light into your liver. With your hand and your attention, you're giving it permission to cleanse.

If you have more than a few seconds, move on and envision your liver as your dearest, closest friend—a long-lost friend who knows you better than anyone else. Your hand is an offer of compassion and reassurance. Connect yourself with your peaceful nature and then send that message of peace to your liver. Acknowledging your liver with this hands-on flushing technique makes a profound difference in connecting the dots of all the steps you're taking to care for it.

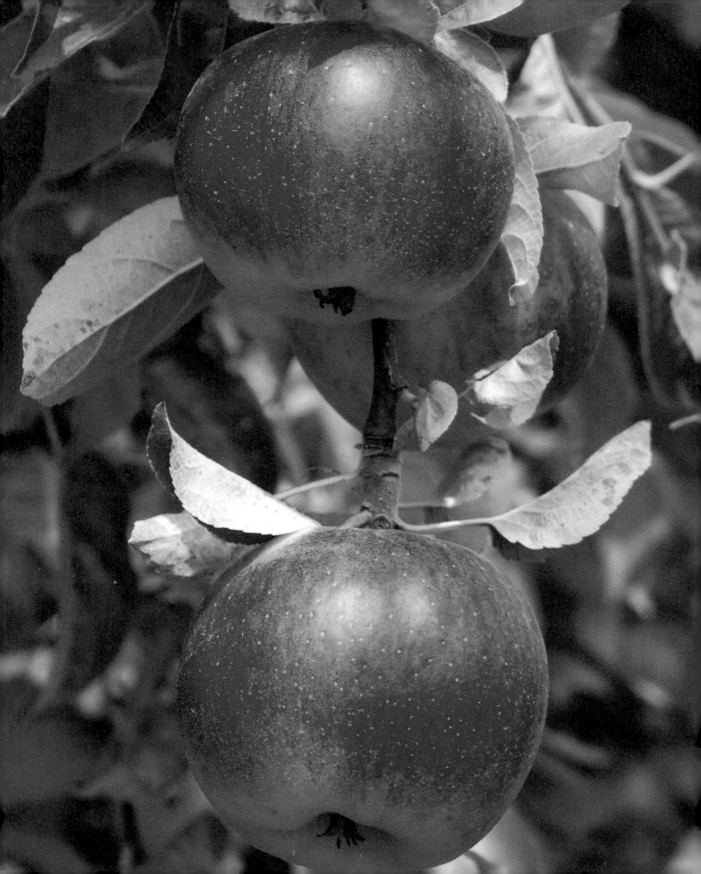

LIVER RESCUE RECIPES

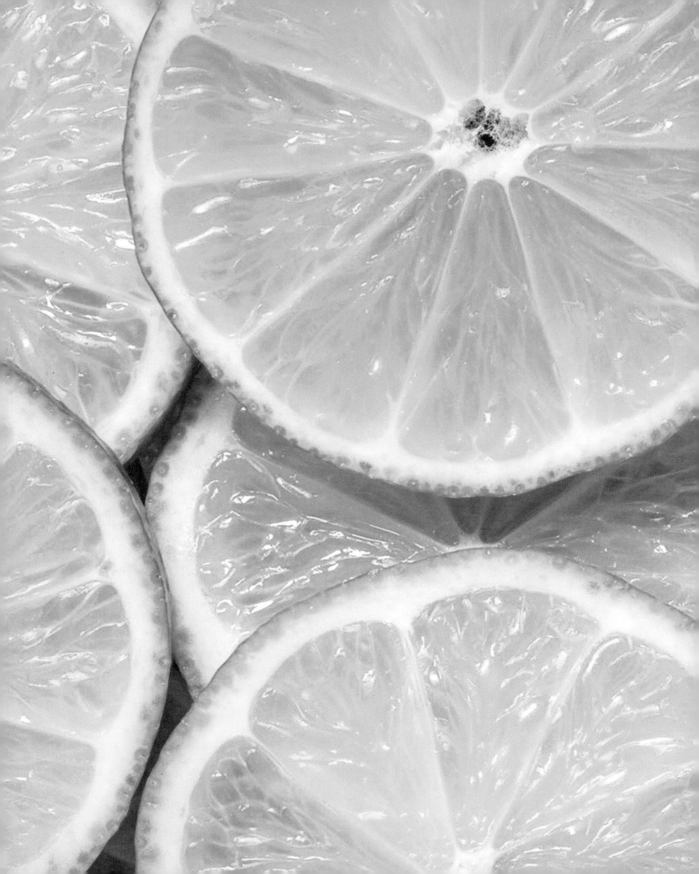

JUICES, TEAS & BROTH

LIVER RESCUE JUICE

Makes 2 servings

Juices are a wonderful way to get in many of the most powerful liver-healing ingredients in a quick and easy-to-digest form. Even better, you can customize this juice until you find your favorite taste combinations. You may find you like an unexpected combination, such as the addition of dandelion greens or radishes!

2 apples

2 cups coarsely chopped pineapple

1 inch ginger

1 bunch celery

1 cup loosely packed parsley

OPTIONAL ADDITIONS

1 cup sprouts

4 small radishes

1 cup loosely packed dandelion greens

Run the apples, pineapple, ginger, celery, and parsley through a juicer.

Choose any or all of the optional additions and run them through the juicer as well. Enjoy immediately for best results, and store any leftover juice in an airtight container in the fridge.

TIPS

- Alternatively, blend all of the ingredients together in a high-speed blender until liquefied and then strain through a nut milk bag or cheesecloth.

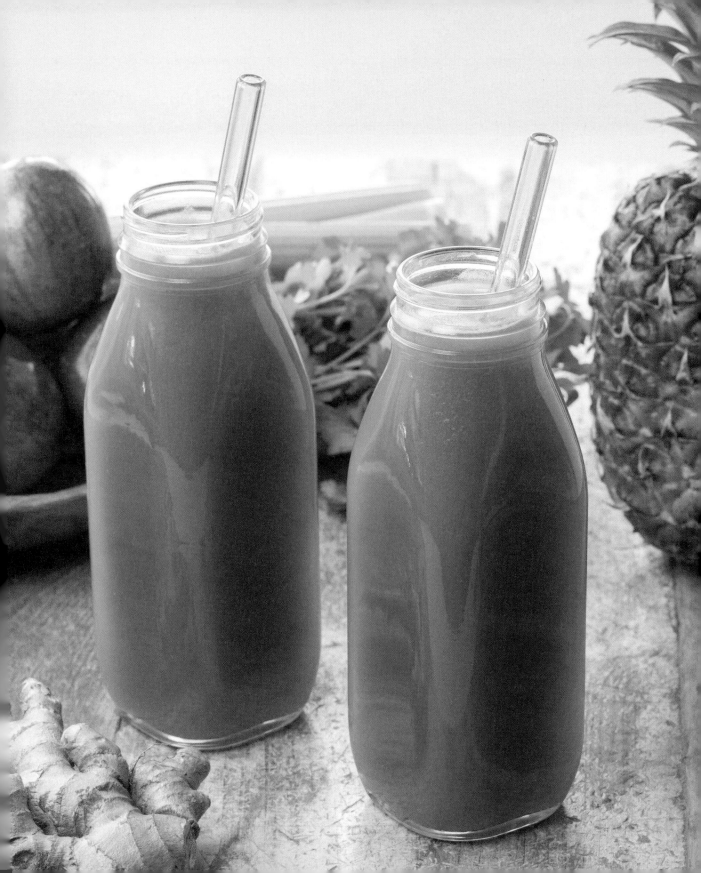

HIBISCUS LEMONADE

This hibiscus lemonade is just as gorgeous as it is delicious. It's the perfect show-stopping beverage for your next gathering, and it's also simple enough to enjoy anytime. Try freezing it into ice cubes and keeping them on hand to make a beautiful hibiscus-infused water on demand.

4 cups water, divided

2 teaspoons dried hibiscus (see Tips)

½ cup fresh lemon juice

4 tablespoons raw honey (see Tips)

Bring 1 cup of water to a boil in a small saucepan. Remove the water from the heat and add the dried hibiscus. Allow the resulting hibiscus tea to steep for at least 10 minutes, and then strain the tea into a mug and place it in the fridge to cool.

In a medium bowl, whisk together the remaining 3 cups of water with the lemon juice and honey until the honey has completely dissolved and a smooth lemonade has formed.

When the hibiscus tea has cooled, stir it into the lemonade base and enjoy!

TIPS

- Store-bought tea bags can be used as well when loose dried hibiscus is not available. Use 1 hibiscus tea bag in place of 1 teaspoon of dried hibiscus.

- Alternatively, maple syrup can be used in place of honey. Start by using 3 tablespoons of maple syrup and adjust until the desired sweetness is reached.

- The recipe above is for a beautiful, light lemonade that anyone can enjoy. If you're looking for even more medicinal benefits, try using up to 2 more tablespoons of dried hibiscus for a stronger hibiscus lemonade with a powerfully tart flavor.

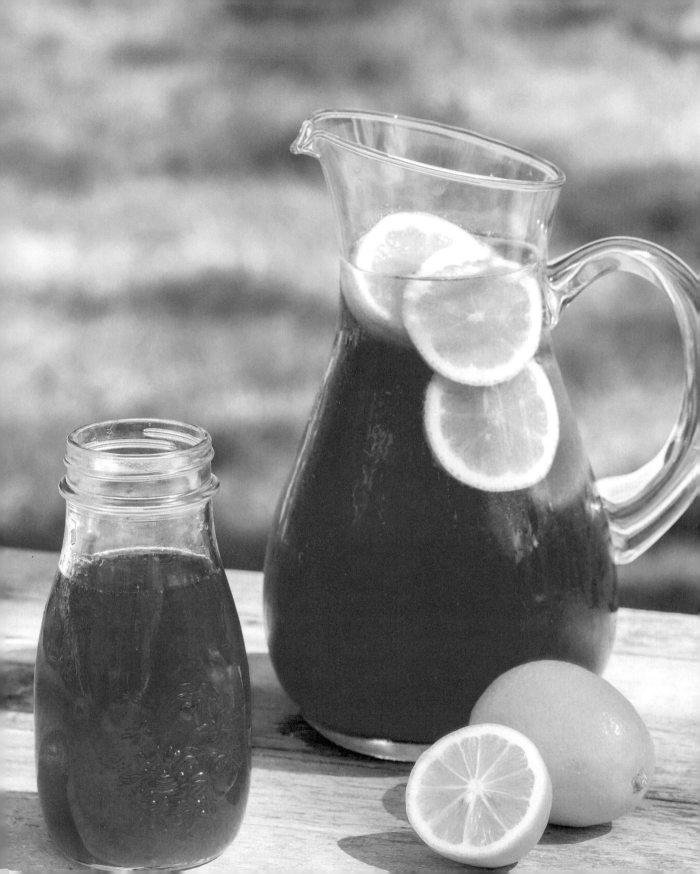

LIME WATER

Makes 1 serving

While it sounds simple, don't let that make you overlook lime water as part of your daily routine. This powerful hydration takes only seconds to prepare and is extremely beneficial for everyone. It not only brings your water to life; it tastes great, too!

2 limes
2 cups water

Squeeze the juice of both limes into the water. Sip and enjoy!

TIPS

- Limes travel well. When you're on the road, you can always throw a few limes into your bag so that you can make this hydrating drink anytime!

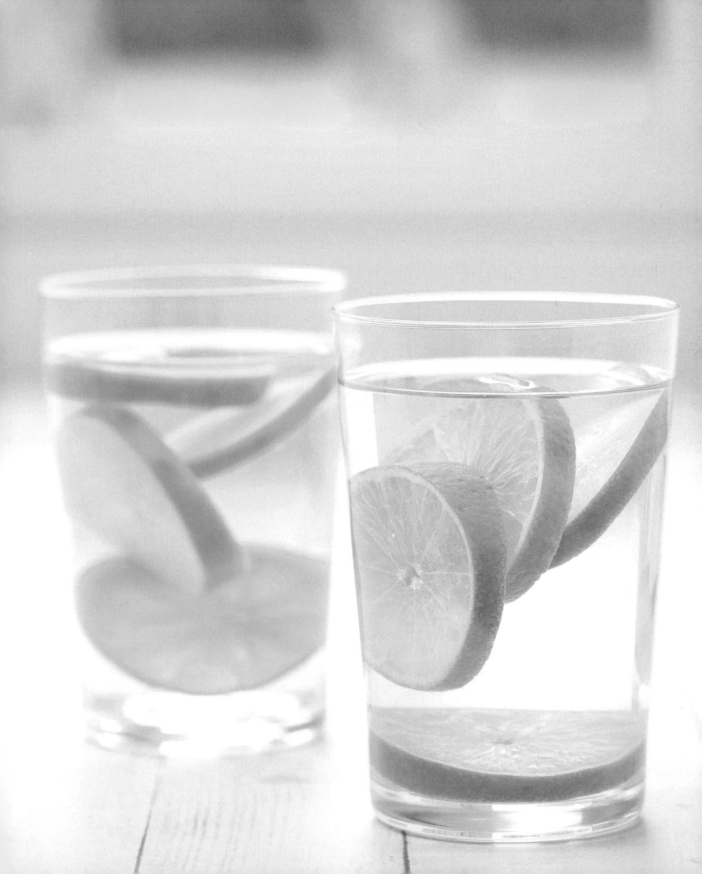

CRANBERRY WATER

This cranberry water is a simple and perfect balance of tart and sweet. It's easy to make, beautiful to look at, and a delicious way to bring the amazing properties of cranberries into your day.

4 cups water
1 cup fresh cranberries
3 tablespoons lime juice
2 tablespoons raw honey

Blend the water and cranberries together until well combined. Strain the resulting cranberry water through a sieve or nut milk bag and into a medium-sized bowl.

Whisk the lime juice and raw honey into the cranberry water until the raw honey has completely dissolved. Serve and enjoy!

TIPS

- Frozen cranberries may be used in place of fresh cranberries. Simply thaw them beforehand and use ½ cup of thawed frozen cranberries in place of the fresh ones.

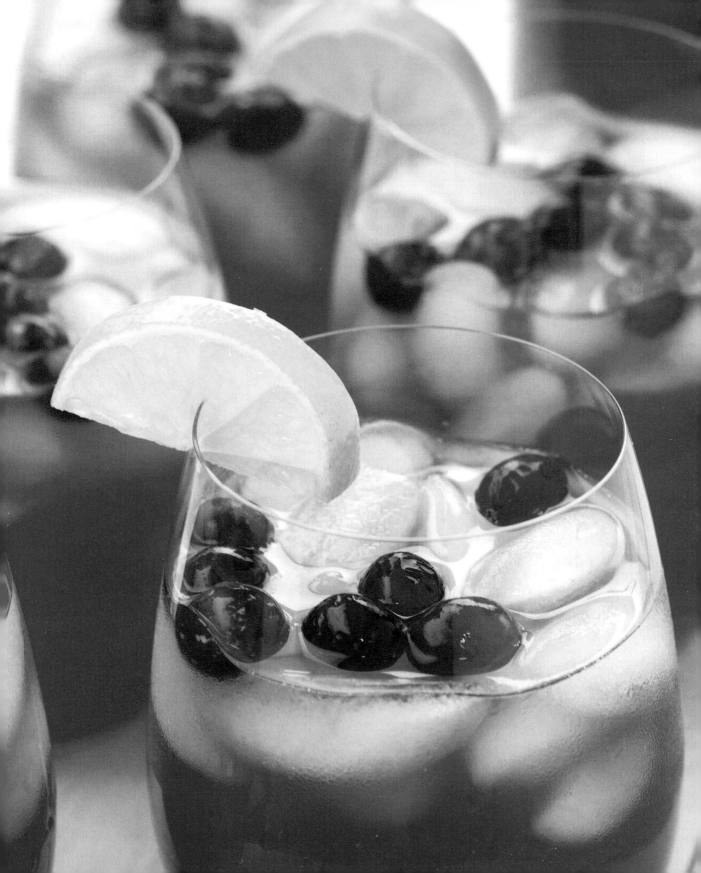

LIVER RESCUE TEA

This earthy tea is just strong enough to bring together all of the incredible properties of burdock, clover, dandelion, and nettle, and it's also mild enough for anyone to consume. Adjust the honey until the sweetness is just to taste. It's a great idea to make a batch of this tea in the morning and leave it in the refrigerator to sip warm or cold throughout the day.

2 cups water

1 teaspoon dried burdock root

1 teaspoon dried red clover

1 teaspoon dried dandelion

1 teaspoon dried nettle leaves

2 teaspoons raw honey (optional)

Bring the water to a boil in a small saucepan or kettle.

Remove the water from the heat and add the herbs. Allow the tea to steep for 15 minutes or more.

Strain the tea and pour it into a mug. Stir in the raw honey if desired and enjoy!

TIPS

- Store-bought tea bags can be used as well when loose tea is not available. Use one tea bag each of burdock root, red clover, dandelion, and nettle.

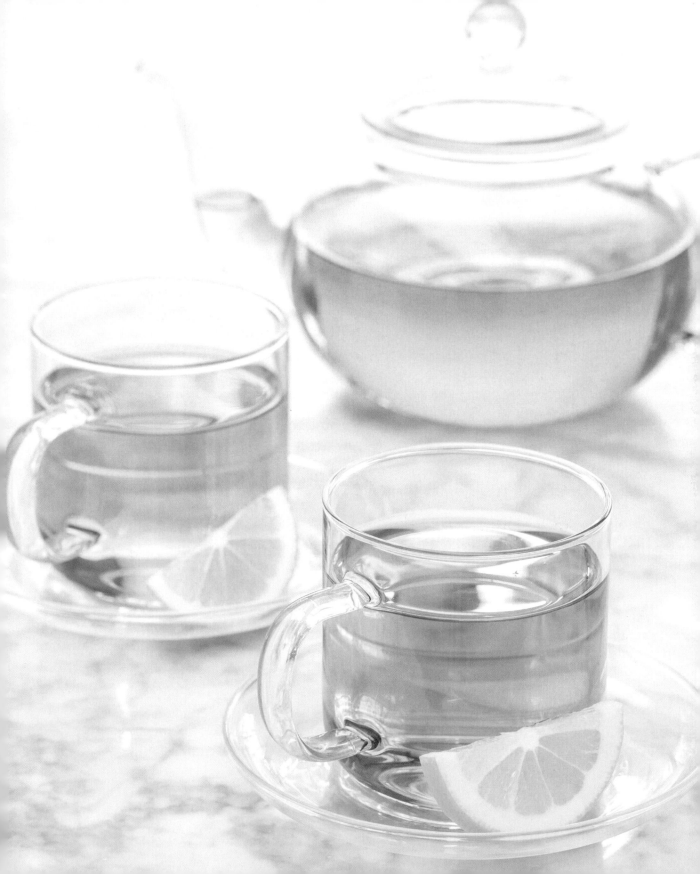

LIVER RESCUE BROTH

This broth is warming liquid gold that you can sip all day long. Sometimes it can seem like a lot of effort to make broth, especially when you're looking at all those beautiful vegetable scraps that get left over at the end. This recipe contains a bonus coconut curry recipe that you can make out of those leftovers so everything gets put to use. Check it out in the Tips. As an alternative, you can blend the broth with the vegetables for a pureed soup.

1 bunch celery, diced

6 carrots, diced

**1 winter squash
(such as butternut), cubed**

2 yellow onions, diced

**1 inch ginger root,
peeled and minced**

**1 inch turmeric root,
peeled and minced**

**1 cup peeled and sliced
burdock root**

1 cup loosely packed cilantro

6 garlic cloves, peeled

12 cups water

Place all the ingredients in a large stock pot.

Cover the pot and bring the water to a boil over high heat, and then reduce the heat and simmer for at least 1 hour and up to 4 hours.

Strain and enjoy as a warm, nourishing broth any time of the day.

TIPS

- This recipe may also be enjoyed as a chunky vegetable soup by leaving the vegetables whole within the broth.

- Make a large batch of this broth and freeze the leftovers for use throughout the week. Try freezing the broth in an ice cube tray for easy thawing later.

- After the broth is strained away, use the leftover veggies to make an indulgent curry soup to share with loved ones. Just return the pot to the heat and stir in 2 cups of coconut milk, 2 teaspoons of yellow curry powder, 1 tablespoon of maple syrup, and 1 teaspoon of sea salt. Cook until everything is warmed through and combined, and then use an immersion blender to partially blend the veggies and make a thick, yellow curry soup. Enjoy!

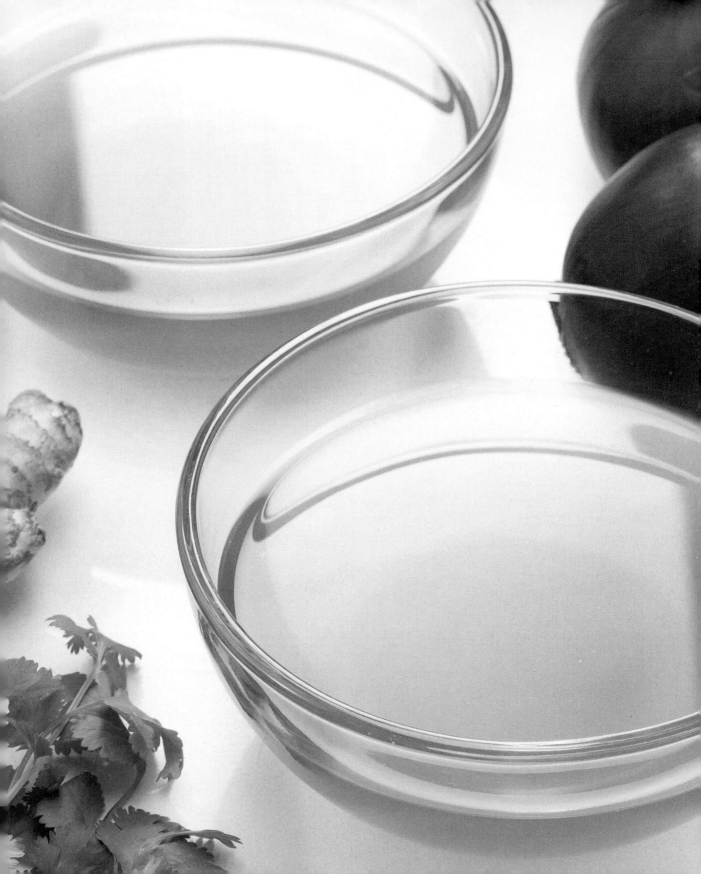

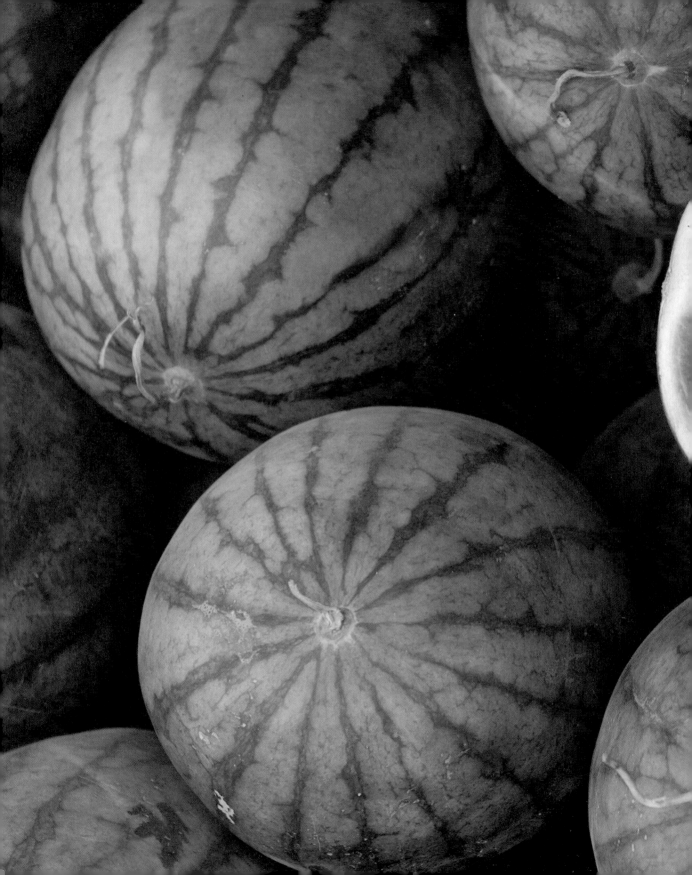

BREAKFAST

LIVER RESCUE SMOOTHIE

Makes 1 to 2 servings

The first smoothie option below is a fast, simple, antioxidant-rich tonic to add to your life for deep liver healing. The second smoothie option is a light, cheery alternative that brings together greens and fruit. If you've never thought of adding sprouts to your smoothie before, now is a perfect time to try it out. They're powerful and mild, and they blend perfectly into this smooth, tropical treat.

OPTION A

2 bananas or
½ Maradol papaya, cubed
½ cup fresh, 1 packet frozen, or 2 tablespoons powdered red pitaya (dragon fruit)
2 cups fresh or frozen or 2 tablespoons powdered wild blueberries
½ cup water (optional)

OPTION B

1 banana or
¼ Maradol papaya, cubed
1 mango
½ cup fresh, 1 packet frozen, or 2 tablespoons powdered red pitaya (dragon fruit)
1 celery stalk
½ cup sprouts (any variety)
½ lime
½ cup water (optional)

Combine all ingredients in the blender.

Blend until smooth. If desired, stream in up to ½ cup of water until desired consistency is reached.

TIPS

- If you don't have access to pitaya and/or wild blueberries, substitute blackberries, cultivated blueberries, or cherries.
- Try adding at least one frozen element to your smoothie. This ensures that your smoothie stays nice and cold!

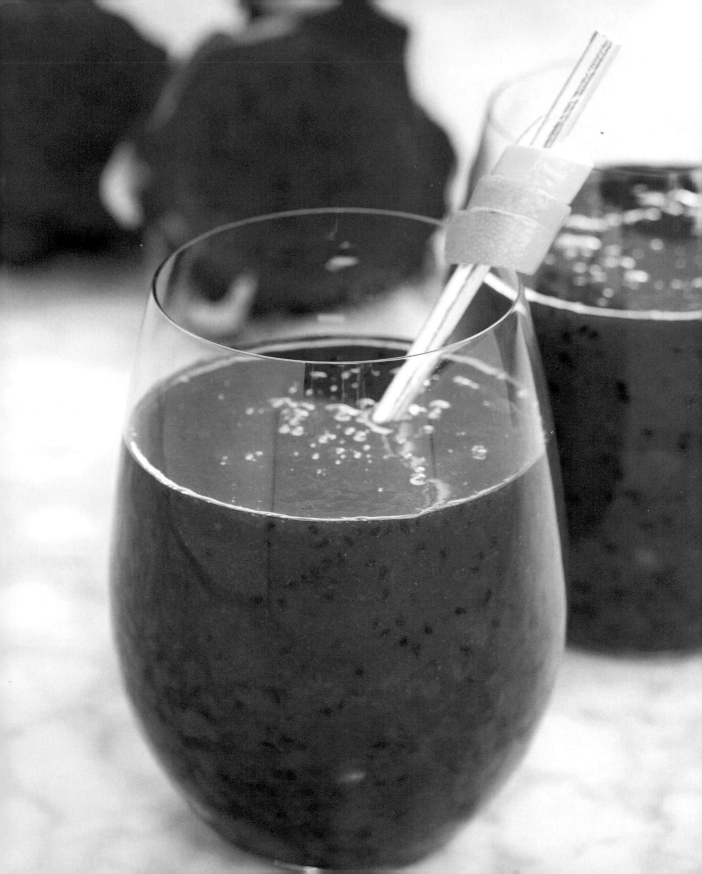

WATERMELON SLUSHY

Makes 2 servings

This slushy is a cold and delicious way to start your morning off right. Friends and family members alike will delight in it, too. Freeze some watermelon the night before so that you're ready to go first thing, or cut some up and leave it in the freezer for at least 2 hours beforehand.

2 cups fresh watermelon cubes

2 cups frozen watermelon cubes

1 lime, juiced

Blend the fresh and frozen watermelon together with the lime juice until smooth. Serve and enjoy!

TIPS

- Adjust the iciness of the slushy by substituting more fresh watermelon in place of frozen if you desire a less frosty beverage.

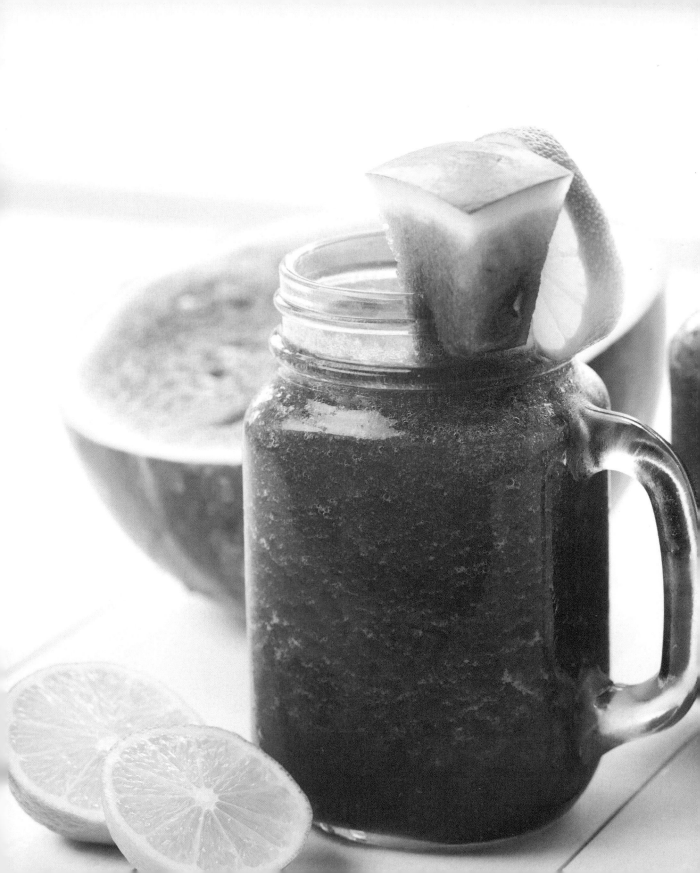

CARAMEL APPLE RINGS

Makes 4 servings

Coming up with fun, easy ideas for families can feel hard sometimes, and that's when you can turn to these caramel apple rings. They're a perfect breakfast idea for kids and adults alike. Try setting out all the different toppings "build your own" style and let everyone decorate the caramel apple rings with their own favorite choices!

1 lemon, juiced, divided
3 red apples
1 cup Medjool dates, pitted
1 inch vanilla bean (optional)
½ cup water

OPTIONAL TOPPINGS

1 cup raspberries
¼ cup raisins
¼ cup dried mulberries
¼ cup shredded coconut
2 tablespoons raw honey

Fill a large bowl with cold water and pour half of the lemon juice into it.

Turn each apple sideways and carefully cut it into slices about ¼ inch thick. Use a small cookie cutter or bottle cap to punch the core out of the center of each apple slice. Place the finished rings immediately into the bowl of lemon water to prevent browning.

Blend the dates, vanilla bean, ½ cup water, and remaining lemon juice together until a thick, smooth "caramel" forms.

Remove the apple rings from the water. Spread caramel along the top of each ring and add any desired toppings!

TIPS

- If the dates you're using are dry, try soaking them in warm water for a few minutes prior to blending.

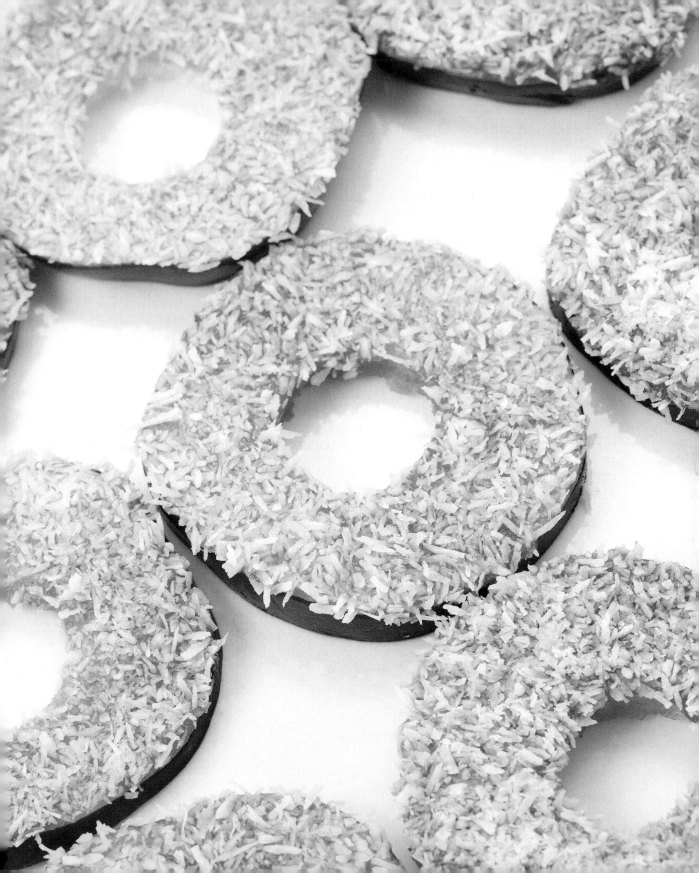

WILD BLUEBERRY MINI MUFFINS

Makes 16 muffins

These bite-sized blueberry morsels come out of the oven warm, fluffy, and ready to enjoy for breakfast or any time of day. They make a great addition to any packed lunch or afternoon snack. The batter comes together in the blender in minutes, making this a quick and easy option whenever you need one.

¼ cup white chia seeds
1 cup mashed banana
½ cup gluten-free oat flour
½ teaspoon baking soda
¼ teaspoon sea salt
¼ cup maple syrup
1 tablespoon lemon juice
½ cup frozen wild blueberries

Preheat the oven to 375°F.

Place the white chia seeds in the blender alone and blend them on high until finely ground.

Add the mashed banana, oat flour, baking soda, sea salt, maple syrup, and lemon juice into the blender and blend until smoothly combined into batter.

Pour the batter into a bowl and stir in the frozen wild blueberries.

Line a mini muffin pan with 16 mini parchment baking cups and fill each with 1 heaping tablespoon of batter.

Place the mini muffin pan into the oven and bake for 20 minutes until the tops of the muffins are turning golden brown and an inserted toothpick comes out clean. Remove the muffins from the oven and allow them to cool before eating. They will continue to firm up inside as they cool.

TIPS

- Make sure to seek out aluminum-free baking soda, available in the natural section of grocery stores, in natural foods stores, or online.

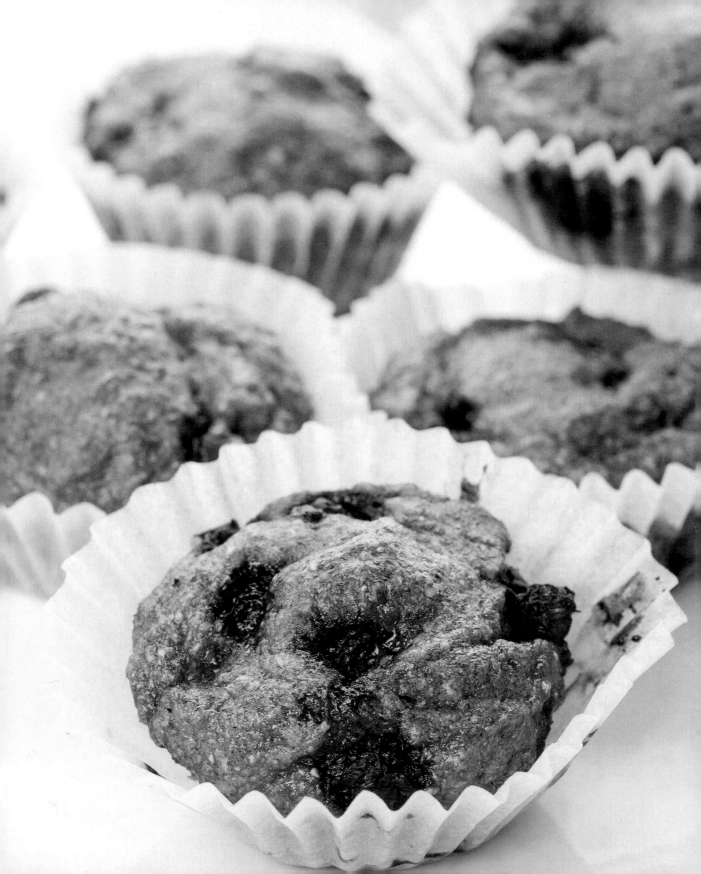

CHICKPEA QUICHE

Makes 6 to 8 servings

This chickpea quiche is portable and stores well in the refrigerator. Try baking one up on Sunday and munching it throughout the week for an easy breakfast or lunch option. It tastes wonderful on its own and also tastes amazing topped with an herby tomato sauce, such as the Ratatouille Tomato Sauce recipe on page 400.

4 cups small broccoli florets

4 cups halved cherry or grape tomatoes

4 cups diced red onion

8 garlic cloves, skins on

2 cups water

3 cups chickpea flour

4 tablespoons fresh lemon juice

2 teaspoons poultry seasoning

2 teaspoons sea salt

Preheat the oven to 400°F.

Spread the broccoli florets, tomatoes, red onion, and garlic cloves on two baking sheets lined with parchment paper and roast for 15 to 20 minutes until tender.

Peel the roasted garlic cloves (being careful not to burn your fingers!) and place them into the blender along with the water, chickpea flour, lemon juice, poultry seasoning, and sea salt and blend until a smooth batter forms.

Pour the batter into a large mixing bowl and stir in all of the roasted vegetables.

Pour this mixture into a quiche dish or pan lined with parchment paper. Alternatively, you can divide the quiche batter into a standard 12-cup muffin pan lined with parchment baking cups and make individual mini quiches.

Bake for 30 to 35 minutes, opening the oven halfway through to release steam. The quiche is done when the top is browned and a toothpick inserted in the middle comes out clean.

Remove the quiche from the oven and allow to cool before serving.

TIPS

- This quiche freezes well, so make two and you'll have one on hand for an easy grab-and-go meal anytime. Remove the parchment lining prior to freezing.

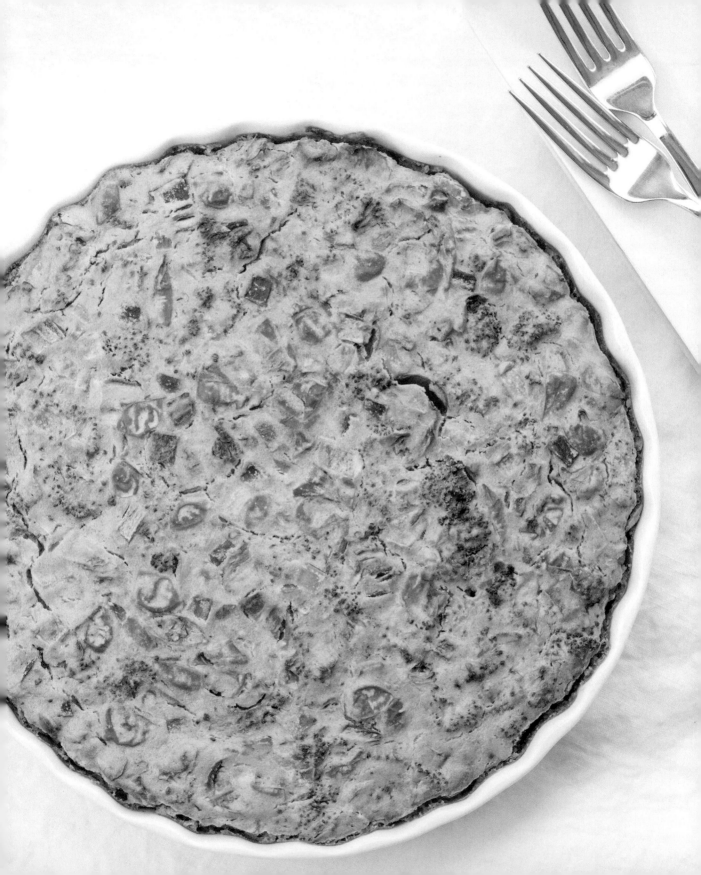

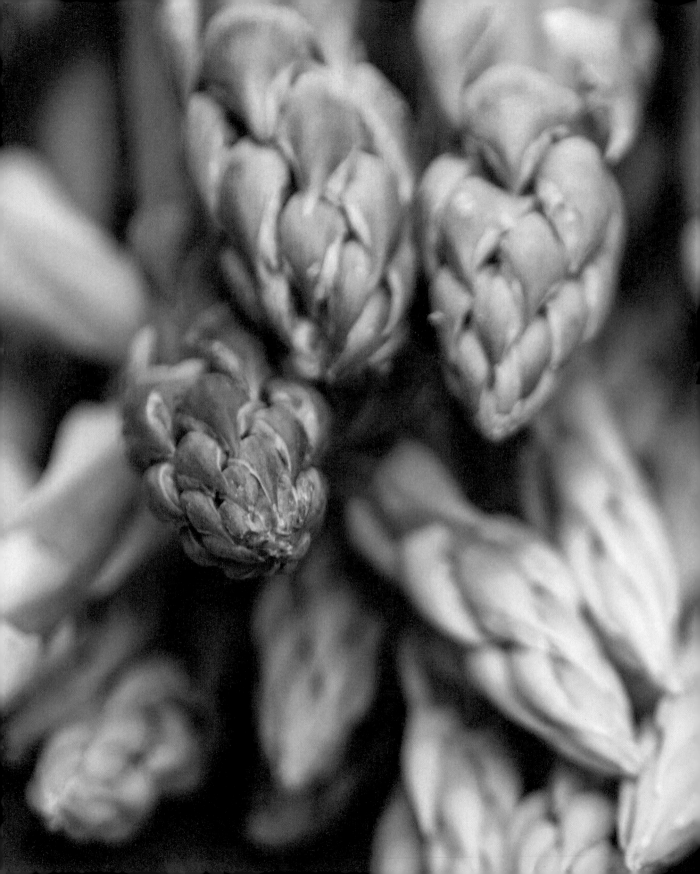

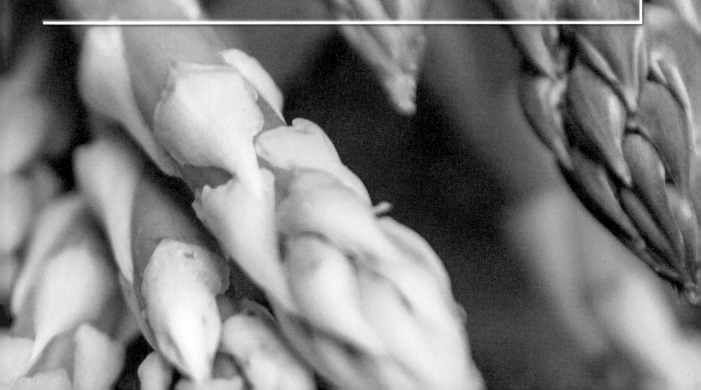

LUNCH

LIVER RESCUE SALAD

These two salad options are brimming with healing properties for your liver. They're great for when you want a lighter meal, and they're also perfect additions to a cooked meal such as the steamed vegetables from the Liver Rescue 3:6:9. You can customize each salad with any of the liver-healing foods from the previous chapter so that you never get bored. If you try the fat-free Orange "Vinaigrette" Dressing, it is sure to become a staple in your kitchen. It's flavorful, sweet, and satisfying for anyone to enjoy.

OPTION A

3 cups chopped tomatoes

1 cucumber, sliced

1 cup chopped celery

1 cup chopped cilantro (optional)

½ cup chopped parsley (optional)

½ cup chopped scallion (optional)

8 cups any variety of leafy greens (spinach, arugula, butter lettuce, etc.)

1 lemon, lime, or orange, juiced

OPTION B

2 cups thinly sliced red cabbage

1 cup diced carrot

1 cup diced asparagus

1 cup diced radish

2 cups diced apples

½ cup chopped cilantro

8 cups any variety of leafy greens (spinach, arugula, butter lettuce, etc.)

1 lemon, lime, or orange, juiced

OPTIONAL ORANGE "VINAIGRETTE" DRESSING

1 cup orange juice

1 garlic clove

1 tablespoon raw honey

¼ cup water

⅛ teaspoon sea salt (optional)

⅛ teaspoon cayenne (optional)

Place the salad vegetables and the leafy greens of your choice in a bowl and mix together to form the base of the salad.

Drizzle the fresh lemon, lime, or orange juice over top to taste. Alternatively, make the Orange "Vinaigrette" by blending all of its ingredients until smoothly combined.

Toss your salad in the straight citrus juice or Orange "Vinaigrette" Dressing until well mixed.

If you're sharing with another or saving some for later, divide the salad into two bowls. Enjoy!

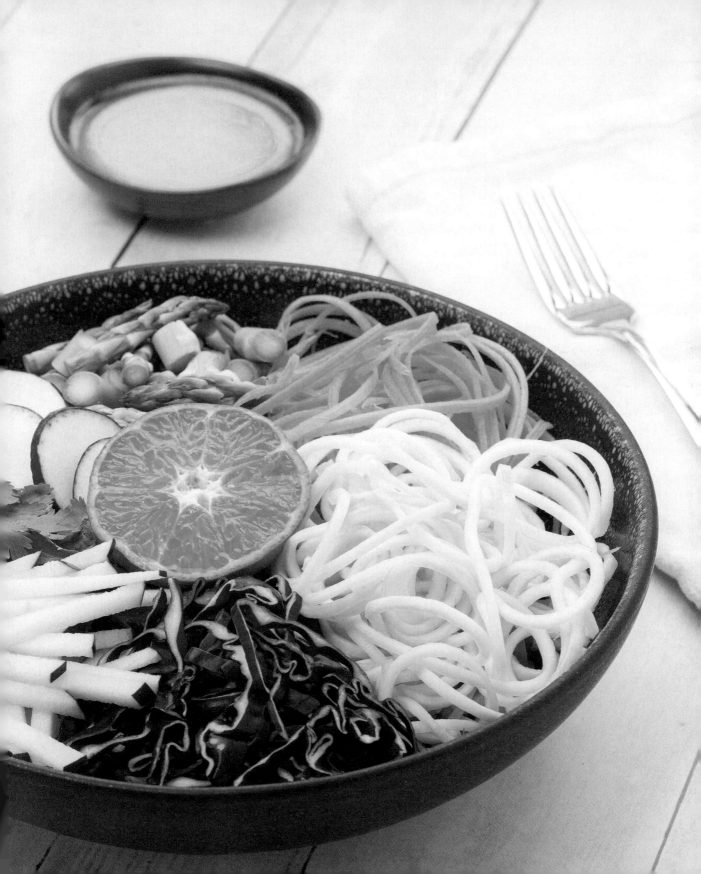

YELLOW CURRY NOODLES TWO WAYS

Makes 2 servings

These days, the best recipes are the ones that can be customized to meet everyone's needs. These curry noodles can be eaten raw or cooked, fat-free or with coconut milk added, and no matter how you choose to prepare it, this dish is easy and delicious. This is an ideal option if you are juggling the necessity of cooking for others.

2 zucchinis, peeled
1 carrot
1 red bell pepper, finely sliced
¼ onion, finely sliced
3 cups kelp noodles
1 ½ cups coconut milk (optional)
½ teaspoon sea salt (optional)
1 lime
¼ cup basil
¼ cup cilantro

YELLOW CURRY SAUCE

3 cups diced zucchini
4 Medjool dates, pitted
1 garlic clove
½ cup cilantro leaves
2 tablespoons lime juice
2 tablespoons coconut aminos (optional, see Tips)
½ tablespoon minced ripe jalapeño
½ teaspoon curry powder

Using a julienne peeler or spiralizer, turn the zucchinis and the carrot into "noodles." Place these noodles into a large bowl along with the red bell pepper, onion, and kelp noodles.

Prepare the Yellow Curry Sauce by blending all the sauce ingredients until smooth and slightly warmed.

For raw curry noodles, pour the Yellow Curry Sauce over the prepared vegetable and kelp noodles, tossing well to combine.

For cooked curry noodles, combine the Yellow Curry Sauce, prepared vegetable and kelp noodles, coconut milk, and sea salt in a large pot. Cook over medium heat for 10 to 15 minutes, until the vegetable noodles are tender and well combined.

Serve the yellow curry noodles topped with basil, cilantro, and a squeeze of fresh lime juice.

TIPS

- Coconut aminos are available in many natural food stores and online. If you prefer, you can leave them out altogether and substitute ⅓ cup chopped dulse or ¼ teaspoon sea salt instead.

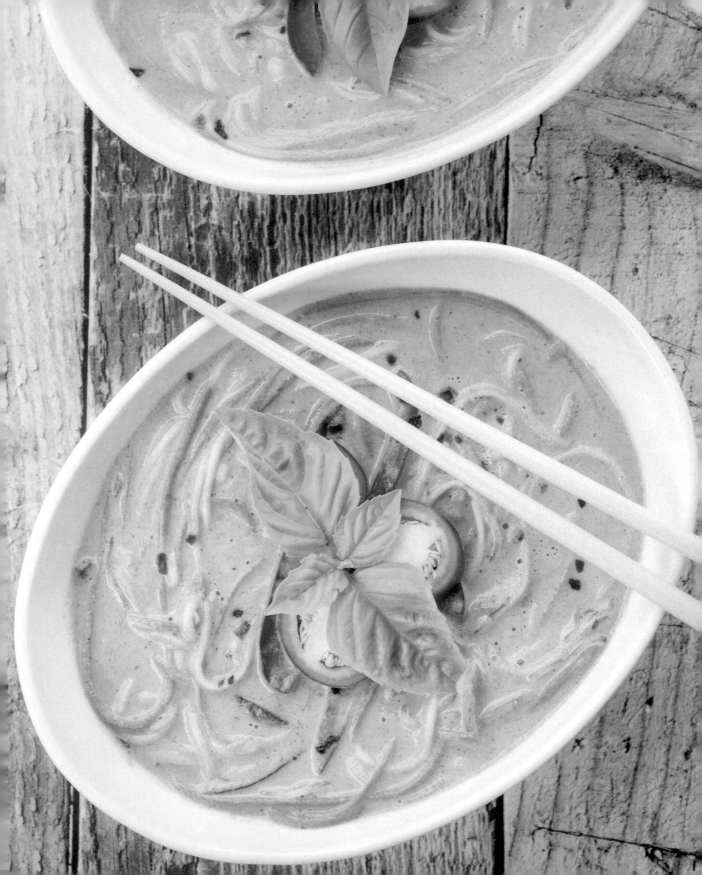

SWEET POTATO AND BLACK BEAN SALAD WITH SPICY LIME "VINAIGRETTE"

Makes 2 to 4 servings

This salad is hearty and full of vibrant flavor from cilantro, limes, and optional jalapeños. It will keep well in the fridge, so make a double batch and you'll be able to enjoy it all week long. You can also try this salad scooped into lettuce cups or wrapped up in gluten-free, corn-free tortillas.

2 sweet potatoes, diced
6 garlic cloves, unpeeled
½ red onion, finely diced
1 red bell pepper, diced
2 cups cooked black beans
¼ cup chopped cilantro
8 cups leafy greens (optional)
Salt to taste

SPICY LIME "VINAIGRETTE"

½ cup loosely packed cilantro
2 tablespoons lime juice
2 tablespoons raw honey
¼ teaspoon sea salt
2 garlic cloves
½ ripe jalapeño (optional)
½ cup water

Preheat the oven to 425°F.

Spread out the sweet potatoes and the garlic cloves on a baking tray lined with parchment paper and place in the oven. Roast the sweet potatoes and garlic for 20 to 30 minutes, until the sweet potatoes are fork-tender.

Peel and mince the roasted garlic cloves (taking care not to burn your fingers).

Place the roasted sweet potatoes, red onion, red bell pepper, minced roasted garlic, and black beans into a mixing bowl and stir to combine.

To make the Spicy Lime "Vinaigrette," place all the dressing ingredients in the blender and blend until a smooth, thin sauce forms.

This salad can be eaten warm or chilled. Immediately prior to serving, toss the sweet potato and black bean mixture in the Spicy Lime "Vinaigrette." Serve garnished with chopped cilantro and over a bed of leafy greens. If desired, add an extra sprinkle of sea salt to taste.

TIPS

- It's best to taste a small bite of the jalapeño you're using to determine how spicy it is. For a spicier dressing, add a larger piece of the jalapeño. For a milder dressing, use a smaller piece of the jalapeño and even remove the seeds, which contain most of the spiciness. If you can't find red, ripe jalapeños, substitute with a different type of ripe hot pepper.

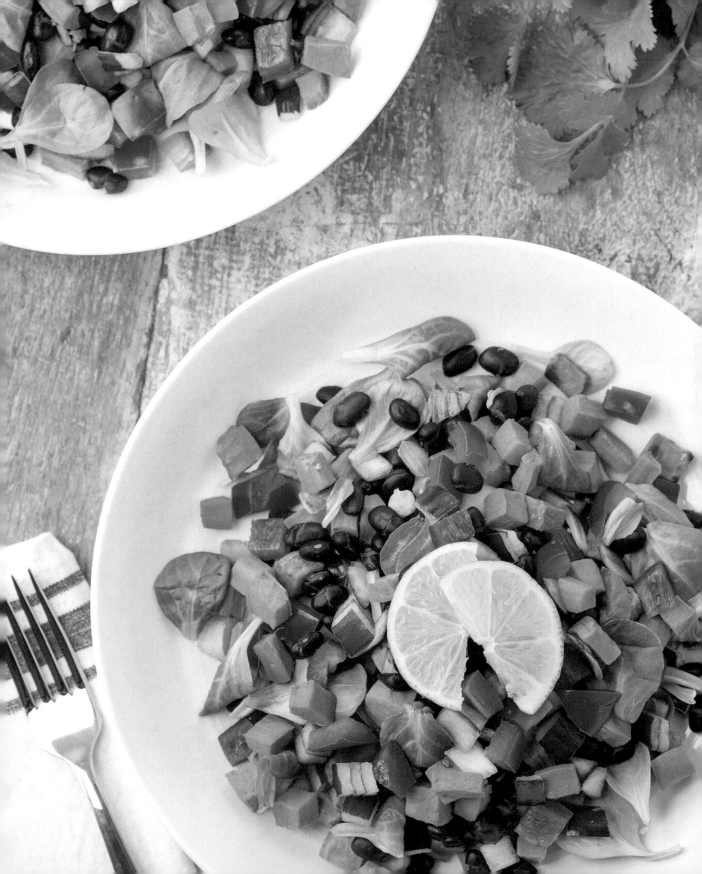

BAKED FALAFEL
WITH MINT TAHINI SAUCE

Makes 2 to 4 servings

This recipe will leave even the hungriest lunch eaters satisfied. Tender, baked falafel are wrapped in lettuce and loaded with a rainbow of vegetables, and then dunked into the complex flavors of the Mint Tahini Sauce. If mint doesn't appeal to you, feel free to substitute any fresh herb that does, such as basil, cilantro, parsley, or tarragon.

3 cups cooked chickpeas
1 cup roughly diced red onion
4 garlic cloves
½ cup loosely packed parsley
½ cup loosely packed cilantro
½ teaspoon sea salt
2 teaspoons cumin
2 heads of butter lettuce
(optional, see Tips)

OPTIONAL TOPPINGS

½ cucumber, sliced
½ cup halved cherry or
grape tomatoes
½ cup shredded red cabbage
½ cup shredded carrot

MINT TAHINI SAUCE

1 cup diced zucchini
½ Medjool date, pitted
2 garlic cloves
2 tablespoons tahini
2 tablespoons lemon juice
2 tablespoons fresh dill
2 tablespoons fresh mint
¼ teaspoon sea salt
½ cup water

Preheat the oven to 350°F.

Place half of the chickpeas into the bottom of the food processor. Then add the diced onion, garlic cloves, parsley, cilantro, and sea salt. On top, add the remaining chickpeas. Pulse all of the ingredients together in the food processor until they are well combined.

Line two baking trays with parchment paper. Using a tablespoon measure, scoop out the chickpea mixture, shape it into balls, and place them on the baking trays spaced 2 inches apart. Gently pat the tops of the balls to flatten them into a falafel shape.

Bake the falafel for 35 to 40 minutes, until the tops are turning golden brown and they are firm on the outside while still tender in the middle. Handle them gently!

To make the Mint Tahini Sauce, blend all of the ingredients together until smoothly combined.

Serve the falafel on top of a salad of butter lettuce or in individual butter lettuce cups topped with veggies and Mint Tahini Sauce.

TIPS

- These falafel can also be served in a gluten-free, corn-free tortilla of your choice.

- If you'd prefer to keep this dish completely fat-free, skip the Mint Tahini Sauce and try pairing the falafel with the Spicy Lime "Vinaigrette" on page 388 instead.

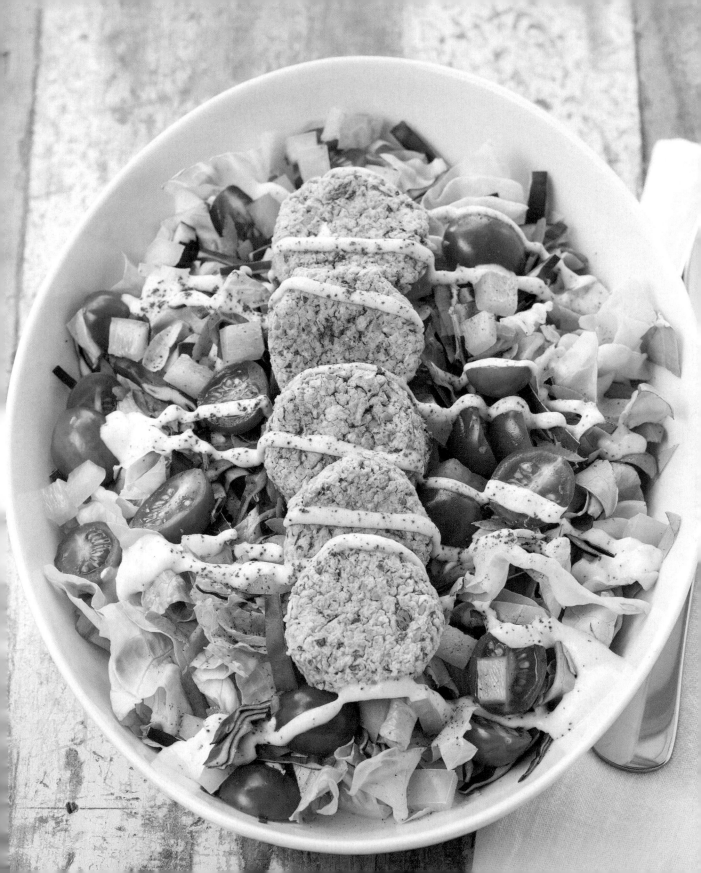

KABOCHA SQUASH SOUP

Makes 2 to 4 servings

This soup is like a hug inside a bowl. It's creamy, warm, and comforting. The nourishing rich flavor of kabocha squash blends beautifully with the warmth of garlic, onions, and curry. This is a great one to make ahead and freeze so that you have an instant satisfying option on hand whenever you need it.

1 medium kabocha squash (see Tips)

3 cups vegetable broth (see Tips)

1 cup diced onion

4 garlic cloves, minced

1 teaspoon curry powder

½ teaspoon sea salt

½ lime, juiced

¼ teaspoon red pepper flakes (optional)

Bring a large pot of water to a rapid boil and submerge the whole kabocha squash, stem and all. Boil the squash for 10 minutes, flipping it upside down halfway through. Remove the squash carefully and set aside to cool.

When the squash is cool enough to handle comfortably, peel it, slice it in half, and remove the seeds. Cut the squash into cubes; this should yield about 4 cups.

Place the cubed kabocha squash into a pot along with the vegetable broth, diced onion, garlic cloves, curry powder, sea salt, and lime juice. Bring the broth to a boil and then reduce to a rapid simmer, stirring frequently.

Continue to simmer for 15 to 20 minutes, until the squash is tender and cooked through.

Transfer the entire contents to a blender and blend until smooth, slowly at first, allowing an opening for steam to escape through the top of the blender.

Serve warm, topped with red pepper flakes if desired.

TIPS

- Make your own broth using the Liver Rescue Broth recipe on page 368. Alternatively, you can find low-sodium vegetable broth at the grocery store (make sure it doesn't have canola oil, citric acid, natural flavors, or other sneaky additives) or replace the broth with water in a pinch.

- If kabocha squash is unavailable where you live, try substituting butternut squash, acorn squash, or even sweet potato instead. You'll need about 6 cups cubed squash of any variety.

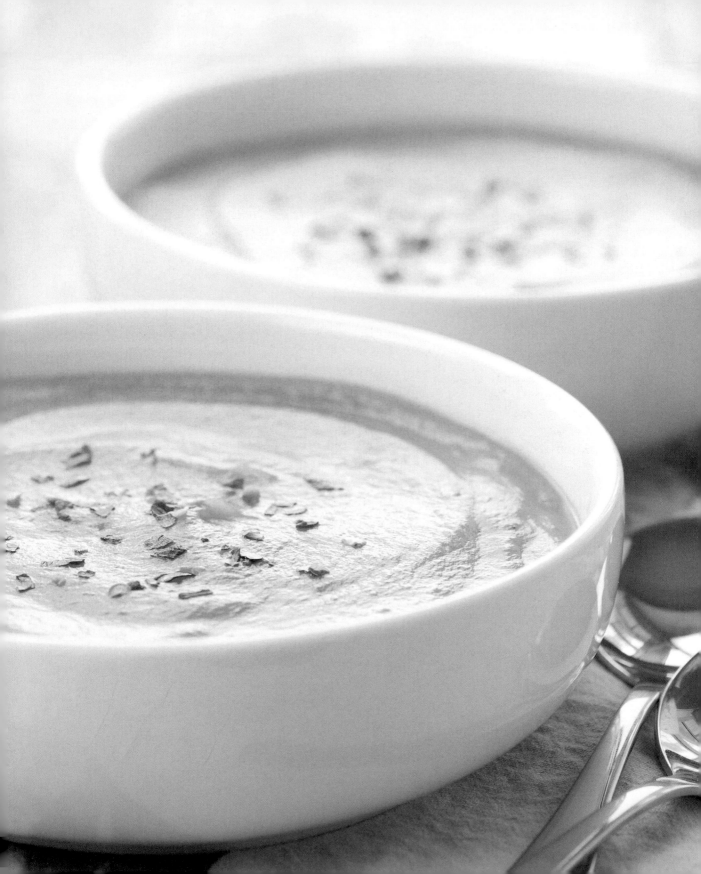

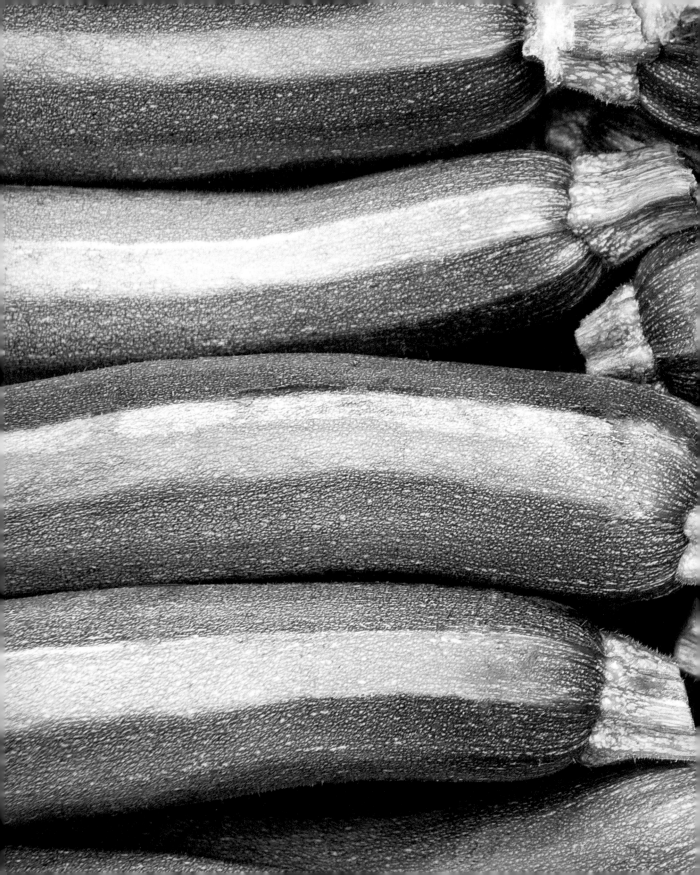

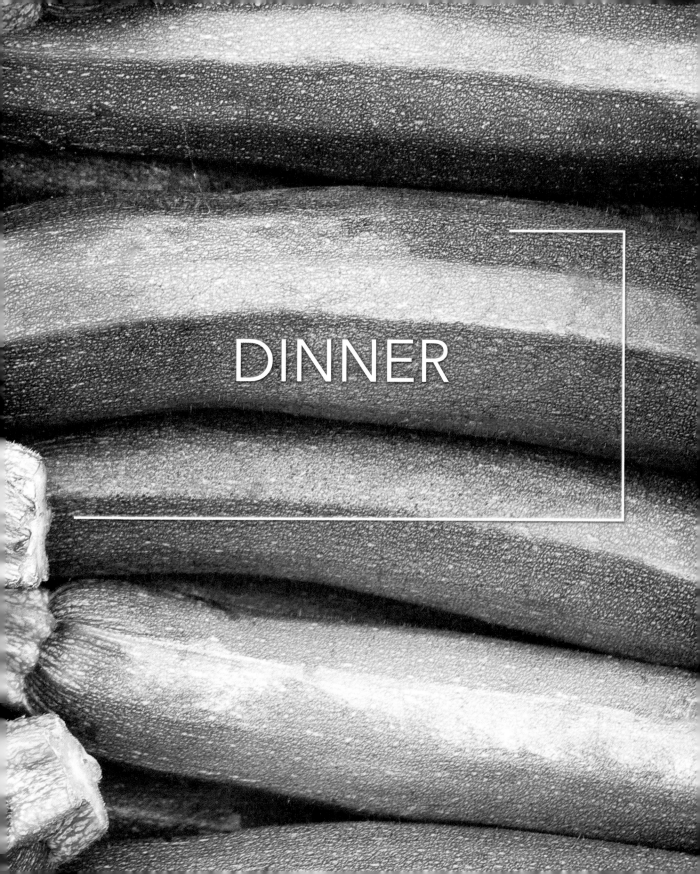

DINNER

LENTIL TACOS

Makes 3 servings

Who doesn't love tacos? The lentil filling for these romaine lettuce tacos can be enjoyed warm or cold according to your preference. If you're looking for something a little heartier, feel free to try gluten-free, corn-free tortillas instead. For an extra kick, this recipe would pair well with the Spicy Lime "Vinaigrette" on page 388 or even the Mint Tahini Sauce on page 390.

1 cup diced onion

½ cup vegetable broth (see Tips)

1 cup diced mushrooms (optional)

4 garlic cloves, minced

3 cups cooked lentils (see Tips)

1 teaspoon poultry seasoning

½ teaspoon chili powder

1 teaspoon cumin

½ teaspoon paprika

½ teaspoon chipotle powder

¼ teaspoon honey or maple syrup (optional)

½ teaspoon sea salt

¼ teaspoon cayenne (optional)

2 heads romaine or butter lettuce

OPTIONAL TOPPINGS

1 cup cherry or grape tomatoes, sliced

1 avocado, sliced

½ cup chopped cilantro

½ cup sliced radish

½ cup shredded red cabbage

½ cup shredded carrots

3 lime halves

1 ripe jalapeño, thinly sliced

Sauté the onion in 2 tablespoons of vegetable broth over medium-high heat for approximately 5 minutes until tender. Continue to add vegetable broth by the spoonful as needed to prevent sticking.

Add the mushrooms, garlic, lentils, poultry seasoning, cumin, paprika, chipotle, honey, and sea salt to the sauté pan. If spiciness is desired, add the cayenne as well. Continue to cook everything over medium-high heat for 5 minutes or until the mushrooms are tender and cooked through.

Serve the lentil mixture in individual romaine leaves as "taco shells" and top with any or all of the optional toppings.

TIPS

- The Liver Rescue Broth found on page 368 can be used for this recipe, or you can use store-bought. As in the previous recipe, make sure it doesn't contain canola oil, citric acid, natural flavors, or other sneaky additives. Water can also be substituted when vegetable broth is unavailable.

- Brown or green lentils work best for this recipe. Prepare 1 cup of dried lentils according to the directions on the packaging.

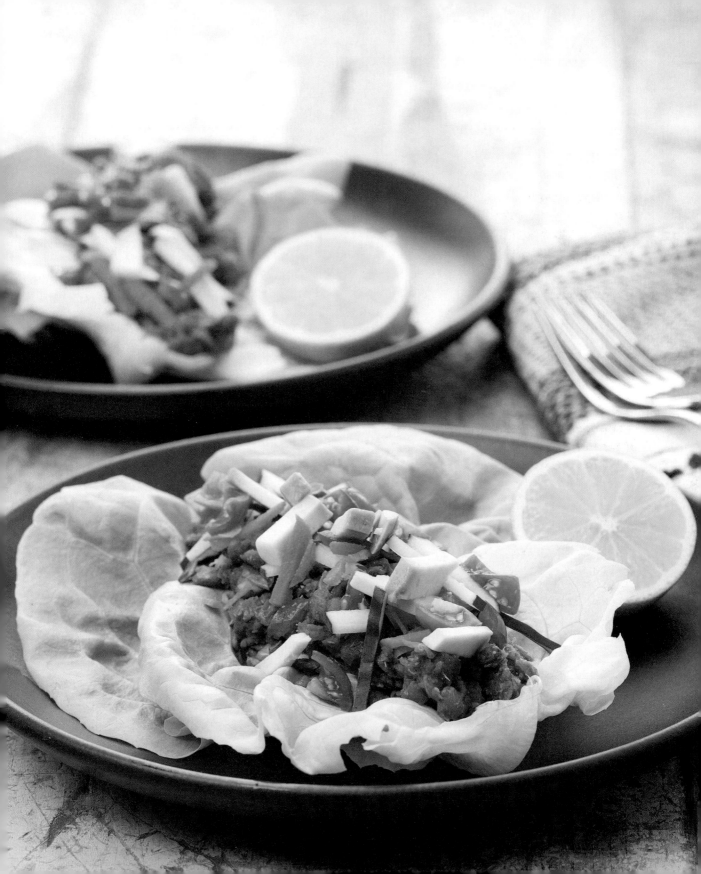

CAULIFLOWER SUSHI WITH THAI CHILI SAUCE

Makes 2 servings

This dish can be made with either raw or cooked cauliflower rice. While it may seem intimidating to think of making your own sushi rolls, it's surprisingly easy. They don't have to look perfect in order to taste great! The options for filling your sushi rolls are endless. Try incorporating fresh herbs like mint, basil, and cilantro for a fresh twist, or branch out into other liver-healing vegetables like radishes, asparagus, or sprouts. You can even incorporate cooked vegetables like sweet potatoes or any variety of squash.

½ cauliflower
6 toasted nori sheets

OPTIONAL FILLINGS

1 cucumber, thinly sliced
1 carrot, thinly sliced
1 red bell pepper, thinly sliced
1 cup thinly sliced red cabbage
1 avocado, thinly sliced
½ cup water

THAI CHILI SAUCE

1 cup cherry or grape tomatoes
1 cup cold water or fresh-squeezed orange juice
¼ cup sun-dried tomatoes
1 garlic clove
2 tablespoons lemon juice
2 tablespoons honey
¼ teaspoon red pepper flakes
1 tablespoon minced Thai red chili or ripe jalapeño

Cut the cauliflower into florets (it should yield approximately 6 cups of florets). Place the florets into a food processor and pulse until a rice-like texture forms. Place the cauliflower rice in a medium bowl and set to one side.

If you'd prefer to have cooked cauliflower rice, cook the processed cauliflower in a sauté pan over medium heat, stirring frequently for 5 to 7 minutes until tender. There is no need to add oil or water to the pan, as the cauliflower itself should remain moist enough to avoid sticking. When the cauliflower rice is tender, set it aside in a medium bowl to cool.

Place one sheet of nori on a cutting board. Scoop about ¾ cup of cauliflower rice onto the end of the nori sheet closest to you and spread it into an even layer covering the bottom half of the nori.

Arrange the desired filling vegetables in the middle of the cauliflower rice. Carefully lift the nori from the bottom edge close to you and begin rolling it tightly toward the top.

Just before finishing the roll, dip your finger in the water or orange juice and run it along the top edge of the sheet. This will help the nori stick to itself as you complete your roll. Using a sharp knife, slice each sushi roll into even pieces.

To make the Thai Chili Sauce, blend the fresh tomatoes, water, sun-dried tomatoes, garlic, lemon juice, honey, and red pepper flakes together with up to 1 tablespoon of minced Thai red chili or jalapeño according to desired spiciness.

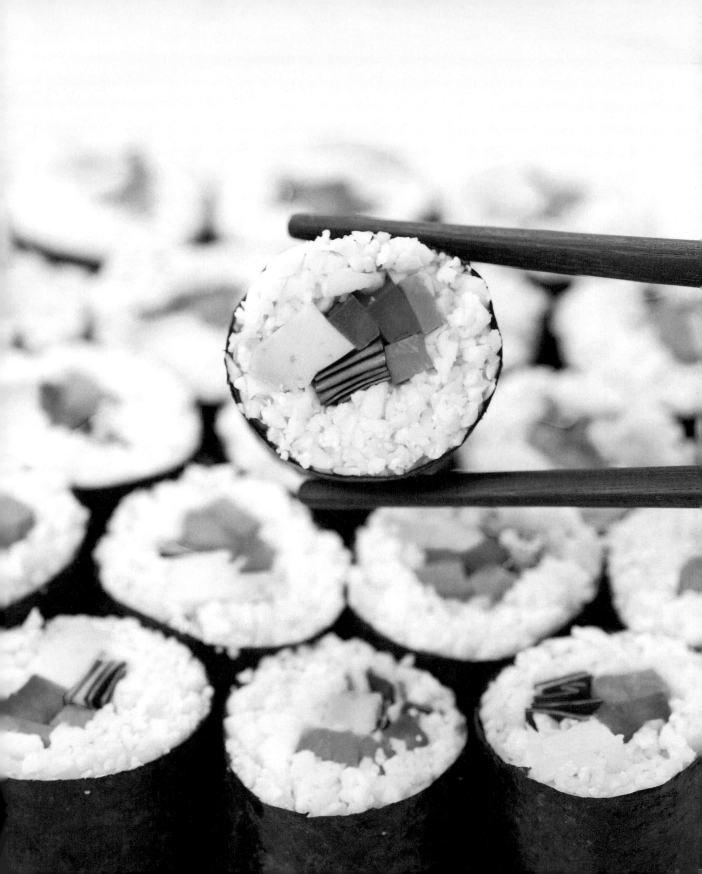

RATATOUILLE

Makes 4 servings

Ratatouille is one of those recipes born of resourcefulness. In late summer, it can be hard to know what to do with the abundance of zucchini, squash, eggplants, and tomatoes bursting out of the garden. This recipe makes a comforting, rustic meal out of these summer vegetables and freezes perfectly to be enjoyed well into fall. Try coming up with your own variations of ratatouille to reflect the seasonal produce in your own area.

1 large zucchini
1 large yellow squash
1 eggplant
1 red bell pepper
4 cups cooked quinoa (optional)

TOMATO SAUCE

4 tomatoes, roughly diced
1 yellow onion, roughly diced
4 garlic cloves, minced
2 tablespoons tomato paste (see Tips)
½ teaspoon sea salt
½ teaspoon dried basil
½ teaspoon poultry seasoning
⅛ teaspoon curry powder

Preheat the oven to 375°F.

Thinly slice the zucchini, yellow squash, eggplant, and red bell pepper into rounds. Set aside.

To make the tomato sauce, combine its ingredients in a saucepan over high heat. Stir frequently for 2 to 3 minutes until the tomatoes have released their juices.

Reduce heat to a simmer and continue stirring occasionally for 15 to 20 minutes until the tomatoes have started to break down. Using an immersion blender, puree the tomatoes until a chunky sauce forms. Alternatively, you can use a standing blender for this step by pulse blending and leaving an opening at the top to allow the steam to escape.

Place a cup of the tomato sauce in the bottom of a baking dish and spread it to coat the bottom. Layer the zucchini, yellow squash, eggplant, and red bell pepper slices in whatever pattern is desired. Cover the baking dish with parchment paper and place in the oven for 45 to 60 minutes, until the vegetables are tender.

Serve the ratatouille topped with the remaining tomato sauce, over a bed of quinoa if desired.

TIPS

- This tomato sauce freezes well and can be kept on hand for quick, easy meals anytime.

- If you use store-bought tomato paste, make sure it doesn't contain citric acid.

- For an even faster version, roughly dice the zucchini, yellow squash, eggplant, and red bell pepper, mix in the tomato sauce, and cook everything in a baking dish for 40 to 60 minutes until all the vegetables are tender.

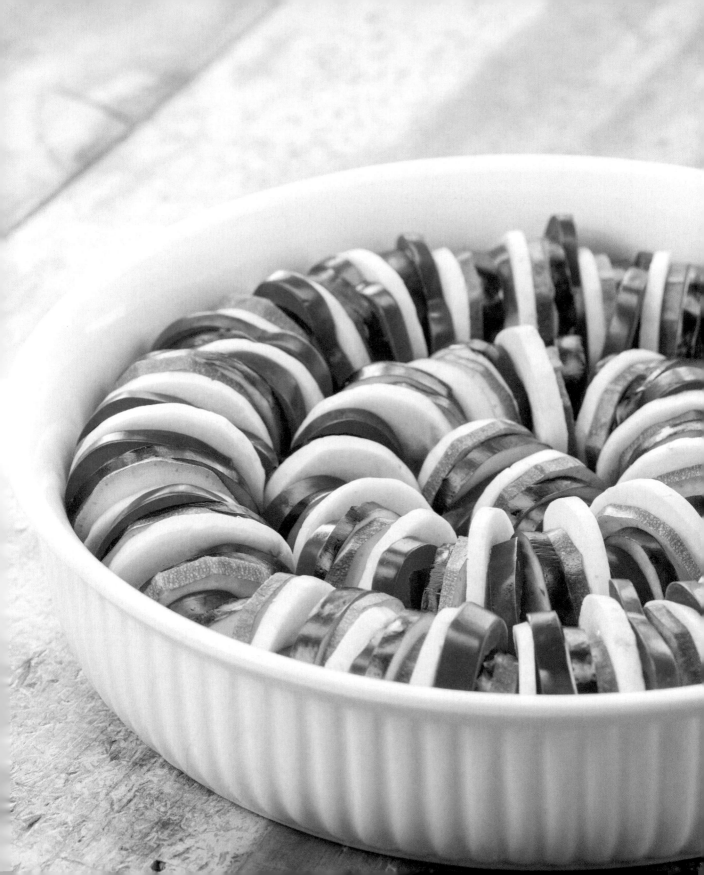

POTATO PANCAKES
WITH CUCUMBER RADISH SALAD

Makes 2 servings

These potato pancakes come out of the oven perfectly crispy and satisfying, and then they're topped off with light, refreshing Cucumber Radish Salad that takes them over the top. Feel free to try other toppings. If you have hungry kids in your life, they may like to try their potato pancakes topped with mashed avocado or black beans!

2 large russet potatoes, peeled and grated

1 tablespoon arrowroot powder

½ teaspoon sea salt, divided

1 cucumber, thinly sliced

6 radishes, thinly sliced

2 teaspoons raw honey

1 tablespoon lemon juice

1 tablespoon dill, minced

¼ cup chopped chives

¼ teaspoon red pepper (optional)

Preheat the oven to 425°F.

Combine the potatoes, arrowroot powder, and ¼ teaspoon sea salt in a mixing bowl and stir to combine.

Line two baking trays with parchment paper. Drop the potatoes onto the parchment paper by the ¼ cup and shape them into circles approximately 3 inches in diameter, using your hands or a cookie cutter as a mold. Press them down until they are approximately ¼ inch thick.

Bake the potato pancakes for 20 minutes. Remove them from the oven and flip the pancakes over by carefully grasping the edges of the parchment paper and flipping the entire sheet. If needed, peel any stuck potato pancakes carefully off the parchment paper and stick them back into the oven on the unlined baking trays for 5 minutes more.

While the potato pancakes are baking, make the Cucumber Radish Salad by combining the sliced cucumber and radishes with the honey, lemon juice, dill, chives, remaining ¼ teaspoon of sea salt, and red pepper in a mixing bowl, tossing gently to combine.

Serve the potato pancakes piping hot and garnished with Cucumber Radish Salad.

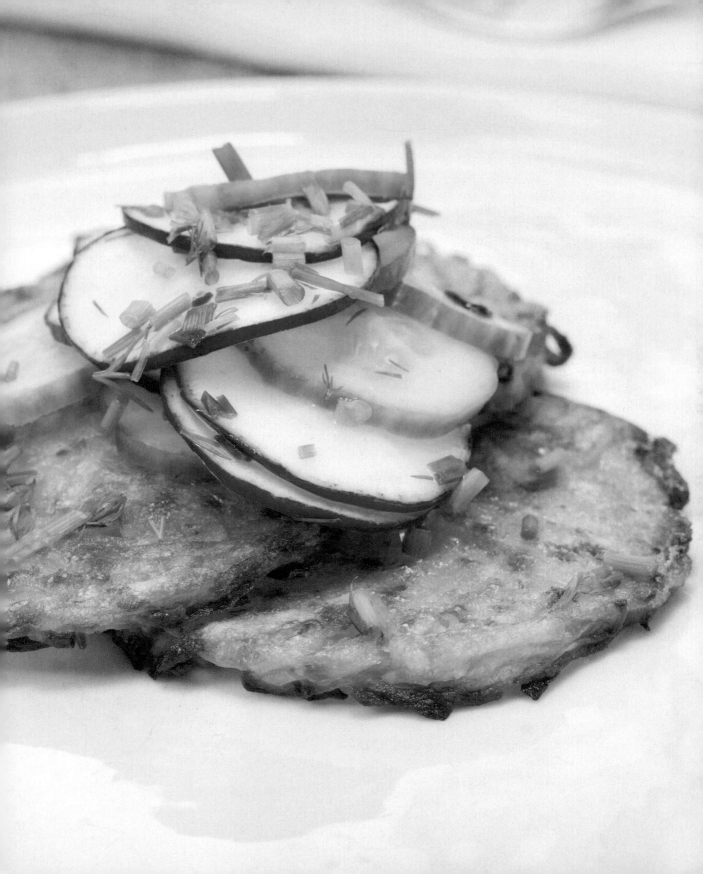

ROASTED VEGGIE PASTA

Makes 2 to 4 servings

This colorful pasta dish is loaded with tender roasted vegetables and tossed together in a light tomato sauce that leaves everything moist and flavorful. It's a great dish to serve when gathered around the table with friends and family, even those who may not eat the same way. If you're serving others, feel free to add a small dash of olive oil to their individual dishes just prior to serving, and they'll never miss a thing!

3 cups cherry or grape tomatoes

1 cup sliced red onion

1 cup diced zucchini

1 cup diced carrot

1 cup diced asparagus

10 garlic cloves, skin on

½ teaspoon lemon juice

¼ teaspoon sea salt

¼ teaspoon red pepper flakes (optional)

12 ounces gluten-free pasta (see Tips)

4 cups arugula (optional)

Additional sea salt, dulse, and/ or black pepper to taste

Preheat the oven to 400°F.

Spread out the tomatoes, red onion, zucchini, carrot, asparagus, and garlic on two baking trays lined with parchment paper and roast the vegetables for 15 to 20 minutes until tender.

Peel all the roasted garlic cloves (being careful not to burn your fingers) and place 4 of them in the blender along with 1 cup of the roasted tomatoes, the lemon juice, sea salt, and the optional red pepper flakes. Blend the ingredients until a light, smooth tomato sauce forms.

Prepare 12 ounces of gluten-free pasta according to the directions on the packaging. Drain the pasta and transfer to a mixing bowl.

Toss the pasta in the tomato sauce. There should be just enough sauce to lightly coat the noodles. Add the remaining roasted tomatoes, red onion, zucchini, asparagus, and garlic cloves. Toss gently to combine.

Serve the pasta over a bed of arugula if desired, and add an extra sprinkle of sea salt, dulse, and/or black pepper to taste.

TIPS

- Look for a gluten-free pasta made from rice, quinoa, beans, or lentils. Try to avoid the varieties that contain corn.

- While this pasta is lightly tossed in a small amount of tomato sauce for flavor, if you want a hearty portion of tomato sauce on top of your pasta, try pairing this recipe with the tomato sauce recipe used in the Ratatouille recipe on page 400.

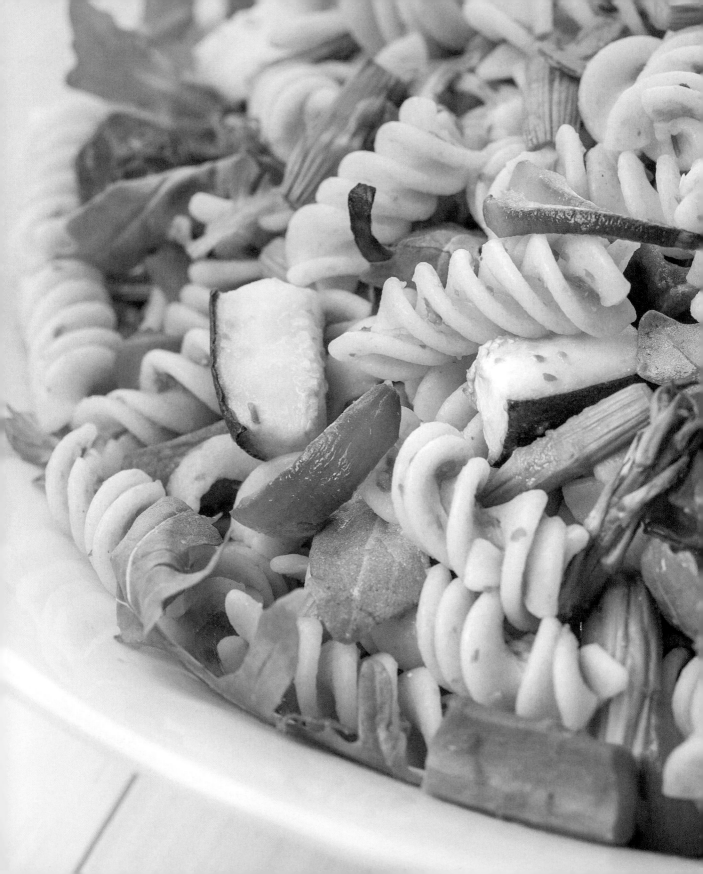

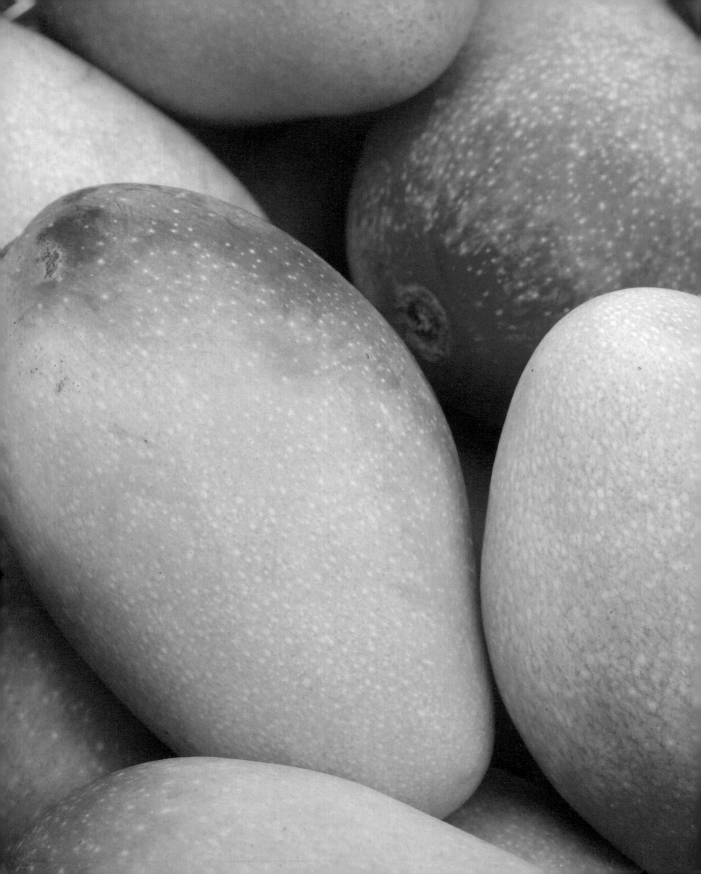

SNACKS

PINEAPPLE AND APPLE CHIPS WITH SPICY MANGO SALSA

Makes 2 servings

Chips and salsa make a classic snack food, and in this version, fruit chips and a flavorful mango salsa are a unique twist on the original. This recipe includes instructions to make either baked apple chips or raw dehydrated pineapple chips. Both are equally delicious.

4 red apples or 1 pineapple
2 cups diced mango
½ cup diced red bell pepper
¼ cup diced red onion
¼ cup finely chopped cilantro
¼ cup finely chopped basil
2 tablespoons lime juice
1 garlic clove, minced
½ teaspoon chili powder
½ tablespoon minced ripe jalapeño (optional)

To make baked apple chips, preheat the oven to 200°F. Thinly slice the apples into rounds no more than ¼ inch thick and arrange the slices on two baking trays lined with parchment paper. Bake the apple slices for 2 hours and then remove from the oven. The apple chips will continue to crisp up as they cool.

To make raw pineapple chips, slice a pineapple into rounds no more than ¼ inch thick and arrange on two dehydrator trays. (Remember: use the sweet bottom ⅔ of the pineapple if you have a sensitive stomach.) Dehydrate at 105°F for approximately 16 hours. The time needed will vary based on how thickly the pineapple is sliced and how humid the environment is.

To make the salsa, combine the mango, red bell pepper, red onion, cilantro, basil, lime juice, garlic clove, and chili powder in a medium bowl and toss to combine. Stir in the jalapeño according to desired spiciness.

Serve the salsa alongside the apple or pineapple chips and enjoy!

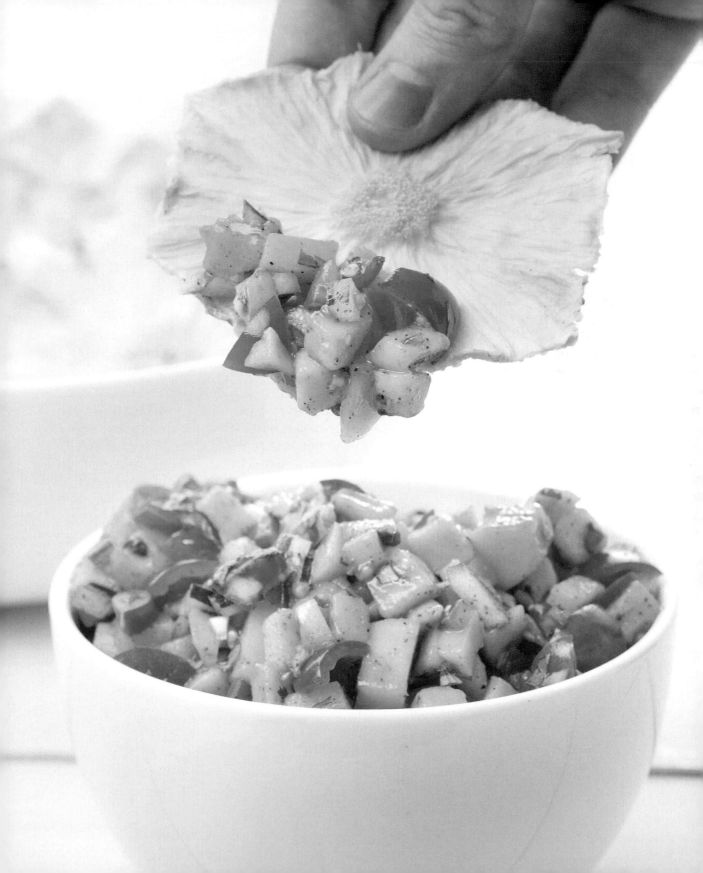

LIVER RESCUE APPLESAUCE

Makes 1 serving

Don't be fooled by this recipe's simplicity—applesauce is one of the most profoundly rejuvenating, revitalizing foods for your liver cells. It truly is a liver rescuer. Plus it's sweet and delicious and easy to whip up anytime.

1 to 2 red apples, diced

1 to 4 Medjool dates, pitted (optional)

1 stalk celery, chopped (optional)

¼ teaspoon cinnamon (optional)

Blend the diced red apple and other desired ingredients in a blender or food processor until a smooth, even applesauce forms. Serve and enjoy immediately or squeeze some fresh lemon juice over the top and seal tightly if you'd like to save it for later.

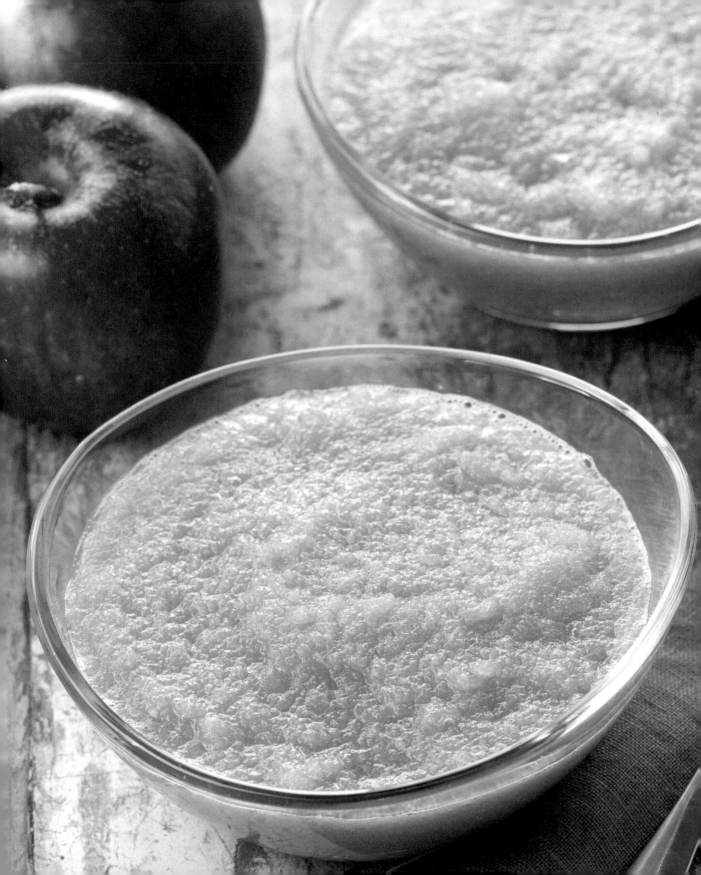

MAPLE ROASTED BRUSSELS SPROUTS

Makes 4 servings

These brussels sprouts are unbelievably appealing. They're sweet and spicy and tangy and rich with flavor. If spicy is not your preference, feel free to leave out the spices for a sweet and salty treat that will keep everyone coming back for more.

2 pounds brussels sprouts
2 tablespoons lemon juice
3 tablespoons maple syrup
1 garlic clove
¼ teaspoon cayenne
¼ teaspoon paprika
¼ teaspoon red pepper flakes
½ teaspoon sea salt, divided

Preheat the oven to 450°F.

Prepare the brussels sprouts by removing the stems and slicing vertically into halves. This should yield about 6 cups of halved brussels sprouts.

Place the lemon juice, maple syrup, garlic clove, cayenne, paprika, red pepper flakes, and ¼ teaspoon of the sea salt into the blender and blend until a smooth marinade forms.

In a large mixing bowl, toss the brussels sprouts in the marinade.

Spread out the brussels sprouts face down on two baking trays lined with parchment paper. Make sure to save the leftover marinade in the mixing bowl.

Roast the brussels sprouts for 15 to 20 minutes, until they start to turn golden brown. For extra crispiness, broil them for 1 minute before removing them from the oven.

Return the roasted brussels sprouts immediately to the mixing bowl and toss them in the leftover marinade. Sprinkle the remaining ¼ teaspoon of sea salt over the top and serve immediately for best results.

TIPS

- Don't skip the step where you reserve the marinade. Tossing the brussels sprouts in the marinade again after roasting causes them to soak up the extra flavor and makes them extra delicious!

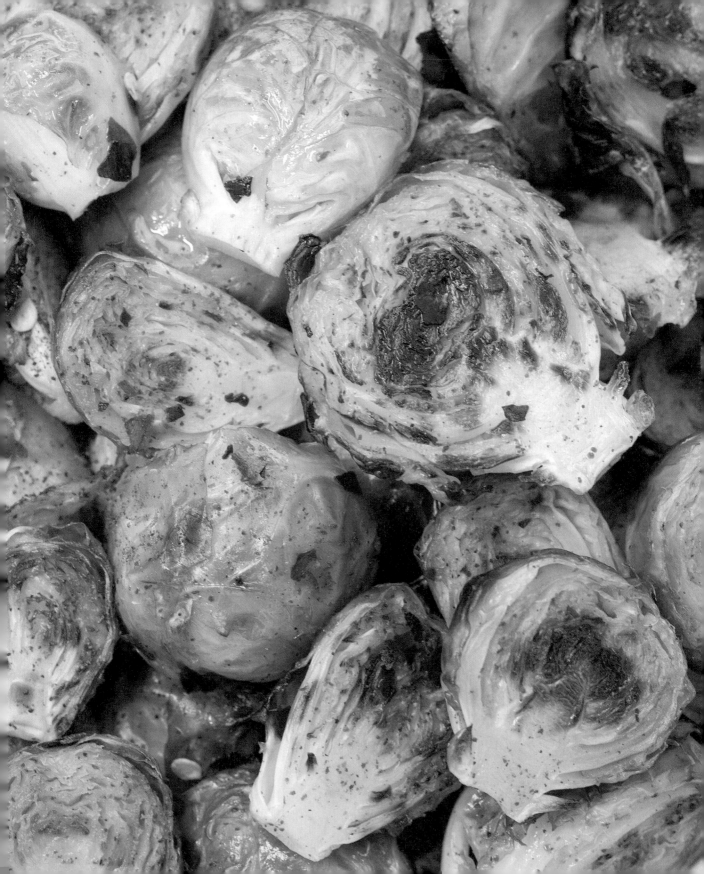

POTATO BRUSCHETTA

No one will miss the crostini with these handheld Potato Bruschetta. The more flavorful your tomatoes, the more bold and wonderful this recipe will be. Diced together with garlic, basil, and sea salt, those tomatoes will sing with the flavors of summer against the tender roasted potato slices.

2 large or 4 small russet potatoes

2 cups diced cherry or grape tomatoes

2 garlic cloves, minced

5 fresh basil leaves, minced

¼ teaspoon sea salt

½ lemon, juiced

1 teaspoon honey (optional)

Additional sea salt, dulse, and/or black pepper to taste

Preheat the oven to 425°F.

Slice the potatoes lengthwise into long ovals about ¼ inch thick and arrange them on a baking tray lined with parchment paper.

Bake the potatoes for 25 to 30 minutes, until the tops are turning golden brown.

Whisk the lemon juice, sea salt, garlic, and honey (if desired) in a small bowl. Add the diced tomatoes and toss to combine.

Arrange the baked potato slices on a serving tray and top them with the diced tomatoes and minced basil. Finish off each bruschetta with an extra sprinkle of sea salt, dulse, and/or black pepper to taste.

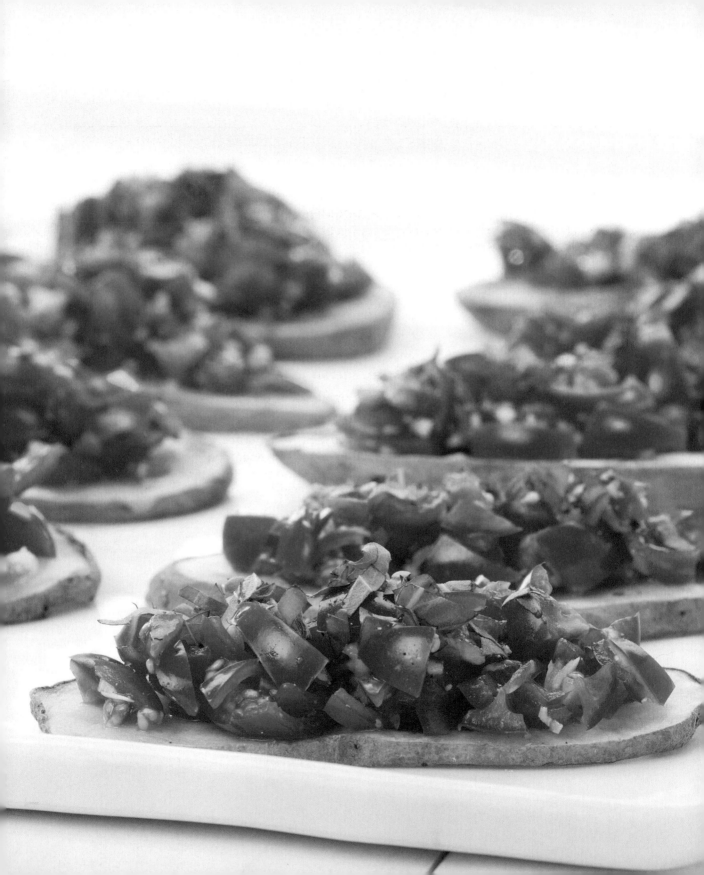

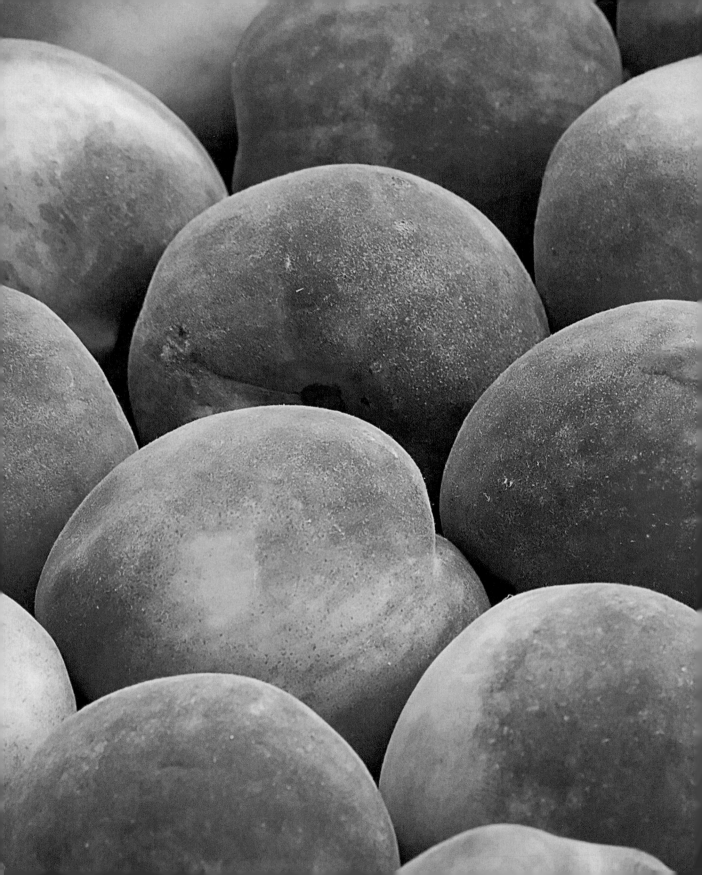

DESSERTS

PEACH GINGER SORBET

Makes 4 servings

This sorbet can be made year-round with frozen peaches from the store or peaches you froze at the height of summer yourself. The sweetness of the peaches goes perfectly with the zing of ginger and the brightness of Meyer lemon juice. If Meyer lemons aren't available, substitute regular lemon juice and adjust the honey until the desired sweetness is reached.

1 thumb knuckle–sized piece of ginger, peeled

4 cups frozen sliced peaches

1 tablespoon Meyer lemon juice

1 tablespoon raw honey (see Tips)

½ cup water

Place the ginger into the food processor and process until finely minced.

Add the frozen peaches, lemon juice, and honey to the food processor and process everything together for 2 to 3 minutes until smoothly combined. Stream in the water slowly, using just enough to keep everything moving. It can also be helpful to stop and scrape down the sides of the food processor.

The sorbet is done when a smooth, even texture has formed. This sorbet will be on the softer side. For a firmer consistency, transfer the sorbet to a container and freeze it for 3 to 4 hours prior to serving.

TIPS

- If using store-bought frozen peaches, make sure they don't contain citric acid.

- If you like things extra sweet, feel free to increase the amount of honey until the taste is exactly what you want it to be!

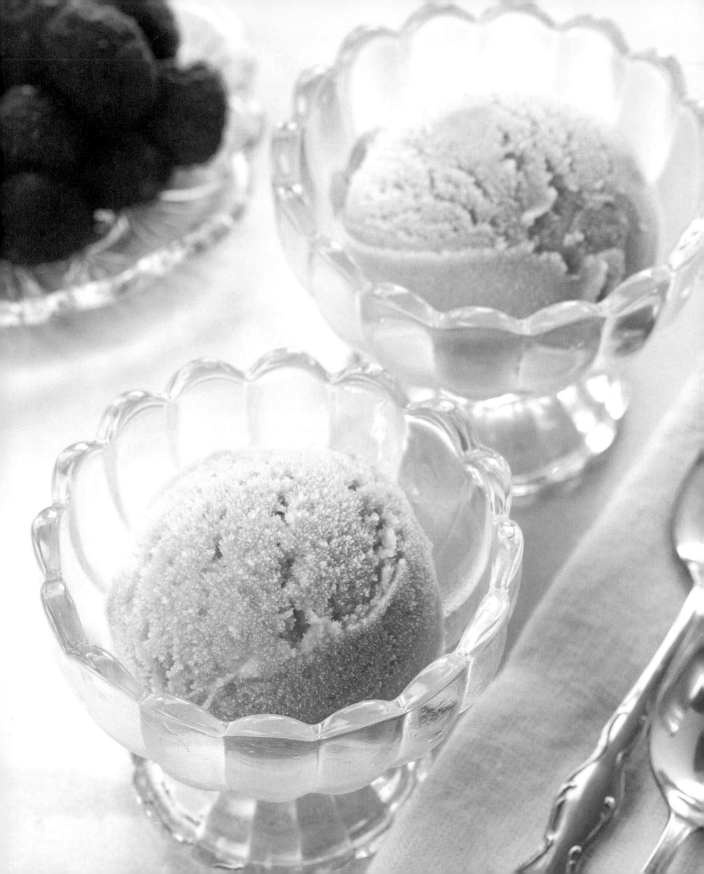

BAKED BANANAS FOSTER

It may feel hard to find fat-free, healthy dessert recipes that are absolutely indulgent and rich. Well, look no further. This Baked Bananas Foster recipe is just as decadent as the original yet full of only the best ingredients for your whole body and soul. Enjoy them plain or serve them with Banana Nice Cream. Either way, you will find yourself swept off your feet.

3 bananas

2 ½ tablespoons maple syrup, divided

½ teaspoon cinnamon

2 teaspoons maple sugar

⅛ teaspoon sea salt (optional)

Preheat the oven to 400°F.

Slice the bananas in half lengthwise and arrange them in a baking dish lined with parchment paper.

In a small bowl, stir together ½ tablespoon of the maple syrup with the cinnamon, maple sugar, and sea salt until well combined.

Brush the banana slices with the remaining 2 tablespoons of maple syrup, making sure to coat both sides.

Spread the cinnamon mixture evenly along the top of the banana slices and bake them in the oven for 15 to 18 minutes, until the bananas are soft and golden brown.

Remove the baked bananas from the oven and serve alongside Banana Nice Cream if desired.

BANANA NICE CREAM

3 frozen bananas

2 tablespoons warm water

Roughly chop the frozen bananas and place them into the food processor. Process the bananas, adding warm water by the tablespoon as needed to prevent sticking. Stop processing once the bananas have reached a smooth, soft-serve consistency.

Enjoy immediately or place in the freezer to set for 2 to 4 hours.

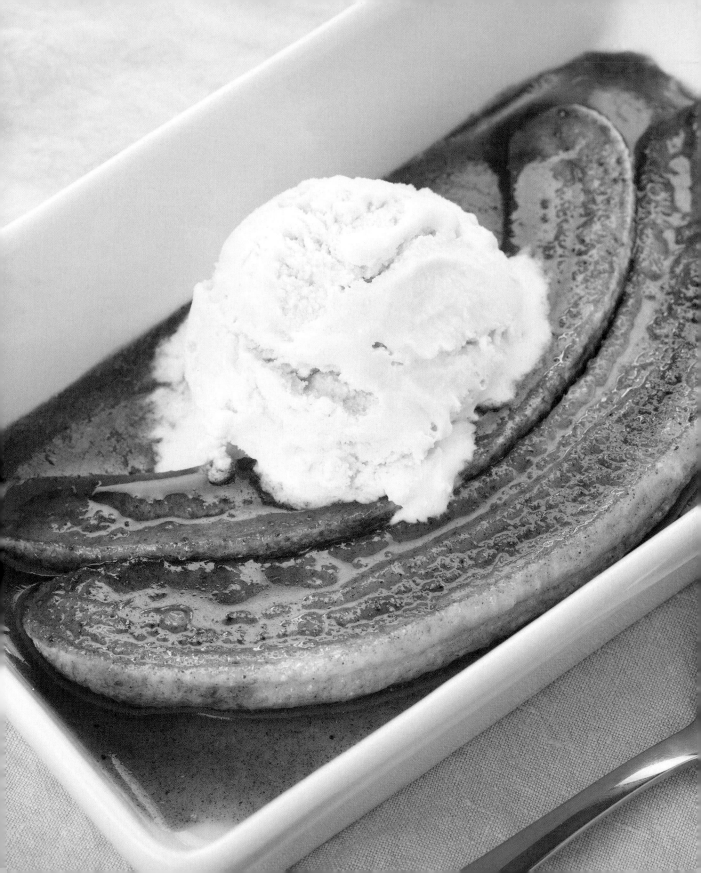

BAKED APPLE ROSES

Baked apple roses are like apple pie filling without the crust, beautifully formed in cups and enjoyed warm right out of the oven. The filling is always the best part anyway, right?

4 red apples

4 tablespoons maple syrup, divided

1 tablespoon fresh lemon juice

¾ teaspoon cinnamon, divided

Preheat the oven to 400°F.

In a large mixing bowl, whisk together 3 tablespoons of the maple syrup, the lemon juice, and ½ teaspoon of the cinnamon until combined.

Using a knife or mandolin, thinly slice the apples, and toss the slices in the maple syrup mixture until well coated.

Arrange the apple slices in 4 small ramekins. Divide the remaining 1 tablespoon of maple syrup over the tops of the ramekins. Finish each one off with a dusting of extra cinnamon.

Bake for 20 to 25 minutes until the apples have softened and gently browned. Remove from the oven and enjoy while still warm!

TIPS

- This healing dessert can also be paired with the Banana Nice Cream recipe on page 420 for an even more satisfying treat.

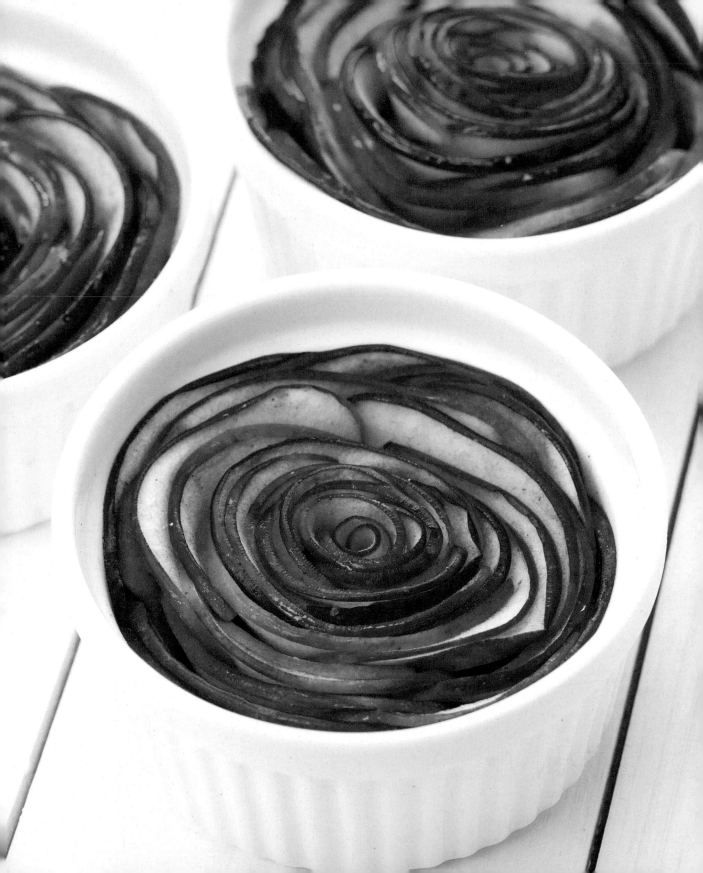

CHAPTER 40

Liver Rescue Meditations

A little goes a long way when it comes to working with and for your liver. When you desire another's attention, all you need to keep going is a pat on the head from a friend, colleague, boss, professor, teacher, mentor, or someone you love—it changes your world when someone you admire sees you in the crowd and recognizes you even for a second. A five-minute break to get some fresh air, clear your head, and find some peace—that's another time when just that little breather can give you all you need. For an organ that gets no care or attention for the most part—it's the brain that gets all the attention—taking a moment to tune in to your liver with the meditations in this chapter can be very powerful. This is no joke. There's a huge difference in your life that comes from knowing what your liver's needs, responsibilities, and struggles are and how hard it works. Once that's in your consciousness, these meditations can activate healing on a whole new level.

If you'd like, you can play music throughout any of these meditations to help relax your liver. Anything that you find soothing will soothe your liver. Liver nerve tension is a topic that doesn't get any attention. It matters greatly, though. One reason is because the state of the liver greatly affects digestion. To put your liver even more at ease, try playing music once a day as you're preparing to eat a meal. As long as the music is relaxing to you, it will calm your digestive tract and reduce conflict and tension in your liver, allowing it to assist the digestion process with much greater ease, which benefits your liver in a virtuous cycle.

Rather than your liver serving your needs 24/7 every single day, these techniques are here to help you serve your liver. Meditating for your liver can be an incredible process. Your liver deems these meditations extremely valuable. Trying them for just a few minutes gives your liver the attention, acknowledgment, recognition, care, and respect that it craves; plus it stabilizes, balances, and strengthens it at the same time. Providing your liver with an understanding of what it goes through gives it the peace it needs to heal so you can finally find relief.

PEACEFUL LIVER BATH MEDITATION

Fill your bathtub with water that's a comfortable temperature for you, not blazing hot and not cold, either. Add one to three tablespoons of sea salt and two tablespoons of kelp powder, and float a natural sea sponge in the water. Enter the bath, close your eyes, and envision yourself in an ocean eddy, a calm little saltwater whirlpool at an out-of-the-way beach where you can relax. If you're adventurous, you can even envision you're inside your liver, though that's not a requirement by any means. The kelp powder will turn your bath into an oceanlike environment, bringing life to the water and creating a bathing tonic that the liver will recognize as practically seawater. Reach for the sponge—when your hand connects to it, your liver will immediately know it really came from the ocean.

The liver is always trying to find balance within the body. It fights our battles for us and protects us in all the ways you've read about—and this bath gives it a break. While the meditation's purpose is to serve your liver, it does that by putting the body, mind, and spirit into a calm state so that the liver can drop its guard for a bit. It's a break between battles for both you and your liver. It's a chance for your liver to chill out and say, "Phew, my job is done for the moment. Let me rest."

Another critical aspect of the bath is that it draws negativity out of the entire body, including the liver, because it grounds you to such a high degree. As you soak in the oceanlike water, hold on to the sponge, and see yourself in a peaceful ocean, it de-angers the liver, pulling out that negativity.

This little vacation, which finally gives your liver peace, contributes to its longevity. It also prepares it for all the healing you want it to do and puts the liver in a mode where it can be more receptive to the meditations that follow. Even if you only do this bath meditation once a month or once every six months, the other meditations will still have great value—this oceanic bath will help set it in motion. You can stay in the bathtub

anywhere from 5 to 45 minutes, though ideally 20 to 30. It's not a technique where the longer you stay in the tub, the better the benefits.

If a bathtub isn't accessible, you can do a mini version of this meditation with a footbath for the same amount of time. Fill a large bowl or container with warm water, add a teaspoon each of sea salt and kelp powder, lower your feet into it, and imagine you're soaking them in the ocean. Dip a sea sponge into the footbath and use it on your feet (or ask a helper if you can't reach) for that final touch.

If by chance you can't do either the bath or footbath, don't worry. You can still benefit from the other meditations and attain a peaceful liver.

LIVER REJUVENATION WALKING MEDITATION

Go for a walk at any pace that feels comfortable. On your breaths in while you walk, envision that you're driving oxygen directly into your liver. Normally, we see breath as all about the lungs. Here, see your liver as your lungs, receiving all that fresh oxygen and becoming saturated with it.

This meditation improves circulation within your liver and enhances new liver cell growth so that your liver can rejuvenate itself with healthy cells. It's especially helpful in that three-month period before every third birthday, when your liver cells are in a particular renewal phase. Don't let that stop you from doing it at other times, though; it's beneficial in between, too.

There's no time constraint on this walking meditation. For the person who can only walk for 30 seconds, one minute, or five minutes, it's still valuable. If you can't walk at all, then when you do the Disease Reversal Meditation later in the chapter, ask the angels you're working with for rejuvenation of your liver cells at the same time. If you don't have trouble walking, go for as long as you'd like. It doesn't have to be its own separate walk in a perfectly serene setting. For example, you could be walking back from lunch with a friend, part ways, and then decide to do the meditation as you walk to your car on your own. If you're a smoker not quite ready to quit, try to hold off on smoking during this meditation.

LIVER COOLING MEDITATION

The liver is inherently concerned that we don't even know it's there, since we live our lives cut off from it, accidentally hurting it and not knowing how to care for it. To show your liver your appreciation, talk to it. Either aloud or in your mind, communicate with it as if it's a friend, loved one, or even a soul mate. Say that you want to take care of it. Even if you're not doing that now, say that you want to care for it in the future. Tell your liver you stand behind it and support it. Tell your liver you love it.

What this does is help your liver cool down. It builds up so much heat from the daily confrontations of the workplace, other responsibilities, and struggles, and that toxic heat—not to be confused with the beneficial detox type of heat—puts the liver constantly on the edge of spasm. With detox heat, the liver can release poisons; with toxic heat, the liver is hot without the ability to release poisons. Toxic heat builds upon toxic heat—no one knows how hot the liver gets when we're driving, for example. Dealing with the other cars on the road puts us on the verge of confrontation the entire time, and that can get the liver close to a spasmodic state. (It's the same heat that results in gallstone formation.) The high stress and pressure of our lives

means our livers crave the reassurance, calming, and cooling of this meditation.

You can talk to your liver anytime, anywhere. Turn it into a full meditation if you want, maybe when you have a little more time over a lunch break, or do it on the go when you want to let your liver know you haven't forgotten about it.

STRENGTHENING BILE PRODUCTION MEDITATION

For this one, it's very helpful if you can get ahold of a recording of running water in nature, like from a stream, though if not, you can still do the meditation. Either way, lie flat on your back, whether in bed, on a couch, or on a yoga mat or blanket on the floor, as long as it's an area that feels protected to you. Close your eyes and envision yourself walking up to a river or stream. It has a gentle, relaxing current, and you take a few steps in, pretty soon finding yourself waist deep. The water is pleasantly cool, nothing that would give you a chill.

You start walking toward the other side, your hands floating on the surface, in no rush at all. The water is staying level now, and you take your time with each step, feeling the sand and river-washed stones stimulating pressure points on your bare feet. As you approach the middle of the stream, you reach a deeper spot, and the water starts to travel higher up your waist and ribs until it's just covering your entire liver area. That's as high as the water will get. You keep going on your slow walk, pacing yourself so that traveling from one side to the other will take no less than 20 minutes. The meditation can last longer if you'd like; it can be as long as you want. Keep envisioning yourself stepping toward the bank on the other side, where trees and grass await.

Eventually, the water level will start to lower down to your waist. As you get closer to the bank, it will get lower and lower until it's at your feet and you're walking out and up onto the grass. See yourself lying down in the grass and listen to the water running. When you're ready, come out of the meditation. You've just given your liver support with bile production so it can aid digestion of fats and build its bile reserves.

KILLING VIRUSES AND OTHER PATHOGENS MEDITATION

Sunlight contains mysterious forces, and when we're exposed to it in our everyday lives, it enters into certain organs for access later. The sun's rays are complex. They contain an infinite amount of information to which the human body connects. Medical research and science have no idea that sunlight is full of so much more healing and life force than what's been discovered. If sun rays could be weighed, measured, and analyzed, the discoveries would be profound and even unbelievable.

It's completely unknown that as you've received these rays throughout life, some have gone directly into your liver. Whenever your liver was doing well, it was able to bank the ones it didn't put to use in the moment. Even if your liver's not too healthy right now and unable to bank new rays, it has old rays stored. This meditation is all about activating the unused sunlight your liver has been holding on to and unleashing its raw power.

Pick a quiet time of day and a place to lie or sit down that's out of the sun. As much as the sun can help us and support the immune system at other times, there are a few reasons to stay out of the sun with this one. For one, you're going to imagine that you *are* in the sun, and

that you're opening your eyes wide and looking directly at it. If you really are out in it, you'll have to work on blocking out the real sun; plus you could accidentally open your eyes and damage them by looking into it. You want to be able to let in every last drop of visualized sunlight with this meditation, and being out in the actual sun will prevent that. For another, when you're doing a meditation while lying out in the sun, it's easy to fall asleep and get burned. And by the way, your powers of envisioning are going to do the work here, so this isn't about turning the heat up to 100 degrees or visiting a sauna, either, to emulate the sun's warmth. Let your mind do the work—it will flip the switch to release past sunlight from inside your liver.

As you're lying or sitting in a comfortable spot, envision that you're lying in a secluded place in the sun. If you'd like, it could be a beach. You may prefer to imagine that you're in a field. Whatever makes you feel best. Let the naturist side of you come out, and imagine that you're lying there without any clothes on in your safe, private area. Keeping your actual eyes closed, imagine that you're opening them to the sun, which is looking down at you from the sky and sending its rays deep into your liver. Now see those visualized sunrays radiating, connecting to, and bringing to life real sun rays of the past that your liver has stored inside of it. Envision a switch turning on that activates the stored rays so that they become powerful light that destroys pathogens such as viruses that reside in the liver. As the light beams throughout the organ, see it as a weapon against those symptom-related, disease-related pathogens that can cause everything from acne to SIBO to autoimmune illness to tumors, cysts, and cancerous tissue. Picture a little microbe-sized bug and imagine the light entering, surrounding, and killing it. Every time you take a deep breath in and release it, see the light getting stronger throughout your liver and bringing its power into your liver's dark, hidden crevices, driving out any critters that have taken advantage. With both the inhale and the exhale, see that light grow.

Ideally, this meditation should last between 25 and 45 minutes—any longer and you'll get sunburned. (Kidding—you can't get sunburned if you're doing this meditation right!)

STRENGTHENING YOUR LIVER'S IMMUNE SYSTEM MORNING MEDITATION

Try this meditation anytime between waking and noon. If you can, start out lying on your stomach. (If you can't, lie on your side.) On the inhale, see yourself breathing amethyst or violet light into your liver from the back. Now exhale the same color. Keep breathing the light in and out. Don't force an unusual breathing pattern. For this to stimulate the liver's immune system, your breath needs to be at your normal and natural rhythm. After about five minutes, flip onto your back if you can. Continue to inhale and exhale the amethyst or violet light, this time bringing it in and out of the front of your liver. Once five minutes have passed on your back, flip again so that you're lying on your stomach and breathing the light into your liver from the back, and do that for five more minutes. Flip onto your back one last time and breathe the colorful light in and out of the front of your liver for five final minutes. It's fine if they weren't perfect five-minute intervals. In the end, it should add up to about 20 minutes total.

Finally, slowly stand (or sit, if you can't) and then take in a deep breath of the amethyst or violet light, seeing it enter into your liver from both the front and back at once. As you breathe

out, send the light out from both sides. Stay standing (or sitting) for one to two minutes, continuing to inhale and exhale the light, deeper than before. Once you're finished, you can be off and running, having strengthened your liver's immune system—which is extremely important for guarding you against pathogen-caused illnesses and toxic exposures that hinder your liver's immune system and its ability to function at its best.

LOOSENING LIVER FAT CELLS MORNING MEDITATION

This is a meditation to perform upon waking; the earlier in the morning, the better it works. Lying flat on your back, carefully bend your right leg and bring that knee up toward your chest. If you have swollen joints, RA, a tricky back, or any other limitation, you don't have to bring your knee all the way up to your chest—only do that if it's a position you're used to and works for you. Otherwise, bring your knee wherever's comfortable, maybe up to the point where you can reach it with your hands. If you can't move it at all, that's fine, too. Only do what you're able. Hold for about 30 seconds. Drop the leg back down and lie flat for 30 seconds. Now bend your left leg and bring that knee toward you for 30 seconds. Drop the leg and lie flat for 30 seconds. That's one leg pump sequence. Repeat the sequence for a total of four times. What you'll be doing during this first part of the meditation is loosening up any fluid retention around the liver, relieving pressure in the lymphatic vessels as you pump out the fluid. If you can't do the movements, envision yourself doing them instead.

After the leg pumps, stay relaxed and straightened out on your back. Rest both of your hands, with fingers interlaced if you'd like, over your liver area. Don't strain; relax your elbows. Imagine that your hands are magnets or suctions, loosening and drawing up fat cells from the organ. Envision an energy going upward to your hands, as though they have their own gravitational pull or other force that's freeing stagnant energy trapped inside the liver and drawing it up to them. Picture this any way you need to, whether as particles of sand falling upward or your own mental image. Continue for 10 minutes.

Now return to the leg pumps, doing another four sequences (eight leg pumps total, four on each side, with rests in between, all in roughly 30-second intervals). Follow that with another 10 minutes of lying flat, resting your hands over your liver as you visualize its fat cells awakening and moving around as the organ's energy comes unstuck. Finish with four leg pump sequences. This is a great meditation for pre-fatty, fatty, stagnant, or sluggish liver, to help encourage lymphatic drainage and disperse fats from the liver into the bloodstream and out of the body.

DISEASE REVERSAL NIGHTTIME MEDITATION

This nighttime meditation requires a little angelic work. Specifically, you're going to call upon the Angels of Order, who bring order to diseased, inflamed, or otherwise weakened livers. This angelic power applies to every liver condition. The same rules apply for calling upon angels as I've written in my previous books: namely that you must ask for their help aloud. A whisper is fine, and sign language works if you can't speak. Before you get to bed—maybe as

you're brushing your teeth, putting your kids to bed, or putting on your pajamas—say, "Angels of Order, please come to do a healing sequence on my liver." If you get to bed and realize you forgot to ask earlier, that's fine. Say it now that you're there.

When you're ready, lie down, close your eyes, and envision three angels around your bed. Everyone has a different way of picturing angels. Some people see light and wings. Some see light itself. Some see a figure within light. Some see a complete figure of a woman with wings; some see a complete figure of a woman with no wings. Whatever you see, bring three of them to mind. The angels of disease reversal are female, not male; that much you need to know. Visualize the three angels walking around your bed, spaced evenly, in a circle. If someone else is in bed with you, like a partner or a friend, that's fine. Keep thinking about the angels. You need to focus on them walking around the bed.

See the Angels of Order taking their hands and creating a pressure of light in the circle and applying this pressure of light to your body, so that it pushes into your liver. This light bypasses other parts of your body and is specifically meant for your liver, where it can shroud out disease, saturate and help shrink cysts and tumors, and repair damaged cells. It's angelic light for anything liver-related. If you have any symptom or condition mentioned at all in this book, from autoimmune to acne, this is helpful. Even if it's only a sluggish liver, the light is there to help reverse it.

Keep picturing the angels circling your bed and sending light to your liver for as long as you'd like, whether three minutes, five minutes, half an hour, or until you fall asleep. Do save this meditation for the evening hours.

ELIMINATING TOXINS MEDITATION

Your liver will already be detoxing on a daily basis as you eat the right foods for cleansing, try the Liver Rescue Morning and the Liver Rescue 3:6:9, sample the recipes, and perhaps try the supplements in this book. You can use this technique alongside everything you're already doing to offer an added level of detox.

This meditation is geared to ease the liver of any tension or spasms at the same time it allows the liver to feel safe enough to detoxify without the concern that it will be called to duty in the moment. Have you ever had a task, job, or responsibility of some kind where you just needed to pause and get a breath of fresh air before heading back into the heat of the moment and the chaos, where you may be called upon at any moment to assist someone? Have you ever had your break cut short because you were called into action to perform, whether as a salesperson at a car dealership, a veterinary assistant at an animal hospital, a nurse at a caregiving facility, a cashier at a busy restaurant, or a parent of a young child? The liver needs that full moment of knowing that it's not going to be put under pressure or demanded to perform. This meditation helps allow the liver to release troublemakers in the midst of a busy time in its and your life.

Take a few moments at any time of day, whether morning, afternoon, or evening, and imagine a wall around you. Choose whatever wall works for you to feel safe and not imprisoned, whether that's a wall of light, trees, hedges, rose bushes, a favorite home, or a sacred building. As you're doing this, think privacy and peacefulness, and get into a mind-set of being alone and not being bothered, whether you're actually sitting at a table in a restaurant, with people all around you, or doing this in a quiet, calm space. You can keep your eyes open and sit, lie down, or even stand.

Once you envision that the world is locked out of your life, or at least that the hustle, bustle, and chaos are at a safe distance, tell your liver that you would like it to detox. Your liver will receive the message and it will also sense that no adrenaline will be surging through your veins to saturate and overwork it. In turn, your liver will efficiently release small amounts of toxins alongside a chemical compound to direct and carry them safely out of the body. The meditation can last from 5 minutes to 20 or more if you'd like. Even after you've stopped and returned to the busyness of your life, the special chemical compounds that have been released will take over from there and continue to drive toxins out of your body throughout the rest of the day and night to free you up so you can live your life.

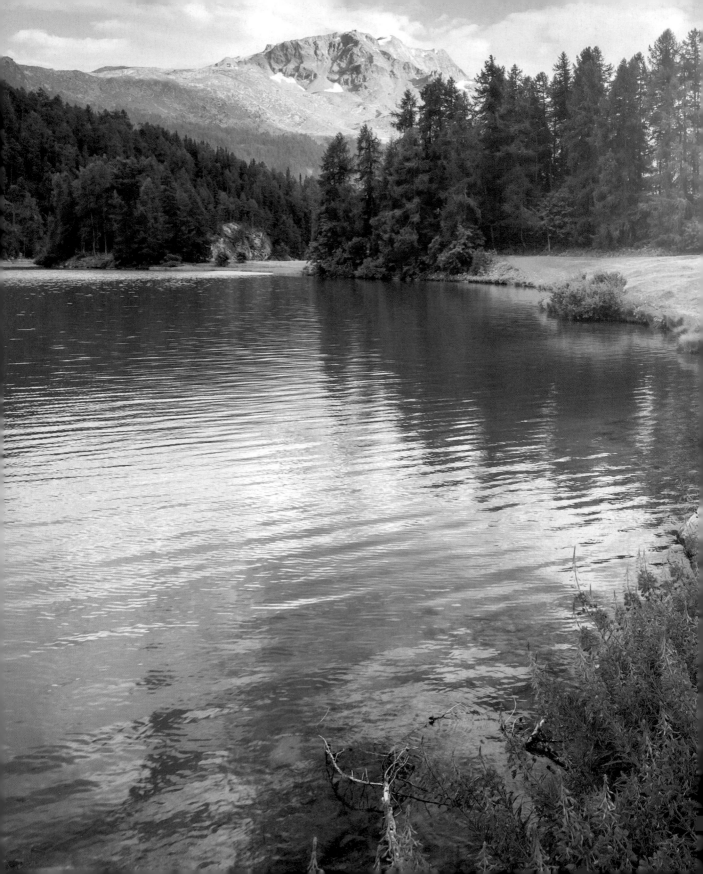

THE STORM WILL PASS

PEACE BE WITH YOU

"When you find peace within yourself by connecting to the living words you've absorbed throughout these pages, you become a beacon that lights the way for others."

CHAPTER 41

The Storm Will Pass

Peace Be with You

If you're dealing with a health challenge, I know that finding peace can be one of your greatest struggles. Though you know now that the liver is the body's peacekeeper, and that bringing peace to your liver can change your life, if you're suffering in the moment, that peace may feel far away. All it takes is losing sleep for one night, having a cold for one week, or suffering with an injury for one month for peace to be disrupted. When you've been faced with a chronic illness that has lasted two, three, five, ten years or more, peace is that much harder to find. That's especially difficult, since it's one of the times you need peace most. It's why so many people who are chronically ill pursue spiritual endeavors to support their well-being, since their bodies remain a mystery.

There are ways to find peace when you're sick. One is knowing what's wrong with you— taking away the mystery and realizing that your body didn't let you down. Another is knowing what to do to heal. A third is knowing that you *can* heal, especially now that you have the truth. The purpose of the words Spirit provides is to offer you each one of those elements. Discovering that troubled livers are behind so much suffering, how to care for our livers the way they're

meant to be cared for, and that we can rescue our livers—this knowledge can instantly put you on the road to peace.

If you're dealing with a symptom, injury, or illness, remind yourself that your physical body is actively working to find peace for you. Even when you're ailing, your liver is orchestrating a peace mission, communicating with other organs and cells and the immune system and even the brain, trying to keep fellowship in the body and bring you to a peaceful internal state. By using the information in this book, you're giving your liver even more tools to keep the peace. Our bodies naturally work toward peace. All we need to do is support them.

THE SOUL OF PEACE

There is another piece of peace, and that's having compassion for yourself. Compassion is the soul of peace, the power of peace, the path to peace, the life of peace, the source of peace, the answer to peace, the creator of peace. We think about peace as an absence—an absence of pain, suffering, disease, hatred, violence, war—when it's also about this presence of compassion.

Why self-compassion and not self-love? Self-love is okay. It's about loving who you are, appreciating who you are, and it can reach into accepting who you are and what you look like. It seems to work perfectly for people when everything is going well. And then . . . what if they go through a hardship? When you're struggling and suffering, that's when the game changes. Self-love doesn't mean you're granting yourself a healing like self-compassion does. Self-love alone cannot grant you peace. When your focus is on loving yourself, it can accidentally bleed over into loving yourself more than anybody around you. Compassion is what wakes us up to the wider world.

Love is not what keeps two people together, either. When you're in the throes of a new romance and the finances are flowing and life is rosy, love can be plenty. When a challenge comes along, love is no longer enough because human love is not the creator of peace. How many relationships are "I love you, I love you, I love you" until the day something goes wrong, and the members of the couple become mortal enemies? Loving another can turn to hating that person very fast, unless compassion's involved. Compassion is the glue-like component in a relationship. It keeps love alive and breathing and stops love from becoming sour and turning to hate. If you look at love as an apple, compassion is its core.

Same goes for self-love—loving yourself without having self-compassion can flip to hating yourself all too easily. If you're suddenly facing chronic illness or an emotional challenge, self-love can vanish and self-hatred can take its place. Self-hatred is one of the greatest obstacles to peace. When an athlete is injured, it can so quickly turn to self-hatred because she feels disconnected from herself and can't achieve like before. The mom who could take care of

everything until symptoms got in her way may start to doubt herself and feel like a failure. The employee who had every answer in the workplace and then suddenly can't do his job anymore because a condition is holding him back may start to despise himself, thinking he's less-than and not needed anymore. It's not just our internal monologues that bring up these feelings. We may also hear from outside sources—in whatever form, whether stated aloud or not—that our illness is our fault. The misguided autoimmune theory of the body attacking itself, the misguided genetic theory that says faulty genes create illness, the misguided attempts to explain illness by saying you manifested it—these can make you hate the very fiber of your being. They're the ultimate peace destroyers of the body, mind, soul, heart, and spirit, if there's no self-compassion there to be a deeply rooted stronghold of peace.

We have no idea that the liver sees us as its baby, an infant it must take care of and feed, and that it uses its compassionate nature to look out for us. We think instead that the body is giving up on us. We lose touch with all compassion for ourselves, if we even held compassion to begin with; it seems to disappear when an ache or pain has been with us too long. The longer the pain or symptom or illness, the further away self-compassion feels. We ask ourselves instead, "What's wrong with me?" In truth, compassion doesn't leave us. While it may seem like it's gone, really, it's closer than ever before, waiting for us to reach out and find it.

Self-hatred can take on a life of its own. It's a beast that can't be tamed with anything other than compassion. That self-compassion must have meaning within it; it can't be an empty word thrown around. There's substance to compassion, and that's what must be tapped into and understood. Having compassion for yourself is a release—a release of judgment, a release of debt, a permission slip allowing you to be forgiven as a human being.

There are two types of forgiveness: normal forgiveness and compassionate forgiveness. Normal forgiveness doesn't bring with it peace. Compassionate forgiveness is real forgiveness; having compassion for yourself *is* the true meaning of being forgiven—forgiven especially for what you might have blamed yourself for that you did not create. Only compassion can free us from the judgments we've placed on ourselves. Even if we think we've made a mistake, and what we feel is a big mistake, compassion can still free us from the greedy beast of self-hatred. Chances are, that mistake is rather small in the big picture. We've all made mistakes. If you feel trapped within the prison of one, that this mistake has somehow locked you in with the beast of self-blame, merely the word *self-compassion* won't release you. Finding true compassion for yourself is what will unlock the cage, free you, and send the beast away.

Self-compassion is a powerful revelation. It's a moment when you've been driven down to your knees and you feel the ultimate blessing of "You've been forgiven" from the highest source above. It's the feeling that being yourself matters, and it's also more than that: It's a connection to the knowledge that God and the heavens care about you. It's tapping into this ultimate kindness that's out there for you at the same time it's within. This revelation kicks out self-hatred, removes the venomous poison from your veins and from your soul.

It is said, "God is love," when God is not love alone. God is *unconditional* love. The human mind will always put conditions upon our love for ourselves and others. We can't help it. We think we can feel unconditional love; what we can really do is tap into compassion alongside our love. Compassion plus love: that's the human version of unconditional love. God's unconditional love is bigger, more powerful. To feel anything approaching that toward ourselves or other people, to experience a sense of peace, it's compassion we need to find.

Often, when people think they have compassion for themselves, it's really confidence. That's what we build the world on now: confidence, not compassion. The minute something goes wrong, confidence, like love, goes away. You can shape a lifetime around confidence, believing in yourself because of your achievements, and in the end, if you can't achieve bigger or better, or if you fail at something, confidence and belief in yourself can disappear with the flick of a switch. With the light off, the darkness of self-doubt takes its place. Confidence is important; we should all hold on to it when we can. It doesn't have the strength of compassion, though. Confidence is not the answer to self-hatred. It's not the home of peace. Confidence comes and goes with the wind. If there's no compassion when your confidence drops away, the damage becomes extreme to the health of your soul and body. If you hold compassion within, on the other hand, you can lose confidence and it won't faze you. You can fail at something, you can get sick, someone you had confidence in can let you down, and compassion remains. Whether you believe in yourself or lose belief in yourself, compassion will hold it all together and keep the peace. Compassion for yourself heals. Its deep healing power can bring you out of your illness so that you gain your confidence back again, and your belief in yourself becomes stronger and stronger.

Still, we don't control the world. There's always going to be not-peace out there. We can't control the free will of the billions of souls on this planet. We *can* gain control over the peace in ourselves. We can work on creating peace within our bodies by tending to the needs of the liver, the body's physical peacekeeper. And we can cultivate compassion, the body's nonphysical peacekeeper. If you fixate on controlling everyone else's free will, you're not going to have peace, nor are you going to bring peace to those around you.

Say an iconic figure lived his life focused on world peace, at the same time giving his child no compassion or peace. The child, who just wanted to be acknowledged and accepted, instead suffered and suffered as his father focused on trying to change the world. It's a classic case of how we can focus in the wrong direction. The plumber who can't get to the plumbing in her own home—that's not her fault; she needs to make her living focused on everyone else's toilets. The proverbial shoemaker whose children have no shoes, so their steps aren't peaceful—that's justifiable; he needs to handcraft and sell every scrap of leather in order to make sure his family has food on the table. What's not justifiable is when the peacemaker's children have no peace. The hobbyist peacemaker, the passion-driven person who follows the delusion that he'll be able to control the free will of over seven billion people—and that this lofty goal exempts him from obligations to those closest to him—is working against his very dream.

That's because there's a difference between passion and compassion. It's passion that we celebrate and even exalt. And just as with love, it does have its value. Yet we get lost, putting everything into our passions, or thinking that passion is a free pass. It's not. If you have passion for someone, it's not the same as having compassion for that person. They're mixed up easily all the time; people believe they're one and the same. If you have passion for a charitable cause, it doesn't mean you're going to

have compassion for it and the people it serves. Maybe you do feel that compassion; it's not automatic if you have passion, though. That's the difference—although so often, passion is seen as compassion, they're two separate forces. If you have a passion for a certain pastime or mission, that doesn't equate to putting compassion into pursuing it, or remembering to look up from your singular focus to take care of yourself. You could be so fixated on passion that you miss out, too, on providing compassion at home so that the ones you love can walk in shoes of peace. We can't mistake passion for compassion; it's an absolute disaster. Just look to the examples throughout history of those who've pursued a passion for world peace while neglecting to tap into compassion. Only when love and confidence and forgiveness and passion come together with compassion can they drive us toward a better world.

THE WILL TO BE FREE

Let's go back to one thought: free will. As important as faith is, faith alone does not create peace around us. Every person's free will allows that soul to choose as she or he wants, and if that's not a peaceful state of some kind, then it's not a peaceful state. We don't have control over other individuals. We don't have control over whether they take care of their livers or experience peace within themselves or take a peaceful route in life. Still, free will is necessary. It grants us the opportunity to be free from others' designs on our lives. It allows us to make mistakes so that we can learn from them. Free will is also essential in our personal searches for peace. Even though free will is what allows some to choose the opposite of peace, if free will did not exist we could not choose to search for peace within ourselves. In this world, we may not get the opportunity to be free from every concern, worry, and problem. We do get our own will to try to find our own peace and freedom.

You don't need to be what you think of as a spiritual person to want peace within yourself; you don't need to be some enlightened being to seek out the basic, responsible direction of finding peace. If you feel you're maybe not a spiritual type of person, it doesn't mean you don't have the power and glory of seeing what's right and wrong around and inside of you. You could be a working mom who doesn't have time to dedicate yourself to spiritual books and classes or the opportunity to head to your favorite sanctuary or church or monument for regular, devoted prayer—don't let this make you feel like you're not enlightened enough. If you're looking around and thinking that another, like maybe a spiritually seeking neighbor, has more peace within herself or himself, don't worry. You don't need to circle the globe and pray on top of a mountain in order to find or sustain peace. Being spiritual is a mind-set that many people choose, and it doesn't mean their hearts are truly in it. People who spend a lifetime searching for peace on retreats and ventures have difficulty finding it. I've seen people come down from their mountaintop retreats after 30 days or six months, and they still don't have peace. Some people use their wealth to put themselves in glorious surroundings, and while, like the travelers, they may find moments of peace, the peace is not *sustained*. Little do they know they've been searching for the wrong thing.

In order to get that peace, they need to be seeking compassion. You could be in a straw shack, in a straw bed, in squalor, starving, with sores all over your body, and you may have more peace than someone with the greatest riches in the most pristine, beautiful environment or someone who has the ability and resources to pray in sanctuaries all over the world. It's all about whether you're tapping into compassion for yourself and others. The same path to peace is available to you as to anyone who's gone on months-long retreats or climbed the highest mountains: compassion.

We often forget about our own bodies, our own organs, and focus instead on what's outside of us. For survival, we're forced in this day and age to pay constant, vigilant attention to the steady stream of updates about what's going on out there. Especially when we're going through a challenging time, or when someone is challenging us, we're forced to pay vigilant attention to what's going on around us. If we spend all our time like this, worrying about others, whether they're around us or far away, we lose ourselves. We give away our own peace from heart, soul, and physical body when we try to die out fires that we can't control. This doesn't mean we should be narcissists. It doesn't mean caring only about ourselves or loving only ourselves. It doesn't mean we shouldn't fight for the causes we believe in or shouldn't fight for our loved ones. It means that we must bring awareness to what we choose to pursue. The more you think you can control what's happening in the world, the more you lose yourself and the more you give up your inner state of peace. Much of what we try to avoid is unavoidable. You must use your free will to draw on self-compassion, and use that self-compassion to choose wisely which fires to put out, what you feel you really can control if you want to keep your physical and emotional state safe and peaceful.

ALL STORMS PASS

Self-compassion—how do we find it? When you're up against a judgment, a crisis, a hardship, the loss of a loved one, an ailing friend or family member, a financial challenge, an injury, an illness, or any of life's other storms, how do you tap into kindness for yourself? First, you see it as that: a storm. Disruptive as hurricanes and blizzards and other storms can be when they come, they do eventually go. When we have "bad weather" in our personal lives that threatens to rob us of our peace, and then we recognize that all storms pass no matter what, we can hold on to some peace as we're going through that storm. No matter what we think or believe or fear, whether we like it or not, *all storms pass, everything changes, nothing ever stays the same.* It's law.

What we often find most peace-disrupting about life's storms is that we have no control over their swirling of darkness onto the radar. Our free will doesn't govern the weather or the weather of life's storms. And yet it's in that lack of control that we can gain our peace. Even if it's a long storm, and you've been in it for years, it will still pass because nothing stays the same. Nothing. The fact that this law is out of our hands—that's where the peace lies.

If you're in a storm and you think things are going to get worse, know that the winds may shift—it may get better instead. If it hasn't gotten better yet, it will, because guess what? Everything changes. And if the storm in your life is getting worse instead of better in the moment, find peace in the fact that it can't stay worse because it has to change; it can't stay the same. Even if you *wanted* it to stay worse, you couldn't keep it that way. Even if you hated someone so badly that you wanted that person's situation to stay worse, it would change. Even if you had

a subliminal desire to be sick—which does not exist anyway—that desire couldn't keep you feeling unwell. Even if you were attracting your illness—which you can't anyway—you couldn't attract it forever. Why? All storms pass, everything changes, nothing ever stays the same.

We lose our peace thinking something bad is going to happen to us. We lose our peace when something bad does happen to us. We lose our peace when we think we caused the something bad that happened to us. Yet we have to be seers. We must look past the storm, even while it's happening, by knowing that the storm is ruled by law and will eventually pass. We must see through and beyond the darkness of the storm. We must look ahead. If you fear something bad happening to or around you, let your comfort be that even if it does, it can't define you because it will leave. *You are not what the bad is. No matter what you think or believe, the bad is not you.*

All too often, we think we deserved the bad in some way because we're somehow bad. When we realize that the bad is a storm, we can see that *we're not part of the storm.* Even if the storm seems to call your name with judgment and finger-pointing—a diagnosis, for example, that lays the blame on your body attacking itself or a trendy theory that tells a mother with a sick child that she's taking the wrong steps for him to get better—whatever it is, the storm is not you. Find compassion for yourself in that knowledge, and then use the peace that self-compassion gives you to separate yourself from the storm. Know that the storm wouldn't stay even if you wanted it to, that you have no control over the fact that it will pass because the storm isn't you, the bad isn't you, the bad doesn't define you, the struggle that's happening isn't who you are. If sickness is your storm, find compassion and peace in knowing that your body would never attack itself and that it loves you unconditionally. Even when it comes to overloading the liver, the problem still isn't you. You didn't know what your liver needed. The world hasn't given you support for your liver.

Understanding all this, you can navigate your ship through the storm and the darkness. When the rain starts to come down and the waves start to tip you from side to side, you can be a visionary, witnessing the wonders that still live beneath the surface and seeing that you'll find safe harbor again. In the meantime, your boat is keeping you sheltered and bringing you peace—and that boat is the knowledge that the storm will pass. Someone's picking on you? Everything changes; nothing stays the same. Going through heartbreak? Everything changes; nothing stays the same. You lose your soul mate, and you think you'll go soul mate-less forever? Everything changes; nothing ever stays the same. All storms pass. From that wisdom, you can see that you are not the source of your suffering. It's life's weather, and you get to take steps to protect yourself from it.

LIVING WORDS

Because the words you've read throughout this book come from Spirit of the Most High, the Spirit of Compassion, they're alive. That's right; there are words that are dead and words that have life to them. Anyone who puts heart and soul into their writing doesn't write dead words. If you're speaking from your heart and soul, those words are not dead. Then there are words that are regurgitated or taken from another source or meant to manipulate—those words can be dead.

And then there are words that live forever. The words here really are living words. It's not just because I put my heart and soul into writing them; it's because they come from a spiritual source. These words will always be here for generations to come; they will always shine, no matter the times. They will never grow old and useless, because what Spirit gives me to document is health scripture, and Spirit is the living essence of the word *compassion*. Even if there are moments when you feel you cannot persevere, these words will persevere for you. They're here for you to grab on to; they're the hands that reach out to pull you up when you're hanging from a cliff.

Living words hold light; dead words can hold darkness. Because of their source, the living words throughout this book hold light and purge the sickness, which is darkness, out of people. Dead words can take people into the darkness. They can lead us to dead ends, whether we realize it in the moment or not. Sometimes they deceive us with smoke and mirrors or mirages. If we follow them, in the end we'll find ourselves disillusioned. Not that dead words can't have meaning. We can still learn from them, the same way we can learn from studying pressed flowers, careful not to touch or hold them and turn them to dust. Living words are like the flowers still in the field.

Even if trust has been broken and the hope inside your heart and soul is diminished from your journeys, living words can be the hope you feel you've lost. When you're blinded by struggle, living words can see for you until you're ready to see the light through your own eyes. While dead words, wherever they come from, whether health literature or elsewhere, can become a part of you over time that keeps you weighted down, living words elevate you. They have the power to release you.

BE THE BEACON

When we throw the word *peace* around without focusing on what it truly means, we lessen its value to the point that it registers as a throwaway rag, a crumpled tissue, a used paper cup. It becomes a pop word that holds no real power. Spoken aloud, it doesn't enter the heart or the soul of the person who hears it; it bounces off us because it doesn't hold the meaning it once did, long ago.

When we reengage with peace's meaning, we find a feeling that takes us over and takes our breath away for a moment—peace that's like being bundled in a warm blanket, like sunlight on the skin, like a hot, home-cooked meal on a cold night, all of it connected to a benevolent force above that's somehow telling us that no matter what happens it's going to be okay in the end. True peace holds power and gives you relief, a window into freedom from what this world puts us through and sometimes takes from us—freedom you can use to heal.

The minute you have compassion for yourself, you've connected yourself to what's behind the stars. You've connected yourself to the heavens. You've connected yourself to God. From that comes peace.

As someone who has experienced hardship, you can have more peace, even if you're still struggling, than someone you'd think has the ultimate freedom: someone who's never been thwarted along the way, who's never had to stop and look inside. What you've endured in your heart, spirit, soul, body, and being has brought you to the place where everything else falls away and you can see that compassion is the truest part of who we are. You've gotten to witness that even through trials and setbacks, you are still worthy.

While your compassion doesn't mean that you can snap your fingers and fix the world, it does mean you can change others' worlds—not by trying to control them; simply by being. When you find peace within yourself by connecting to the living words you've absorbed throughout these pages, you become a beacon that lights the way for others. Let me tell you truly: the light you hold rids the darkness, for the darkness cannot exist with light present.

With your compassion, you can instill peace in loved ones and others who come to you for help. Even if they haven't overcome their emotional, physical, or spiritual struggles yet, the experience of compassion from you can grant instant moments of peace that may even stay and become a part of them. It's a power within you granted from above by the Spirit of Compassion and the Angel of Peace for you to do your divine, holy work on this planet. Let me tell you truly: you hold great power within.

Peace be with you.

INDEX

NOTE: Page references in *italics* refer to photos of recipes.

A

Abscesses (liver), individualized support for, 322
A1C, 52
Acid reflux, infant, 187–188
Acne, 155–160
    antibiotics for, 156–157
    formation of, 158–159
    hormones and, 157–158
    immunity from, 160
    individualized support for, 311
    strep as cause of, 155–156
Acorn squash, 298
Actinic keratosis, 151
Adaptogenic liver
    fat processing and, 11–15
    pancreas protected by, 16–17
Adrenal glands
    adrenaline neutralization and, 131–134
    adrenal problems, 127–134
    bloating, constipation, and IBS, 171
    diabetes and, 110–111
    excess adrenaline as liver troublemaker, 280
    extreme cleanse and effect on, 127–131, 133
    high blood pressure and, 115
    hunger and, 88–89
    individualized support for, 311
    job of, 127, 134
    Liver Rescue 3:6:9 for, 340
    mood and, 182
    weight gain and, 82–84

Aerosol can air fresheners, 273
Aftershave, 273
Age spots, 151
Aging, 93–96
    DNA indicators and, 95–96
    fear of, 93–94
    individualized support for aging liver, 322
    liver health and, 94–95, 96
    weight gain and, 84–85
Air fresheners, 273
ALA (alpha lipoic acid), 299–300
Alanine transaminase (ALT), 56
Albumin, 56
Alcohol
    autoimmune liver, hepatitis, and, 195
    glucose and, 91
    liver scar tissue and, 199
    as liver troublemaker, 8, 269
    reducing intake of, 285
    sugar in, 248
Alcohol, in toiletries and medications, 277
Aldolase B isoenzyme, 235–236
Alert levels, of liver, 13–15
Alkaline phosphatase (ALP, enzyme), 56
Alkalinity
    alkaline water, 243–245
    in stomach, 239
Allergies, chronic and seasonal, 63, 156, 166, 180
Allergies, food, 149
Aloe vera, 300
Aluminum
    brain fog and, 177

    as liver troublemaker, 279
Aminotransferase (AST), 56
Amla berry, 300
Ammonia permeability, 172
Amphetamines, 276
Angiogenesis, 206
Antibiotics
    acne and, 155–160
    as liver troublemakers, 276
    SIBO and, 166–167
Antidepressants
    as liver troublemakers, 276
    SAD and, 183
Antifungals, 156
Anti-inflammatories, 276
Antioxidants
    aging and, 95
    diet and, 38
    hyperantioxidants, 204
Anxiety. *See* Mood struggles
Appendix, 166, 173–174
Apples
    apple cider vinegar vs., 238–240
    Baked Apple Roses, 422, *423*
    Caramel Apple Rings, 376, *377*
    cucumber-apple juice, for Liver Rescue 3:6:9, 350
    glucose and, 90–91
    as healing food, 285–286
    Liver Rescue Applesauce, 410, *411*
    during Liver Rescue 3:6:9, 343–344
    Pineapple and Apple Chips with Spicy Mango Salsa, 408, *409*
    sensitivity to, 140
Apricots, 286
Arrhythmias, 121–125

Arsenic, 279
Artichokes, 286
Artificial sweeteners, 267
Arugula, 286
Ashwagandha, 300
Asparagus, 286
Aspartame, 267
Atlantic dulse, 67
Atlantic sea vegetables, 286–287
Atrial fibrillation, 121, 125
Autoimmune liver, 193–198
    defined, 197–198
    diagnosis bias and, 194–195
    Epstein-Barr virus and, 40–41
    hepatitis, future of, 197
    hepatitis causes, 196–197
    individualized support for, 312
    individualized support for
        hepatitis, 319
    inflammation, 193–194
    regaining control of, 198
    spleen inflammation and, 198
Avocados
    benefits of, 23
    high-fat diet trend and, 253
    sugar and fat in, 188

B

Baby liver, 187–192
Bacteria. See also Candida
    E. coli, 211
    as liver troublemakers, 272
    Streptococcus (See Strep)
Bacterial vaginosis (BV)
    individualized support for, 329
    misdiagnosis of, 155–156
Baked Apple Roses, 422, 423
Baked Falafel with Mint Tahini Sauce,
    390, 391
Bananas
    Baked Bananas Foster, 420, 421
    Banana Nice Cream, 420, 421
    as healing food, 287
Barium, 279
Barley grass juice powder, 300
Bath Meditation, Peaceful Liver,
    425–426
B-complex, healing properties of,
    300–301
Beets, 242–243
Berries, 287
Bile
    alkaline water and, 244

bile duct white blood cells, 41
    bloating, constipation, and IBS,
        171
    fat intake and, 11–15
    gallbladder and, 209–217
    ox bile, 227–230
    SIBO and, 161
    Strengthening Bile Production
        Meditation, 427–428
Bilirubin, 56, 214
Bilirubin stones, 212
Bioactive water molecules, 65
Biofilm, 35
Biologics, 276
Biotics, elevated, 26
Bird's eye peppers, 291
Birth control pills, 277
Black walnut, 301
Bloating, 171–174
    causes of, 171–172
    from constipation, 173–174
    gut healing for, 174
    IBS and, 174
    individualized support for, 312
Blood
    angiogenesis, 206
    blood fat, 75–79
    liver flushes and, 233
    natural thinning of, 125
    purification by liver, 33–38
    thick blood and fatty liver, 75–79
Blood sugar. See Diabetes and
    blood sugar imbalance
Blueberries, wild
    as healing food, 297
    Wild Blueberry Mini Muffins, 378,
        379
Brain, fat and, 254
Brain fog, 175–178
    descriptions of, 175
    gut health beliefs about, 175–177
    individualized support for, 313
    reasons for, 176–177
    understanding, 177–178
Breakfast recipes, 371–381
    Caramel Apple Rings, 376, 377
    Chickpea Quiche, 380, 381
    Liver Rescue Smoothie, 372, 373
    Watermelon Slushy, 374, 375
    Wild Blueberry Mini Muffins, 378,
        379
Broccoli, 287
Broth, Liver Rescue, 368, 369
Bruschetta, Potato, 414, 415
Brussels sprouts

    as healing food, 287
    Maple Roasted Brussels Sprouts,
        412, 413
Burdock root, 301
Butternut squash, 298
B_{12} vitamin
    healing properties of, 307
    methylation and, 142–145

C

Cabbage, red, 295–296
Cadmium, 279
Caffeine
    avoiding, during Liver Rescue
        3:6:9, 337
    from coffee enemas, 241–242
    as liver troublemaker, 270
Cancer of liver. See Liver cancer
Candida
    acne and, 156
    SIBO and, 163–165
Candles, scented, 273
Canola oil, 271
Caramel Apple Rings, 376, 377
Carbohydrates
    critical clean carbohydrates (CCC),
        defined, 88–91 (See also
        Critical clean carbohydrates
        (CCC))
    fatty liver and, 77
    high-fat diet trend and, 250–252
    need for, 23–24
Cardamom, 301
Carpet chemicals, 265
Carrots, 288
Castor oil packs, 214
Cat's claw, 301
Cauliflower Sushi with Thai Chili
    Sauce, 398–399, 399
Cayenne peppers, 291
Celery
    benefits of celery juice, 230
    celery juice for digestive
        hypersensitivities, 338
    celery juice and Liver Rescue
        3:6:9, 335, 346
    as healing food, 288
    for strep, 168–169
Celiac, 174, 189, 197–198, 235
Cell regeneration, 225–277
Cellulitis, 151
Central nervous system
    chemical sensitivity and, 139

fatty liver and, 78
Chaga mushroom, 301
Cheese
    acne and, 159
    as liver troublemaker, 268
Chemical and food sensitivities,
    135–140. *See also* Chemical
    neuroantagonists as liver
    troublemakers; Chemicals (in
    homes) as liver troublemakers
    causes of chemical sensitivities,
        137–139
    causes of food sensitivities,
        139–140
    compassion for, 135
    individualized support for, 313
    skin conditions and, 152
    variety of, 135–137, 140
Chemical fertilizers, 265
Chemical neuroantagonists as liver
    troublemakers, 265–267
    chemical fertilizers, 265
    chlorine, 267
    DDT, 266
    fluoride, 267
    fungicides, 266
    insecticides/pesticides, larvicides,
        herbicides, 265–266
    smoke exposure, 266–267
Chemicals (in homes) as liver
    troublemakers, 273–275
    aerosol can air fresheners, 273
    cologne and aftershave, 273
    conventional cleaners, 275
    conventional laundry products,
        275
    conventional makeup, 274
    dry cleaning chemicals, 275
    hair dye, 274
    hairspray, 273–274
    nail chemicals, 275
    perfumes, lotions, creams, gels,
        273
    plug-in air fresheners, 273
    spray-bottle air fresheners and
        mists, 273
    spray tan, 274–275
    talcum powder, 274
Chemical solvents/solutions/agents,
    as liver troublemakers, 264
Cherries, 288
Chickpea Quiche, 380, *381*
Chicory root, 301
Children
    baby liver, 187–192

child liver, defined, 190
child liver, individualized support
    for, 314
dirty blood syndrome in, 67, 68
glucose and glycogen stores in
    pregnancy, 88
PANDAS, jaundice, and baby liver
    in, 187–192
Chlorine, 267
Cholecystitis, 210
Cholesterol
    heart health and, 117–119
    high cholesterol and individualized
        support, 320
    stones, 212
Chronic dehydration, 63–66
Cilantro, 288–289
Cirrhosis
    individualized support for, 314
    liver scar tissue and, 199–202
    pericirrhosis, 199–200
Cleaners, in homes, 275
Cleanse. *See also* Liver Rescue 3:6:9
    adrenal glands and effect of,
        127–131, 133
    cell regeneration and, 227
    for skin conditions, 153
    time needed for cleansing
        troublemakers, 260
Coconuts
    fat in, 251
    healing properties of, 289
"Code alert" levels, of liver, 13–15
Cofactor water, 336
Coffee, drinking, 65
Coffee enemas, 240–242
Colitis, 190
Cologne, 273
Compassion
    finding it for self, 353, 439–441
    liver's need for, 332, 353
    living essence of, xxi, xxii, 439, 441
    power of, xxii, 433, 442
    as soul of peace, 435–438, 442
Constipation, 171–174
    bloating and, 171–172
    causes of, 173–174
    gut healing for, 174
    IBS and, 174
    individualized support for, 314–
        315
Copper
    as liver troublemaker, 279
    skin conditions and, 148–153
CoQ$_{10}$ (Coenzyme Q$_{10}$), 301

Corn, 271
Cortisol, 131
Cosmetic products, 273–275
Cranberries
    Cranberry Water, 364, *365*
    as healing food, 289
Creams, 273
Critical clean carbohydrates (CCC)
    defined, 88–91
    diabetes and, 105
    high-fat diet trend and, 252
Cruciferous vegetables, 289
Cucumbers
    cucumber-apple juice, for Liver
        Rescue 3:6:9, 350
    for dark under-eye circles, 67
    as healing food, 289
    Potato Pancakes with Cucumber
        Radish Salad, 402, *403*
Curcumin, 301
Curry, Yellow, Noodles Two Ways,
    386, *387*
Cysts (liver), individualized support
    for, 324

D

Dairy
    acne and, 159
    constipation from, 173
    lactose and, 235
    as liver troublemaker, 268
Dandelion greens, 289–290
Dandelion root, 301
Dark under-eye circles
    from dirty blood syndrome, 67–68
    individualized support for, 315
Dates
    as healing food, 290
    during Liver Rescue 3:6:9, 343–344
DDT, 9, 122–123, 148, 151, 266
Dehydration
    dirty blood syndrome and, 63–66
    Liver Rescue 3:6:9 for, 335
    sinuses and, 180
Delicata squash, 298
Depression. *See* Mood struggles
Dermatitis, 151
Dermatoxin effect, 149–153
Dessert recipes, 417–423
    Baked Apple Roses, 422, *423*
    Baked Bananas Foster, 420, *421*
    Banana Nice Cream, 420, *421*
    Peach Ginger Sorbet, 418, *419*

Detergent, laundry, 275
DHA (docosahexaenoic acid), 302
Diabetes and blood sugar
    adrenals and, 110–111
    blood sugar support for, 107–109
    diet and, 103–104
    dirty blood syndrome and, 70
    fat in diet and, 106–107
    fructose intolerance and, 235
    glucose and, 105–106
    heart health affected by, 110
    imbalance, 101–111
    individualized support for, 315
    pancreas and, 101–102
    types of diabetes, 102–103
    viruses and, 103
Diagnosis bias, hepatitis and,
    194–196
Diesel, 263
Diet. See also Liver support
    for acne, 160
    cholesterol and, 117
    diabetes and blood sugar
        imbalance, 103–104
    dirty blood syndrome and, 70–71
    eating liver, 230–232
    fat processing and, 11–15
    fatty liver and, 75
    food-borne toxins as liver
        troublemakers, 272
    food chemicals as liver
        troublemakers, 267–268
    food sensitivities, 135–140
    healing with, 38
    liver cancer and, 204
    problematic foods group as liver
        troublemakers, 268–271
    SAD and, 183–185
Digestion. See also Intestines;
    Stomach
    of babies and children, 187–192
    bloating, constipation, and IBS,
        171–174
    strep and, 167–168
Dinner, 395–405
    Cauliflower Sushi with Thai Chili
        Sauce, 398–399, 399
    Lentil Tacos, 396, 397
    Potato Pancakes with Cucumber
        Radish Salad, 402, 403
    Ratatouille, 400–401, 401
    Roasted Veggie Pasta, 404, 405
Dioxins, 264
Dirty blood syndrome, 63–74
    chronic dehydration and, 63–66

dark under-eye circles from,
    67–68
defined, 66
energy issues of, 66–67
gout from, 69–71
healing for, 74
individualized support for, 316
inflammation from, 72–73
insomnia from, 73–74
methylation and, 145–146
Raynaud's syndrome from, 68–69
thick blood and, 71
varicose veins from, 71–72
Diverticulitis, 211
Diverticulosis, 211
D-mannose, 302
Dosage guidelines, for individualized
    support, 308–310
Dragon fruit, 38, 205, 242, 243,
    294–295, 346
Drugs
    autoimmune liver, hepatitis, and,
        195
    liver scar tissue and, 199
    recreational, as liver
        troublemakers, 278
Dry cleaning chemicals, 275
Dryer sheets, 275
Dulse, 67, 286–287
Dye, hair, 274

E

E. coli, 211
Ear infections, 155
Ectopic heartbeat, 121, 125
Eczema
    causes of skin problems, 148–151
    dermatoxin effect, 149–150
    healing, 153
    individualized support for, 316
    symptom cycles, 152–153
    types of skin problems, 147–148
Eczema and psoriasis, 147–153
Eggplant, 290
Eggs
    constipation from, 173
    as liver troublemaker, 268
    sensitivity to, 139–140
Eliminating Toxins Meditation, 431
Emotions. See Mood struggles
Energy issues and fatigue
    of dirty blood syndrome, 66–67
    individualized support for, 317

Engine oil and grease, 263
Enzymes, testing of, 55–61
EPA (eicosapentaenoic acid), 302
Epstein-Barr virus (EBV)
    autoimmune conditions and,
        40–41
    autoimmune liver, hepatitis, and,
        196
    brain fog and, 176–178
    chemical sensitivity and, 138
    dirty blood syndrome and, 68–70,
        72
    hunger and, 88–89
    liver cancer and, 203–208
    methylation and, 145
    mystery heart palpitations from,
        122–125
    skin conditions and, 149–153
    thyroid and, 5
Exercise
    dehydration and, 65
    for diabetes and prediabetes, 109
Exhaust fumes, 263
Eyebright, 302

F

Falafel, Baked, with Mint Tahini
    Sauce, 390, 391
Fasting, Liver Rescue 3:6:9 vs., 334
Fat (body). See also Weight gain
    in liver, 89 (See also Fatty liver)
    Loosening Liver Fat Cells Morning
        Meditation, 429–430
    nutrients in, 79
Fat (dietary)
    diabetes and blood sugar
        imbalance, 106–107
    high-fat diet trend, 247–257
    Liver Rescue 3:6:9 and, 335, 340,
        344
    lowering, 108–109
    measuring, 15
    processing of, 11–17
    reducing fat intake, 284–285
    toxins stored in, 231
"Fat-free" foods, 248
Fatty liver
    blood thickness and, 75–79
    fruit and, 21
    hunger and, 88–89
    individualized support for, 317
    mood and, 181
    weight gain and, 85

Fermented foods, 239–240
Fertilizers, 265
Fibrillation, atrial, 121, 125
Fibrolamellar hepatocellular
    carcinoma (FHCC), 203
Figs, 290
Five-MTHF
    (5-methyltetrahydrofolate), 299
Fluoride
    dental treatments, 115
    as liver troublemaker, 267
Flushes
    gallbladder, 214–216, 232
    liver, 232–234
    Liver Rescue 3:6:9 flushing
        technique, 352–353
Food belief systems, 333–334
Food-borne toxins, as liver
    troublemakers, 272
Food chemicals as liver
    troublemakers, 267–268
    aspartame and artificial
        sweeteners, 267
    formaldehyde, 267
    MSG (monosodium glutamate),
        267
    preservatives, 267–268
Food labels, 15, 251–252
Food poisoning, 210–212
Food sensitivities. See Chemical and
    food sensitivities
Formaldehyde, 267
Free will, 438–439
Fructose intolerance, 234–236
Fruit
    "fear" of, 253–254
    gallbladder and, 217
    glucose and glycogen storage, 21
    high-fat diet trend and, 253–254
Fumes, exhaust, 263
Fungicides, 57, 265–266

G

Gallbladder
    baby liver and, 188
    flushes, 232
    gallstones, 212–216, 233, 318
    individualized support for, 318
    sickness, 209–217
Gamma-glutamyl transpeptidase
    (GGT), 56
Garlic, 290–291
Gas grills/stoves/ovens, 264

Gasoline, 262
Gels (cosmetic products), 273
Genetics
    aging and, 95–96
    methylenetetrahydrofolate
        reductase (MTHFR) gene
        mutation and, 141, 142,
        144–146
    weight gain and, 86
Ginger
    as healing food, 302–303
    Peach Ginger Sorbet, 418, 419
Glucose and glycogen, 19–24
    blood sugar balance and, 19–20
    carbohydrate need and, 23–24
    children and, 190
    diabetes and blood sugar
        imbalance, 105–106, 110
    fat processing and, 11, 1416
    glucose as fuel, 20–23
    hunger and, 88–91
    for liver support, 285
    sugar needs and, 252–254
Glutathione, 303
Gluten
    constipation from, 173
    inflammation and, 73
    as liver troublemaker, 271
GMO (genetically modified) foods,
    242–243
Goldenseal, 303
Gout
    from dirty blood syndrome, 69–71
    individualized support for, 318
    liver enzymes and, 60
Grapes, 291
Grazing, benefits of, 111, 285, 337
Grills, gas, 264
Gut health. See Digestion; Intestines

H

Habeñero peppers, 291
Hair dye, 274
Hairspray, 273–274
HDL (high-density lipoproteins), 117
Healing foods, 285–298. See also
    Liver Rescue 3:6:9; individual
    recipes
    apples, 285–286 (See also Apples)
    apricots, 286
    artichokes, 286
    arugula, 286
    asparagus, 286

Atlantic sea vegetables, 67,
    286–287
bananas, 287
berries, 287
broccoli, 287
brussels sprouts, 287
carrots, 288
celery, 288
cherries, 288
cilantro, 288–289
coconut, 251, 289
cranberries, 289
cruciferous vegetables, 289
cucumbers, 289 (See also
    Cucumbers)
dandelion greens, 289–290
dates, 290
eggplant, 290
figs, 290
garlic, 290–291
grapes, 291
hot peppers, 291
Jerusalem artichokes, 291
kale, 292
kiwis, 292
leafy greens, 292
lemons and limes, 292 (See also
    Lemon (lime) water)
mangoes, 292
maple syrup, 292–293
melons, 109, 293
mushrooms, 293
onions and scallions, 293
oranges and tangerines, 293
papayas, 294
parsley, 294
peaches and nectarines, 294
pears, 294
pineapple, 294
pitaya (dragon fruit), 38, 205, 242,
    243, 294–295, 346
pomegranates, 295
potatoes, 295
radishes, 295
raw honey, 295
red cabbage, 295–296
spinach, 296
sprouts and microgreens, 296
sweet potatoes, 296–297
tomatoes, 217, 297
turmeric (fresh), 297
wild blueberries, 297
winter squash, 298
zucchini, 298

Healing herbs and supplements,
298–308. *See also* Vitamins;
individual recipes
ALA (alpha lipoic acid), 299–300
aloe vera, 300
amla berry, 300
ashwagandha, 300
barley grass juice powder, 300
B-complex, 300–301
black walnut, 301
burdock root, 301
cardamom, 301
cat's claw, 301
chaga mushroom, 301
chicory root, 301
CoQ$_{10}$ (Coenzyme Q$_{10}$), 301
curcumin, 301
dandelion root, 301
D-mannose, 302
EPA and DHA (eicosapentaenoic
acid and docosahexaenoic
acid), 302
eyebright, 302
five-MTHF
(5-methyltetrahydrofolate), 299
ginger, 302–303
glutathione, 303
goldenseal, 303
hibiscus, 303
lemon balm, 303
licorice root, 303
L-lysine, 303–304
magnesium glycinate, 304
melatonin, 304
milk thistle, 304
MSM (methylsulfonylmethane), 304
mullein leaf, 304
NAC (N-acetyl cysteine), 304
nascent iodine, 305
nettle leaf, 305
olive leaf, 305
Oregon grape root, 305
overview, 298–299
peppermint, 305
raspberry leaf, 305
red clover, 305–306
rose hips, 306
schisandra berry, 306
selenium, 306
spirulina, 306
turmeric (supplement form),
306–307
vitamin B$_{12}$ (as adenosylcobalamin
with methylcobalamin), 307
vitamin C, 307

vitamin D$_3$, 307–308
yellow dock, 308
zinc (as liquid zinc sulfate), 308
Heart health
cholesterol and, 117–119
diabetes and blood sugar
imbalance, 110
heart palpitations, 121–125
heart palpitations, individualized
support for, 319
high blood pressure, 113–116
mystery heart palpitations and,
121–125
Heat, liver, 51, 234
Heavy metals
aluminum, 177
children and, 191–192
Liver Rescue 3:6:9 for heavy metal
detox, 352
mercury, 177
as part of "Unforgiving Four," 9
toxic heavy metals as liver
troublemakers, 278–279
Hepatic artery white blood cells, 40
Hepatic ducts, 234
Hepatic portal vein
fatty liver and, 77, 79
significance of, 33
white blood cells, 40
Hepatic vessel white blood cells, 40
Hepatitis
autoimmune liver and, 193–198
individualized support for, 319
Hepatocellular carcinoma (HCC), 203
Hepatocytes, 36–37, 287, 292, 307
Herbal tinctures, 299. *See also*
Healing herbs and supplements
Hereditary fructose intolerance (HFI),
235
HHV-6
children and, 191–192
human herpes virus 6, defined, 41
skin conditions and dermatoxins,
151
Hibiscus, 303
Hibiscus Lemonade, 360, *361*
High blood pressure, 113–116
hidden factors of, 113–115
individualized support for, 319
solving, 115–116
High cholesterol. *See* Cholesterol
High-fat diet trend, 247–257
animal protein in, 248, 254–257
background of, 247–249
fruit and, 253–254

high-fat foods as liver
troublemaker, 269
hybrid diets, 249–250
sugar, carbohydrates, protein, and
hidden fat in "high-protein"
foods, 250–252
sugar needs and, 252–253
Hives, 147, 149
Homes, chemicals in, 273–275
Honey, raw, 295
Hormones. *See also* Adrenal glands
acne and, 157–158
cortisol, 131
from food, as liver troublemaker,
268–269
heart palpitations and, 121, 122
hormonal problems,
individualized support for, 320
hormone medications as liver
troublemaker, 277
hormone replacement therapy
(HRT), 31, 52, 93, 122, 213
melatonin, 304
Hot flashes, individualized support
for, 321. *See also* Menopause
Hot peppers, 291
Hunger, 87–91
critical clean carbohydrates and,
88
glucose obstacles and, 90–91
liver stressors and, 88–89
mystery hunger, individualized
support for, 326
Hybrid diets, 249–250
Hydrobioactive water, 336
Hydrochloric acid, 161–169, 188, 239
Hyperantioxidants, 204
Hypertension (high blood pressure),
113–116

I

IBS (irritable bowel syndrome),
171–174
bloating and constipation,
171–174
causes of, 174
gut healing for, 174
individualized support for, 321
Ileum, 26, 141–146
Immune system
adrenal glands and, 131
autoimmune liver and hepatitis,
193–198

Strengthening Your Liver's Immune System Morning Meditation, 429
white blood cells and, 33, 36, 39–43
Immunosuppressants, 276
Individualized support, 308–329
acne, 311
adrenal problems, 311
autoimmune liver (viral-caused autoimmune disorders and diseases), 312
bloating, 312
brain fog, 313
chemical and food sensitivities, 313
child liver, 314
cirrhosis and pericirrhosis, 314
constipation, 314–315
dark under-eye circles, 315
diabetes and blood sugar imbalance, 315
dirty blood syndrome, 316
dosage, 308–310
eczema and psoriasis, 316
emotional liver and mood struggles, 317
energy issues and fatigue, 317
everyday liver and health maintenance, 310
fatty liver, 317
gallbladder infections, 318
gallstones, 318
gout, 318
heart palpitations, 319
hepatitis, 319
high blood pressure, 319
high cholesterol, 320
hormonal problems, 320
hot flashes, 321
IBS, 321
inflammation, 321–322
jaundice, 322
liver abscesses, 322
liver aging, 323
liver cancer, 323
liver insomnia, 323
liver scar tissue, 323–324
liver tumors and cysts, 324
liver worms and parasites, 324–325
methylation problems, 325
mystery hunger, 326
PANDAS, 326
Raynaud's syndrome, 326

SAD, 327
SIBO, 327
sinus infections, 328
skin conditions, 316
sluggish liver, 317
strep throat and sore throat, 328
supplement list explanations, 309–310
UTIs, yeast infections, and BV (bacterial vaginosis), 329
varicose and spider veins, 329
weight gain, 330
Infant acid reflux, 187–188
Inflammation
autoimmune liver and hepatitis, 193–198
from dirty blood syndrome, 72–73
gene mutation tests and, 142, 145
individualized support for, 321–322
Inherited toxins, 47
Insecticides, as liver troublemakers, 265–266. See also Pesticides
Insomnia
causes of, 73–74
individualized support for, 323
Insulin
diet and insulin resistance, 16–17
fructose intolerance and, 235
Intestines
baby liver and, 187–188
bloating, constipation, and IBS, 171–174
chemical sensitivity and, 139
ileum, 26, 141–146
SIBO (small intestinal bacterial overgrowth), 161–169
Irritable bowel syndrome. See IBS

J

Jalapeño peppers, 291
Jaundice, 187–192
baby liver and, 187–188
causes of, 188–189
child liver and, 190
individualized support for, 322
PANDAS and, 191–192
Jerusalem artichokes, 291
Juice, Liver Rescue, 358, 359
Juice, tea, and broth recipes, 355–369
Cranberry Water, 364, 365
Hibiscus Lemonade, 360, 361

Lime Water, 362, 363
Liver Rescue Broth, 368, 369
Liver Rescue Juice, 358, 359
Liver Rescue Tea, 366, 367

K

Kabocha squash
as healing food, 298
Kabocha Squash Soup, 392, 393
Kale, 292
Kelp, 286–287
Kerosene, 263
Killing Viruses and Other Pathogens Meditation, 428–429
Kiwis, 292
Kupffer cells, 33–38, 287, 292

L

Labels, food, 15, 251–252
Lactose, 235
Larvicides, 265–266
Latent autoimmune diabetes in adults (type 1.5 diabetes, LADA), 103
Laundry products, 275
LDL (low-density lipoproteins), 117
Lead, 279
Leafy greens, 292
"Lean" protein, 250
Lectin, 236–237
Lemonade, Hibiscus, 360, 361
Lemon balm, 303
Lemon (lime) water
drinking, in morning, 65
Lime Water (recipe), 362, 363
for Liver Rescue 3:6:9, 335, 343
Lemons/limes, as healing food, 292
Lentil Tacos, 396, 397
Lettuce, 292
Lichen sclerosus, 151
Licorice root, 303
Lighter fluid, 263–264
Lime Water, 362, 363
Liquid zinc sulfate, 308
Liver. See also Dirty blood syndrome; Symptoms and conditions
abscesses, 322
as adaptogenic, 11–17
aging and, 93–96, 323
awareness about, 3–9
blood purification by, 33–38

as body's peacemaker, 221–224
enzyme testing, 55–61
fatty liver, 75–79
glucose and glycogen storage, 19–24
hunger and, 87–91
immune system and, 33, 36, 39–43
jelly-like byproduct of, 123–125
liver heat, 51, 234
lobules of, 22, 31, 33–38, 40–41, 339
myths about (See Myths about liver)
protection by, 29–32
protective membranes, 201
sluggish, 47–54
spasms, 182
transplants, 182, 183
troublemakers to (See Liver troublemakers)
vitamin and mineral storage by, 25–27
Liver cancer, 203–208
avoiding, 207–208
formation of, 205–206
individualized support for, 323
as primary vs. secondary, 206–207
viruses and, 203–205
Liver lymphocytes, 41–42
Liver Rescue Applesauce, 410, 411
Liver Rescue Broth, 368, 369
Liver Rescue Juice, 358, 359
Liver Rescue meditations, 425–442
Disease Reversal Nighttime Meditation, 430
Eliminating Toxins Meditation, 431
Killing Viruses and Other Pathogens Meditation, 428–429
Liver Cooling Meditation, 427
Liver Rejuvenation Walking Meditation, 426–427
Loosening Liver Fat Cells Morning Meditation, 429–430
Peaceful Liver Bath Meditation, 425–426
playing music for, 425
Strengthening Bile Production Meditation, 427–428
Strengthening Your Liver's Immune System Morning Meditation, 429

Liver Rescue Salad, 384–385, 385
Liver Rescue Tea, 366, 367
Liver Rescue 3:6:9, 331–353
The 3, 339, 342–345
The 6, 345–348
The 9, 339, 348–352
for adrenals, 127–131, 133
for cell regeneration, 227
fasting vs., 334
flushing technique, 352–353
food belief systems and, 333–334
heavy metal detox with, 352
Liver Rescue Morning, overview, 332–338
mono eating and, 338–341
overview, 332–333
for relief, 331–332
for skin conditions, 153
time needed for, 260 (See also Liver troublemakers)
transition time, 351–352
Liver support, 283–329
balancing diet for, 284–285
fuel needed for, 283
healing foods for, 285–298 (See also Healing foods)
healing herbs and supplements for, 298–308 (See also Healing herbs and supplements)
individualized support for, 308–329 (See also Individualized support)
liver storage and, 283–284
Liver troublemakers, 259–281
chemical industry domestic invasion, 273–275
chemical neuroantagonists, 265–267
excess adrenaline, 280
food chemicals, 267–268
overview of list, 261
pathogenic group, 271–272
petrochemicals, 261–265
pharmaceuticals, 275–278
problematic foods, 268–271
radiation, 279–280
rainfall exposure, 280–281
three depths of liver and, 259–261
time needed for cleansing of, 260
toxic heavy metals, 278–279
L-lysine, 237, 303–304
Lobules
blood purification by, 33–38
defined, 22

lobule white blood cells, 40–41
perime cells and, 31
shape of, 339
Lotions, 273
"Low-fat" foods, 248
Lunch recipes, 383–393
Baked Falafel with Mint Tahini Sauce, 390, 391
Kabocha Squash Soup, 392, 393
Liver Rescue Salad, 384–385, 385
Sweet Potato and Black Bean Salad with Spicy Lime "Vinaigrette," 388, 389
Yellow Curry Noodles Two Ways, 386, 387
Lupus, 147, 149, 151
Lymphatic system
constipation and, 173
lymphedema and weight gain, 85
lymphocytes, 131, 158

M

Magnesium glycinate, 304
Makeup, 274
Malabsorption, fructose, 235
Mangoes
as healing food, 292
Mango Salsa, Spicy, Pineapple and Apple Chips, 408, 409
Maple Roasted Brussels Sprouts, 412, 413
Maple syrup, 292–293
Medical Medium (William), 21
Medical Medium Life-Changing Foods (William), 21
Medical Medium Thyroid Healing (William), 5
Medications
antibiotics, 155–160
antidepressants, 183
antifungals, 156
pharmaceuticals as liver troublemakers, 275–278
statins, 119
steroids, 152
Meditations. See Liver Rescue meditations
Melatonin, 304
Melons, 109, 293
Menopause
acne and, 158

gallbladder and, 213
heart palpitations and, 122
hormone replacement therapy (HRT), 31, 52, 93, 122, 213
hot flashes, individualized support for, 321
Menstruation
constipation and, 173
gallbladder and, 213
Mercury
brain fog and, 177
as liver troublemaker, 278–279
skin conditions and, 148–153
Metabolism, 67, 81, 82, 85
Methylation, 141–146
B$_{12}$ vitamin and, 142–145
defined, 26, 141–142
individualized support for problems of, 325
methylation problems, individualized support for, 325
methylenetetrahydrofolate reductase (MTHFR) gene mutation, 141, 142, 144–146
Microadhesions, 36, 103, 201
Microgreens, 296
Milk thistle, 304
Mineral salts
in celery juice, 230
glucose and, 16, 20
Mineral storage, 25–27
Mint Tahini Sauce, Baked Falafel with, 390, 391
Mists, air freshener, 273
Mold, 272
Mono eating, 338–341
Mood struggles, 179–185
antidepressants and, 183, 276
diet and, 183–185
emotional liver and, 182–183, 185
individualized support for, 317, 327
seasonal affective disorder (SAD), 179–181
Morning meditations
Loosening Liver Fat Cells Morning Meditation, 429–430
Strengthening Your Liver's Immune System Morning Meditation, 429
"Mother," 238
MSG (monosodium glutamate), 267
MSM (methylsulfonylmethane), 304

MTHFR (methylenetetrahydrofolate reductase) gene mutation, 141, 142, 144–146
Muffins, Mini, Wild Blueberry, 378, 379
Mullein leaf, 304
Mushroom, chaga, 301
Mushrooms, 293
Myths about liver, 225–245
alkaline water, 243–245
apple cider vinegar, 238–240
beets, 242–243
cell regeneration and, 225–277
coffee enemas, 240–242
eating liver, 230–232
fructose intolerance, 234–236
lectin, 236–237
liver flushes, 232–234
"liver stones," 234
ox bile, 227–230

N

NAC (N-acetyl cysteine), 304
Nail chemicals, 275
Nascent iodine, 305
Nectarines, 294
Nettle leaf, 305
Neurotoxins, 59
brain fog and, 176–178
children and, 191–192
Nice Cream, Banana, 420, 421
Nickel, 279
Nighttime Meditation, Disease Reversal, 430
Noodles, Yellow Curry, Two Ways, 386, 387
Nutrient conversion, 25–27
Nutrition labels, 15, 251–252
Nuts, fat in, 251

O

Oil, for gallbladder flushes, 214–216
Oils
canola oil, 271
olive oil for gallbladder flushes, 214–216
Olive leaf, 305
Onions, 293
Opioids, 276
Oranges, 293
Oregon grape root, 305

Ovens, gas, 264
Ox bile, 227–230
Oxygen
from exercise, 109
oxygen saturation tests, 124
thick blood and fatty liver, 76–79

P

Paint, 264–265
Paint thinner, 265
Palpitations, mystery, 121–125
Pancreas
diabetes and blood sugar imbalance, 101–102 (See also Diabetes)
enzymes and, 56, 58
fat processing and protection of, 16–17
fatty liver and, 79
pancreatitis, 79, 103, 215–216
sluggish liver and, 51–52
PANDAS (pediatric autoimmune neuropsychiatric disorders associated with streptococcal infections), 187–192
antibiotics for, 156–157
baby liver and, 187–188
child liver and, 190 defined, 191–192
individualized support for, 326
jaundice and, 188–190
Papayas, 294
Parasites, individualized support for, 324–325
Parsley, 294
Pasta, Roasted Veggie, 404, 405
Pathogens. See also Bacteria; Toxins; Viruses
bacteria, 272
food-borne toxins, 272
Killing Viruses and Other Pathogens Meditation, 428–429
as liver troublemakers, 271–272
mold, 272
viruses and viral waste matter, 271–272
Peace
finding, 435
free will and, 438–439
self-compassion, finding, 439–441
self-compassion as soul of, 435–438, 442

Spirit and, 441
spirituality for, 439
Peaceful Liver Bath Meditation,
425–426
Peach Ginger Sorbet, 418, *419*
Peaches, 294
Pears, 294
Pelvic inflammatory disease (PID), 166
Peppermint, 305
Peppers
    Cauliflower Sushi with Thai Chili
      Sauce, 398, *399*
    as healing food, 291
Perfumes, 273
Pericirrhosis
    individualized support for, 314
    liver scar tissue and, 199–200
Perime cells, 31
Pesticides
    DDT, 122–123, 148, 151, 266
    liver enzymes and, 57
    as liver troublemakers, 265–266
    skin conditions and, 148, 151
Petrochemicals as liver
    troublemakers, 261–265
    carpet chemicals, 265
    chemical solvents, solutions, and
      agents, 264
    diesel, 263
    dioxins, 264
    engine oil and grease, 263
    exhaust fumes, 263
    gas grills, stoves, ovens, 264
    gasoline, 262
    kerosene, 263
    lighter fluid, 263–264
    paint, 264–265
    paint thinner, 265
    plastics, 262
Pharmaceuticals as liver
    troublemakers, 275–278
    alcohol in toiletries and
      medications, 277
    antibiotics, 276
    antidepressants, 276
    anti-inflammatories, 276
    biologics, 276
    birth control pills, 277
    blood pressure medications, 277
    hormone medications, 277
    opioids, 276
    prescription amphetamines, 276
    recreational drug abuse, 278
    regular immunosuppressants, 276
    sleeping pills, 276

statins, 276–277
steroids, 277
thyroid medications, 277
Pigment stone, 212
Pineapple
    as healing food, 294
    Pineapple and Apple Chips with
      Spicy Mango Salsa, 408, *409*
Pitaya (dragon fruit), 38, 205, 242,
    243, 294–295, 346
Plastics, 262
Platelet issues, thick blood vs., 71
Plug-in air fresheners, 273
Poblano peppers, 291
Polycystic ovarian syndrome (PCOS),
    81, 173
Pomegranates, 295
Pork products, 271
Potato Bruschetta, 414, *415*
Potatoes, 295
Potato Pancakes with Cucumber
    Radish Salad, 402, *403*
Prediabetes, 102–103
Preeclampsia, 145
Preservatives, food, 267–268
Problematic foods group, as liver
    troublemakers, 268–271
    caffeine, 270
    canola oil, 271
    cheese, 268
    corn, 271
    dairy, 268
    eggs, 268
    excessive salt use, 270–271
    excessive vinegar use, 269–270
    gluten, 271
    high-fat foods, 269
    hormones from food, 268–269
    pork products, 271
    recreational alcohol, 269
Processed foods, avoiding during
    Liver Rescue 3:6:9, 337
Protective membranes of liver, 201
Protein
    high-fat diet trend and, 247–257
    Liver Rescue 3:6:9 and, 336–337
Psoriasis, 147–153
    causes of skin problems, 148–151
    dermatoxin effect, 149–150
    healing, 153
    individualized support for, 316
    symptom cycles, 152–153
    types of skin problems, 147–148
Puberty, acne and, 157–158
Purpose-plus stress, 131

Q

Quiche, Chickpea, 380, *381*

R

Radiation
    as liver troublemaker, 279–280
    as part of "Unforgiving Four," 9
Radishes
    as healing food, 295
    Potato Pancakes with Cucumber
      Radish Salad, 402, *403*
Rainfall exposure, as liver
    troublemaker, 280–281
Raspberry leaf, 305
Ratatouille, 400–401, *401*
Raw honey, 295
Raynaud's syndrome, 68–69
    defined, 68–69
    individualized support for, 326
Recipes, breakfast, 371–381
    Caramel Apple Rings, 376, *377*
    Chickpea Quiche, 380, *381*
    Liver Rescue Smoothie, 372, *373*
    Watermelon Slushy, 374, *375*
    Wild Blueberry Mini Muffins, 378,
      379
Recipes, desserts, 417–423
    Baked Apple Roses, 422, *423*
    Baked Bananas Foster, 420, *421*
    Banana Nice Cream, 420, *421*
    Peach Ginger Sorbet, 418, *419*
Recipes, dinner, 395–405
    Cauliflower Sushi with Thai Chili
      Sauce, 398–399, *399*
    Lentil Tacos, 396, *397*
    Potato Pancakes with Cucumber
      Radish Salad, 402, *403*
    Ratatouille, 400–401, *401*
    Roasted Veggie Pasta, 404, *405*
Recipes, juices, teas, and broth,
    355–369
    Cranberry Water, 364, *365*
    Hibiscus Lemonade, 360, *361*
    Lime Water, 362, *363*
    Liver Rescue Broth, 368, *369*
    Liver Rescue Juice, 358, *359*
    Liver Rescue Tea, 366, *367*
Recipes, snacks, 407–415
    Liver Rescue Applesauce, 410, *411*
    Maple Roasted Brussels Sprouts,
      412, *413*

Pineapple and Apple Chips with
Spicy Mango Salsa, 408, *409*
Potato Bruschetta, 414, *415*
Red cabbage, 295–296
Red clover, 305–306
Regeneration, of cells, 225–277
Roasted Veggie Pasta, 404, *405*
Rosacea, 147, 149, 151
Rose hips, 306

S

Salt, excessive use of, 270–271
Scallions, 293
Scarring of liver
blood purification and, 36–37
cirrhosis and, 199–202
individualized support for,
323–324
microadhesions, 36, 103, 201
Scented candles, 273
Schisandra berry, 306
Scleroderma, 151
Sea vegetables, 67, 286–287
Seasonal affective disorder (SAD),
179–181, 326. *See also* Mood
struggles
Seborrheic dermatitis, 151
Selenium, 306
SIBO (small intestinal bacterial
overgrowth), 161–169
antibiotics and, 166–167
balance for, 168–169
Candida vs., 163–165
digestion and, 167–168
gastric juices and, 161–163
individualized support for, 327
Sinuses
sinus cavity sensitivity, 180
sinus infections and cause, 156
sinus infections and individualized
support, 327
Skin conditions
acne, 155–160
actinic keratosis, 151
age spots, 151
cellulitis, 151
dermatitis, 151
eczema and psoriasis, 147–153
individualized support for, 316
lichen sclerosus, 151
lupus-style rashes, 149, 151
rosacea, 149, 151
scleroderma, 151

seborrheic dermatitis, 151
vitiligo, 151
Sleep
insomnia and, 73–74
sleeping pills, 276
Sluggish liver, 47–54
five areas of, 53–54
individualized support for, 317
mood and, 181
symptoms of, 47–53
Slushy, Watermelon, 374, *375*
Smoke exposure, 266–267
Smoothie, Liver Rescue, 372, *373*
Snacks, recipes, 407–415
Liver Rescue Applesauce, 410, *411*
Maple Roasted Brussels Sprouts,
412, *413*
Pineapple and Apple Chips with
Spicy Mango Salsa, 408, *409*
Potato Bruschetta, 414, *415*
Sorbet, Peach Ginger, 418, *419*
Spasms
gallbladder, 214
liver spasms, defined, 74, 182
Spider veins
defined, 71–72
individualized support for, 329
Spinach, 296
Spinach soup, 349
Spirit, 333–334, 338, 441
Spirituality, 439
Spirulina, 306
Spleen, inflammation of, 198
Spray-bottle air fresheners and
mists, 273
Spray tan, 274–275
Sprouts, 296
Statins
for cholesterol, 119
as liver troublemakers, 276–277
Steroids
as liver troublemakers, 277
for skin conditions, 152
Sties, 166
Stomach
alkalinity in, 239
in babies, 188
fatty liver and, 78–79
gastric juices of, 161–169, 239
Stones
gallstones, 212–216, 233, 318
"liver stones," 234
Stoves, gas, 264
Strengthening Bile Production
Meditation, 427–428

Strep
acne and, 155–160
children and, 191–192
classification of, 166
gallbladder and, 210–211
individualized support for, 328
SIBO and, 164–169
in sinuses, 180
skin conditions and, 151
Stress
adrenal glands and, 131
excess adrenaline as liver
troublemaker, 280
high blood pressure and, 115
Subcutaneous tissue, 158–159
Sugar
in alcohol, 248
blood sugar imbalance, 107–109
(*See also* Diabetes and blood
sugar imbalance)
fatty liver and, 77
glucose and glycogen storage,
19–24
high blood pressure and, 114
high-fat diet trend and, 250–253
hunger and glucose, 90–91
Sunchokes, 291
Super chili peppers, 291
Supplements. *See* Healing herbs and
supplements
Sushi, Cauliflower, with Thai Chili
Sauce, 398–399, *399*
Sweeteners, artificial, 267
Sweet Potato and Black Bean Salad
with Spicy Lime "Vinaigrette,"
388, *389*
Sweet potatoes, 296–297
Symptoms and conditions, 99–217.
See also individual symptoms and
conditions
acne, 155–160
adrenal problems, 127–134
autoimmune liver and hepatitis,
193–198
brain fog, 175–178
chemical and food sensitivities,
135–140
cirrhosis and liver scar tissue,
199–202
diabetes and blood sugar
imbalance, 101–111
eczema and psoriasis, 147–153
gallbladder sickness, 209–217
heart palpitations, 121–125
high blood pressure, 113–116

liver cancer, 203–208
methylation problems, 141–146
mood struggles, 179–185
PANDAS, jaundice, and baby liver, 187–192
SIBO (small intestinal bacterial overgrowth), 161–169

T

Tacos, Lentil, 396, *397*
Talcum powder, 274
Tangerines, 293
Tanning products, 274–275
Tea, Liver Rescue, 366, *367*
Testing
 for blood fat, 76
 of liver enzymes, 55–61
 methylenetetrahydrofolate reductase (MTHFR) gene mutation and, 141, 142, 144–146
 oxygen saturation tests, 124
Thai Chili Sauce, Cauliflower Sushi with, 398, *399*
Throat pain, individualized support for, 328
Thrombosis, 146
Thyroid
 chronic illness and, 5
 thyroid medications, 277
 weight gain and, 82
Tomatoes, as healing food, 217, 297
Tonsillitis, 166
Toxins. *See also* Liver troublemakers
 chemical and food sensitivities, 135–140
 dermatoxin effect, 149–153
 detoxification, 33–38
 eating liver and, 230–232
 Eliminating Toxins Meditation, 431
 inherited, 47
 liver enzymes and, 57
 Liver Rescue 3:6:9 for cleansing of, 340
 nutrient conversion and, 26–27
 protection from, 29–32
 symptoms from, 6–7
Transplants, liver, 182, 183
Tumors (liver), individualized support for, 324
Turmeric (fresh), 297
Turmeric (supplement form), 306–307
Type 1 diabetes, 102–103

Type 2 diabetes, 52, 102–103. *See also* Diabetes and blood sugar imbalance
Type 1.5 diabetes (latent autoimmune diabetes in adults, LADA), 103

U

"Unforgiving Four," 9
Uric acid, gout and, 69–71
UTIs
 individualized support for, 329
 misdiagnosis of, 155–156

V

Varicose veins
 defined, 71–72
 individualized support for, 329
Vegetables, sugars in diet and, 109. *See also* Healing foods; *individual recipes*
Vinegar
 apple cider vinegar, 238–240
 blood pressure and, 114
 as liver troublemaker, 269–270
Viruses. *See also* Epstein-Barr virus (EBV); HHV-6
 diabetes and blood sugar imbalance, 103
 hunger and, 88–89
 individualized support for viral-caused autoimmune disorders and diseases, 311–312
 Killing Viruses and Other Pathogens Meditation, 428–429
 liver cancer and, 203–208
 as liver troublemakers, 271–272
 methylation and, 144–146
 mystery heart palpitations from, 122–125
 as part of "Unforgiving Four," 9
 skin conditions and, 149–153
 weight gain and, 82
Vitamins
 B-complex, 300–301
 B$_{12}$ vitamin, 142–145, 307
 C, 307
 D$_3$, 307–308
 storage of, 25–27
Vitiligo, 151

W

Walking Meditation, Liver Rejuvenation, 426–427
Water
 Cranberry Water, 364, *365*
 hydrobioactive and cofactor, 336
 Lime Water, 362, *363*
Watermelon Slushy, 374, *375*
Weight gain, 81–86
 adrenal-liver link to, 82–84
 aging and, 84–85
 genetics and, 86
 individualized support for, 330
 liver enzymes and, 60
 liver storage and, 83–84, 133
 metabolism and, 81, 82, 85
 thyroid-liver link to, 82
 weight and cholesterol, 118–119
White blood cells, immune system and, 33, 38
Wild blueberries
 as healing food, 297
 Wild Blueberry Mini Muffins, 378, *397*
William, Anthony
 Medical Medium, 21
 Medical Medium Life-Changing Foods, 21
 Medical Medium Thyroid Healing, 5
Winter squash, 298
Worms, individualized support for, 324–325

Y

Yeast infections
 Candida, 156, 163–165
 individualized support for, 329
 misdiagnosis of, 155–156
Yellow Curry Noodles Two Ways, 386, *387*
Yellow dock, 308

Z

Zinc (liquid zinc sulfate), 308
Zucchini
 as healing food, 298
 noodles, 349

ACKNOWLEDGMENTS

Thank you to Patty Gift, Anne Barthel, Reid Tracy, Margarete Nielsen, Diane Hill, everyone at Hay House Radio, and the rest of the Hay House team for your faith and commitment to getting Spirit's wisdom out into the world so it can continue to change lives.

Helen Lasichanh and Pharrell Williams, you are extraordinarily kindhearted seers.

Gwyneth Paltrow, Elise Loehnen, and your devoted GOOP crew, your caring and generosity are a profound inspiration.

Dr. Christiane Northrup, your inexhaustible devotion to the health of womankind has become its own star in the universe.

Dr. Prudence Hall, your selfless work to enlighten patients who need answers renews the true, heroic meaning of the word *doctor*.

Craig Kallman, thank you for your support, advocacy, and friendship on this journey.

Chelsea Field and Scott, Wil, and Owen Bakula, how did I get so blessed to have you in my life? You are true crusaders for the Medical Medium cause.

Kimberly and James Van Der Beek, there's a special place in my heart for you and your family. I'm truly thankful to have crossed paths with you in this lifetime.

Nanci Chambers and David James, Stephanie, and Wyatt Elliott, I can't thank you enough for your dear friendship and everlasting encouragement.

Lisa Gregorisch-Dempsey, your acts of kindness have been deeply meaningful.

Grace Hightower De Niro, Robert De Niro, and family, you are precious, gracious beings.

Liv Tyler, it's such a great honor to be a part of your world.

Jenna Dewan, your fighting spirit is an inspiration to behold.

Lisa Rinna, thank you for tirelessly using your influence to spread the message.

Marcela Valladolid, knowing you is a gift in my life.

Kelly Noonan, thank you for always looking out for me. It means so much.

To the following special souls whose loyalty I treasure, my thanks go out: Jennifer Aniston; Calvin Harris; Michael Bernard Beckwith; LeAnn Rimes Cibrian; Hana Hollinger; Sharon Levin; Nena, Robert, and Uma Thurman; Jenny Mollen; Jessica Seinfeld; Jennifer Meyer; Kelly Osbourne; Demi Moore; Kyle Richards; Caroline Fleming; India.Arie; Kristen Bower; Taylor Schilling; Kerri Walsh Jennings; Rozonda Thomas; Peggy Rometo; Debbie Gibson; Carol, Scott, and Christiana Ritchie; Peggy Lipton, Kidada Jones, and Rashida Jones; Naomi Campbell; Jamie-Lynn Sigler; Amanda de Cadenet; Marianne Williamson; Gabrielle Bernstein; Sophia Bush; Maha Dakhil; Bhavani Lev and Bharat Mitra; Woody Fraser, Milena Monrroy, Midge Hussey, and everyone at Hallmark's Home & Family; Morgan Fairchild; Patti Stanger; Catherine, Sophia, and Laura Bach; Annabeth Gish; Robert Wisdom; Danielle LaPorte; Nick and Brenna Ortner; Jessica

Ortner; Mike Dooley; Dhru Purohit; Kris Carr; Kate Northrup; Kristina Carrillo-Bucaram; Ann Louise Gittleman; Jan and Panache Desai; Ami Beach and Mark Shadle; Brian Wilson; Robert and Michelle Colt; John Holland; Martin, Jean, Elizabeth, and Jacqueline Shafiroff; Kim Lindsey; Jill Black Zalben; Alexandra Cohen; Christine Hill; Carol Donahue; Caroline Leavitt; Michael Sandler and Jessica Lee; Koya Webb; Jenny Hutt; Adam Cushman; Sonia Choquette; Colette Baron-Reid; Denise Linn; and Carmel Joy Baird. I deeply value you all.

To the compassionate doctors and other healers of the world who have changed the lives of so many: I have tremendous respect for you. Dr. Alejandro Junger, Dr. Habib Sadeghi, Dr. Carol Lee, Dr. Richard Sollazzo, Dr. Jeff Feinman, Dr. Deanna Minich, Dr. Ron Steriti, Dr. Nicole Galante, Dr. Diana Lopusny, Dr. Dick and Noel Shepard, Dr. Aleksandra Phillips, Dr. Chris Maloney, Drs. Tosca and Gregory Haag, Dr. Dave Klein, Dr. Deborah Kern, Dr. Darren and Suzanne Boles, Dr. Deirdre Williams and the late Dr. John McMahon, and Dr. Robin Karlin—it's an honor to call you friends. Thank you for your endless dedication to the field of healing.

Thanks to David Schmerler, Kimberly S. Grimsley, and Susan G. Etheridge for being there for me.

A very warm, heartfelt thanks to Muneeza Ahmed; Lauren Henry; Tara Tom; Bella; Gretchen Manzer; Kimberly Spair; Stephanie Tisone; Megan Elizabeth McDonnell; Ellen Fisher; Hannah McNeely; Victoria and Michael Arnstein; Nina Leatherer; Michelle Sutton; Haily Cataldo; Kerry; Amy Bacheller; Michael McMenamin; Alexandra Laws; Ester Horn; Linda and Robert Coykendall; Tanya Akim; Heather Coleman; Glenn Klausner; Carolyn DeVito; Michael Monteleone; Bobbi and Leslie Hall; Katherine Belzowski; Matt and Vanessa Houston; David, Holly, and Ginnie Whitney; Olivia Amitrano and Nick Vazquez; Melody Lee Pence; Terra Appelman; Eileen Crispell; Bianca Carrillo-Bucaram; Jennifer Rose Rossano; Kristin Cassidy; Catherine Lawton; Taylor Call; Alana DiNardo; Min Lee; and Eden Epstein Hill.

Thank you to the countless people, including those in the Medical Medium communities, whom I've had the privilege and honor of seeing blossom, heal, and transform.

Thank you to the Practitioner Support Group. Bless you for sharing the value of your experiences and carrying your teachings to others. You are changing the world.

Sally Arnold, thank you for shining your light so brightly and lending your voice to the movement.

Ruby Scattergood, your masterful patience and countless hours of dedication have heroically formed the true spine of this book. The Medical Medium series would not be possible without your writing and editing. Thank you for your literary counsel.

Vibodha and Tila Clark, your creative genius has been astoundingly instrumental to the cause of helping others. Thank you for standing with us throughout the years.

Friar and Clare: *In the midst of the street of it, and on either side of the river, was there the tree of life, which bare twelve manner of fruits, and yielded her fruit every month: and the leaves of the tree were for the healing of the nations.*

Sepideh Kashanian and Ben, thank you for your warm, loving care.

Ashleigh, Britton, and McClain Foster and Sterling Phillips, thank you for all your hard work and devotion. We're blessed to have you by our side.

Jeff Skeirik, thank you for the best pictures, man.

Jon Morelli and Noah, you two are all heart.

Acknowledgments

Robby Barbaro and Setareh Khatibi, your unwavering positivity lifts up everyone around you.

For your love and support, as always, I thank my family: my luminous wife; Dad and Mom; my brothers, nieces, nephews, aunts, and uncles; my champions Indigo, Ruby, and Great Blue; Hope; Marjorie and Robert; Laura; Rhia and Byron; Alayne Serle and Scott, Perri, Lissy, and Ari Cohn; David Somoroff; Joel, Liz, Kody, Jesse, Lauren, Joseph, and Thomas; Brian, Joyce, and Josh; Jarod; Brent; Kelly and Evy; Danielle, Johnny, and Declan; and all my loved ones who are on the other side.

Finally, thank you, Spirit of the Most High, for providing all of us with compassionate wisdom from the heavens that inspires us to keep our heads up and carry the sacred gifts you've been so kind to give us. Thank you for putting up with me over the years and reminding me to keep a light heart with your never-ending patience and willingness to answer my questions in search of the truth.

ABOUT THE AUTHOR

Anthony William, #1 *New York Times* best-selling author of *Medical Medium Thyroid Healing: The Truth behind Hashimoto's, Graves', Insomnia, Hypothyroidism, Thyroid Nodules & Epstein-Barr*; *Medical Medium Life-Changing Foods: Save Yourself and the Ones You Love with the Hidden Healing Powers of Fruits & Vegetables*; and *Medical Medium: Secrets Behind Chronic and Mystery Illness and How to Finally Heal*, was born with the unique ability to converse with the Spirit of Compassion, who provides him with extraordinarily accurate health information that's often far ahead of its time. Since age four, when he shocked his family by announcing that his symptom-free grandmother had lung cancer (which medical testing soon confirmed), Anthony has been using his gift to "read" people's conditions and tell them how to recover their health. His unprecedented accuracy and success rate as the Medical Medium have earned him the trust and love of millions worldwide, among them movie stars, rock stars, billionaires, professional athletes, best-selling authors, and countless other people from all walks of life who couldn't find a way to heal until he provided them with insights from Spirit. Anthony has also become an invaluable resource to doctors who need help solving their most difficult cases.

Learn more at www.medicalmedium.com

CONVERSION CHARTS

The recipes in this book use the standard United States method for measuring liquid and dry or solid ingredients (teaspoons, tablespoons, and cups). The following charts are provided to help cooks woutside the U.S. successfully use these recipes. All equivalents are approximate.

Standard Cup	Fine Powder (e.g., flour)	Grain (e.g., rice)	Granular (e.g., sugar)	Liquid Solids (e.g., butter)	Liquid (e.g., milk)
1	140 g	150 g	190 g	200 g	240 ml
¾	105 g	113 g	143 g	150 g	180 ml
⅔	93 g	100 g	125 g	133 g	160 ml
½	70 g	75 g	95 g	100 g	120 ml
⅓	47 g	50 g	63 g	67 g	80 ml
¼	35 g	38 g	48 g	50 g	60 ml
⅛	18 g	19 g	24 g	25 g	30 ml

Useful Equivalents for Liquid Ingredients by Volume					
¼ tsp				1 ml	
½ tsp				2 ml	
1 tsp				5 ml	
3 tsp	1 tbsp		½ fl oz	15 ml	
	2 tbsp	⅛ cup	1 fl oz	30 ml	
	4 tbsp	¼ cup	2 fl oz	60 ml	
	5⅓ tbsp	⅓ cup	3 fl oz	80 ml	
	8 tbsp	½ cup	4 fl oz	120 ml	
	10⅔ tbsp	⅔ cup	5 fl oz	160 ml	
	12 tbsp	¾ cup	6 fl oz	180 ml	
	16 tbsp	1 cup	8 fl oz	240 ml	
	1 pt	2 cups	16 fl oz	480 ml	
	1 qt	4 cups	32 fl oz	960 ml	
			33 fl oz	1000 ml	1 l

Useful Equivalents for Dry Ingredients by Weight

(To convert ounces to grams, multiply the number of ounces by 30.)

1 oz	1/16 lb	30 g
4 oz	1/4 lb	120 g
8 oz	1/2 lb	240 g
12 oz	3/4 lb	360 g
16 oz	1 lb	480 g

Useful Equivalents for Cooking/Oven Temperatures

Process	Fahrenheit	Celsius	Gas Mark
Freeze Water	32° F	0° C	
Room Temperature	68° F	20° C	
Boil Water	212° F	100° C	
Bake	325° F	160° C	3
	350° F	180° C	4
	375° F	190° C	5
	400° F	200° C	6
	425° F	220° C	7
	450° F	230° C	8
Broil			Grill

Useful Equivalents for Length

(To convert inches to centimeters, multiply the number of inches by 2.5.)

1 in			2.5 cm	
6 in	1/2 ft		15 cm	
12 in	1 ft		30 cm	
36 in	3 ft	1 yd	90 cm	
40 in			100 cm	1 m

Hay House Titles of Related Interest

YOU CAN HEAL YOUR LIFE, the movie, starring Louise Hay & Friends
(available as a 1-DVD program, an expanded 2-DVD set, and an online streaming video)
Learn more at www.hayhouse.com/louise-movie

THE SHIFT, the movie,
starring Dr. Wayne W. Dyer
(available as a 1-DVD program, an expanded 2-DVD set, and an online streaming video)
Learn more at www.hayhouse.com/the-shift-movie

———————

MEDICAL MEDIUM: Secrets behind Chronic and Mystery Illness and How to Finally Heal, by Anthony William

MEDICAL MEDIUM LIFE-CHANGING FOODS: Save Yourself and the Ones You Love with the Hidden Healing Powers of Fruits & Vegetables, by Anthony William

MEDICAL MEDIUM THYROID HEALING: The Truth behind Hashimoto's, Graves', Insomnia, Hypothyroidism, Thyroid Nodules & Epstein-Barr, by Anthony William

All of the above are available at your local bookstore,
or may be ordered by contacting Hay House (see next page).

———————

We hope you enjoyed this Hay House book. If you'd like to receive our online catalog featuring additional information on Hay House books and products, or if you'd like to find out more about the Hay Foundation, please contact:

Hay House, Inc., P.O. Box 5100, Carlsbad, CA 92018-5100
(760) 431-7695 or (800) 654-5126
(760) 431-6948 (fax) or (800) 650-5115 (fax)
www.hayhouse.com® • www.hayfoundation.org

———

Published in Australia by:
Hay House Australia Pty. Ltd., 18/36 Ralph St., Alexandria NSW 2015
Phone: 612-9669-4299 • *Fax:* 612-9669-4144 • www.hayhouse.com.au

Published in the United Kingdom by:
Hay House UK, Ltd., Astley House, 33 Notting Hill Gate, London W11 3JQ
Phone: 44-20-3675-2450 • *Fax:* 44-20-3675-2451 • www.hayhouse.co.uk

Published in India by: Hay House Publishers India,
Muskaan Complex, Plot No. 3, B-2, Vasant Kunj, New Delhi 110 070
Phone: 91-11-4176-1620 • *Fax:* 91-11-4176-1630 • www.hayhouse.co.in

———

<u>Access New Knowledge.</u>
<u>Anytime. Anywhere.</u>

Learn and evolve at your own pace
with the world's leading experts.

www.hayhouseU.com

HAY HOUSE
Online Video Courses

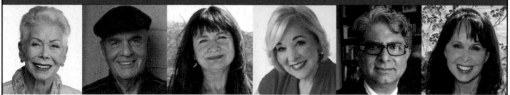

Expand your knowledge with Online Courses from best-selling authors in healing and self-empowerment, including Dr. Wayne W. Dyer, Denise Linn, Louise Hay, Dr. Christiane Northrup, Deepak Chopra, and Doreen Virtue.

LEARN MORE ON:

- fulfilling your one true purpose in life
- learning to clear your energy and your home
- using the mirror to learn how to love YOU
- living agelessly, vibrantly, and healthfully by harnessing the power and beauty of your body
- what it takes to get noticed by a publisher and what publishers are looking for in new authors
- creating healthy boundaries and the importance of assertiveness

For a complete list of Online Courses,
visit www.HayHouse.com/online-courses.

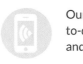

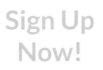